Handbook of Antioxidants

Handbook of Antioxidants

Editor: Grace McCoy

FOSTER
ACADEMICS
www.fosteracademics.com

www.fosteracademics.com

Cataloging-in-Publication Data

Handbook of antioxidants / edited by Grace McCoy.
p. cm.
Includes bibliographical references and index.
ISBN 978-1-63242-873-8
1. Antioxidants. 2. Chemical inhibitors. 3. Antioxidants--Health aspects. 4. Antioxidants--Therapeutic use. I. McCoy, Grace.
RB170 .H36 2020
613.286--dc23

Foster Academics,
118-35 Queens Blvd., Suite 400,
Forest Hills, NY 11375, USA

ISBN 978-1-63242-873-8 (Hardback)

Printed and bound in China.

Contents

Preface

Oxidative stress is considered to be a major contributor to a wide range of diseases, such as cardiovascular disease, Alzheimer's disease, Parkinson's disease, rheumatoid arthritis, neurodegeneration in motor neuron diseases and the pathologies caused by diabetes. Oxidative damage in DNA may cause harmful mutations and cancer, while protein damage may result in protein degradation, enzyme inhibition and denaturation. Organisms have a complex system of antioxidant metabolites and enzymes to prevent oxidative damage to cellular components. Antioxidants are compounds that inhibit oxidation. Antioxidant vitamins can be found in certain foods such as fruits, vegetables, eggs, nuts and legumes. This book is compiled in such a manner, that it will provide in-depth knowledge about antioxidants. It includes some of the vital pieces of work being conducted across the world, on various topics related to this area of study. It is a vital tool for all researching or studying antioxidants as it gives incredible insights into emerging trends and concepts.

This book has been the outcome of endless efforts put in by authors and researchers on various issues and topics within the field. The book is a comprehensive collection of significant researches that are addressed in a variety of chapters. It will surely enhance the knowledge of the field among readers across the globe.

It gives us an immense pleasure to thank our researchers and authors for their efforts to submit their piece of writing before the deadlines. Finally in the end, I would like to thank my family and colleagues who have been a great source of inspiration and support.

Editor

1

Selenoprotein K Increases Efficiency of DHHC6 Catalyzed Protein Palmitoylation by Stabilizing the Acyl-DHHC6 Intermediate

Gregory J. Fredericks [1], FuKun W. Hoffmann [1], Robert J. Hondal [2], Sharon Rozovsky [3], Johann Urschitz [4] and Peter R. Hoffmann [1,*]

1. Department of Cell and Molecular Biology, John A. Burns School of Medicine, University of Hawaii, 651 Ilalo Street, Honolulu, HI 96813, USA; gjf@hawaii.edu (G.J.F.); fukun@hawaii.edu (F.W.H.)
2. Department of Biochemistry, University of Vermont, 89 Beaumont Ave, Given Building Room B413, Burlington, VT 05405, USA; robert.s.hondal@gmail.com
3. Department of Chemistry and Biochemistry, University of Delaware, 136 Brown Laboratory, Newark, DE 19716, USA; rozovsky@udel.edu
4. Department of Anatomy, Biochemistry and Physiology, John A. Burns School of Medicine, University of Hawaii, 651 Ilalo Street, Honolulu, HI 96813, USA; johann@hawaii.edu

* Correspondence: peterrh@hawaii.edu

Abstract: Selenoprotein K (SELENOK) is a selenocysteine (Sec)-containing protein localized in the endoplasmic reticulum (ER) membrane where it interacts with the DHHC6 (where single letter symbols represent Asp-His-His-Cys amino acids) enzyme to promote protein acyl transferase (PAT) reactions. PAT reactions involve the DHHC enzymatic capture of palmitate via a thioester bond to cysteine (Cys) residues that form an unstable palmitoyl-DHHC intermediate, followed by transfer of palmitate to Cys residues of target proteins. How SELENOK facilitates this reaction has not been determined. Splenocyte microsomal preparations from wild-type mice versus SELENOK knockout mice were used to establish PAT assays and showed decreased PAT activity (~50%) under conditions of SELENOK deficiency. Using recombinant, soluble versions of DHHC6 along with SELENOK containing Sec_{92}, Cys_{92}, or alanine (Ala_{92}), we evaluated the stability of the acyl-DHHC6 intermediate and its capacity to transfer the palmitate residue to Cys residues on target peptides. Versions of SELENOK containing either Ala or Cys residues in place of Sec were equivalently less effective than Sec at stabilizing the acyl-DHHC6 intermediate or promoting PAT activity. These data suggest that Sec_{92} in SELENOK serves to stabilize the palmitoyl-DHHC6 intermediate by reducing hydrolyzation of the thioester bond until transfer of the palmitoyl group to the Cys residue on the target protein can occur.

Keywords: palmitic acid; palmitoyl-CoA; palmitoylation; inositol 1,4,5-triphosphate receptor; ANK repeat and PH domain-containing protein 2 (ASAP2); cluster of differentiation (CD36); selenium; thioester

---

1. Introduction

Dietary selenium exerts its biological effects mainly through selenoproteins, which all contain the amino acid selenocysteine (Sec) and exhibit a wide variety of functions [1]. The Sec residue has intrinsic redox potential at physiological pH and the selenium within this amino acid side chain is likely to be more resistant to permanent oxidation compared to the sulfur present in the more common amino acid cysteine (Cys) [2] These chemical properties underly the selective advantages for proteins incorporating Sec over Cys [3]. Many selenoproteins exhibit oxidoreductase activity and serve as cellular antioxidants, regulators of redox tone, reducers of oxidized methionine residues, and deiodinases that regulate thyroid hormone [4]. However, some selenoproteins may not function as enzymes and exactly what their biological roles are remains unclear.

We recently identified a new role for one member of the selenoprotein family, selenoprotein K (SELENOK), which appears to be involved in acyl transferase reactions. In particular, SELENOK was shown to interact with the enzyme, DHHC6 (where single letter symbols represent Asp-His-His-Cys amino acids), in the membrane of the endoplasmic reticulum (ER) to promote protein palmitoylation [5]. DHHC enzymes are protein acyl transferases (PATs) conserved throughout eukaryotes that catalyze the addition of acyl groups (e.g., palmitate) onto cysteine residues of substrate proteins in a process termed S-acylation (a.k.a. palmitoylation) [6]. The addition of the 16-carbon fatty acid, palmitic acid, to the sulfhydryl group of cysteine residues forms a thioester bond resulting in S-acylation of the target protein [7]. SELENOK knockout mice are healthy and fertile, although certain aspects of the immune system are compromised [8].

The enzymes contain the conserved 51 amino acid catalytic domain including a DHHC motif embedded within a cysteine-rich domain [9]. DHHC6 is one of 23 members of this family in humans, but it is the only member that contains a Src-homology 3 (SH3) domain. SELENOK is the only selenoprotein with an SH3 binding element, and our previous work showed that interactions via the SH3/SH3 binding domains are essential for DHCC6 and SELENOK binding and subsequent palmitoylation [5]. The DHHC6/SELENOK complex is required for the palmitoylation of certain proteins such as the inositol 1,4,5-triphosphate receptor (IP3R) [5], ANK repeat and PH domain-containing protein 2 (ASAP2) [10], the oxidized low density lipoprotein (LDL) receptor CD36 [11], and likely other proteins [12]. SELENOK appears to serve as a cofactor for the DHHC6 catalyzed S-acylation reaction, but its specific role in facilitating S-acylation has not yet been determined.

DHHC-catalyzed palmitoylation reactions proceed via a two-step ping-pong mechanism [13]. In the first autopalmitoylation step, a Cys residue within the PAT (likely the conserved Cys within the DHHC catalytic domain) reacts with palmitoyl-CoA to form a palmitoyl-PAT intermediate. In the second step, the palmitoyl group is transferred from the PAT to a Cys residue on the target protein. The first step is rapid, whereas the second is much slower. Thus, after the first step, the unstable thioester bond between Cys on the PAT and the palmitic acid may hydrolyze before transfer of the palmitic acid to a target protein, termed the "futile cycle" [14]. This raises the possibility that SELENOK may function to stabilize the palmitoyl-DHHC6 intermediate thereby reducing hydrolyzation of the thioester bond until transfer of the palmitoyl group to the Cys residue on the target protein can occur. In fact, in yeast such stabilization of a palmitoyl-PAT intermediate by the Ethylene-Responsive Transcription Factor 4 (Erf4) cofactor (γ-Tubulin Complex, GCP16, in mammals) has been shown for the Erf2 PAT (DHHC9 in mammals) [15,16]. There are also intriguing questions of whether Cys instead of Sec in SELENOK would be able to equivalently function to facilitate DHHC6 catalyzed palmitoylation. With these questions in mind, we set out to develop in vitro assays to study molecular mechanisms of S-acylation by the DHHC6/SELENOK complex.

2. Materials and Methods

2.1. Reagents and Mice

Ni-NTA agarose for cytosolic DHHC6 purification from bacteria was purchased from Qiagen (Hilden, Germany). Dynabeads for His-tag isolation and pull-down of DHHC6 during subsequent assays were obtained from ThermoFischer (Waltham, MA, USA). All versions of SELENOK with an N-terminal 8 amino acid StrepII tag (WSHPQFEK) were expressed in bacteria and purified in the laboratory of Dr. Sharon Rozovsky at the University of Delaware as previously described [16,17]. StrepTactin™ beads (Millipore-Sigma, Burlington, MA, USA) were used for SELENOK pull-down. The FITC-labeled fluorescent peptide corresponding to the amino acid sequence surrounding the N-terminal dicysteine palmitoylation consensus site of CD36 (MGCDRNCK) was purchased from

Peptide 2.0 (Chantilly, VA, USA). Palmitoyl-CoA (C16:0) lithium was purchased from Sigma (St. Louis, MO, USA) and NBD-palmitoyl-CoA purchased from Avanti Polar Lipids. Antibodies used to detect DHHC6 and SELENOK were previously described [5]. C57BL/6J wild-type controls were generated from mice originally purchased from the Jackson Laboratory (Bar Harbor, ME, USA). Generation of SELENOK KO mice was previously described [8]. All animal protocols were approved by the University of Hawaii Institutional Animal Care and Use Committee (Animal Welfare Assurance number: A3423-01).

2.2. DHHC6 Preparation

We generated a soluble cytosolic DHHC6 enzyme by cloning the NCBI sequence NM_001033573.1 encoding the two functional cytosolic domains of DHHC6 connected by a flexible linker domain (GGGSGGGSGGGS) into a pET-14b His-tagged expression vector for bacterial expression (GenScript, Piscataway, NJ, USA). His-tagged cytosolic DHHC6 was expressed in *E. coli* BL21(DE3) cells, purified using a Ni-NTA agarose column and stored in aliquots at −80 °C until they were ready to be used. Prior to running the assay, aliquots of cytosolic DHHC6 were thawed and incubated overnight in 50 mM MES, pH 6.4 containing 0.05% DDM and 10 mM DTT.

2.3. Polyacrylamide Based Analyses of S-Acylation of DHHC6

For studies examining the influence of SELENOK on cytosolic DHHC6 autoacylation, His-tagged DHHC6 protein was incubated overnight at a 1:1 molar ratio with three versions of SELENOK (U92A, U92C and U92) that each included an N-terminal streptavidin-tag II as well as 2 mg StrepTactin™ beads (Millipore, Burlington, MA, USA) in 50 mM MES, pH 6.4 containing 0.05% DDM and 10 mM DTT. The following day, beads were washed three times and incubated in 50 mM MES (pH 6.8 or 7.4 or 8.2) containing 0.05% DDM and 10 µM NBD-palmitoyl-CoA at 30°C for 60 min with aliquots collected from the magnetic beads. The beads were re-suspended in sample loading buffer (50 mM Tris–HCl (pH 6.4), 2% SDS, 12.5 mM EDTA, 10% glycerol) and subjected to 10–20% Tris-Tricine SDS–PAGE. Fluorescent bands in the gel were visualized using a UV gel box with DHHC6 acylation represented by fluorescent NBD-palmitoyl-DHHC6. The gel was then stained using Coomassie Brilliant Blue (Thermo Fisher Scientific, Waltham, MA, USA) per manufacturer's instructions to validate equivalent quantities of SELENOK as well as equivalent DHHC6 pull-down. Western blots were performed and analyzed using an Odyssey scanner (Li-Cor, Lincoln, NE, USA) as previously described [18].

2.4. TLC-Based Fluorescent Peptide Microsomal PAT Assay

Spleens were collected from WT and SELENOK KO mice and leukocytes separated as previously described [19], and ER microsomes isolated from splenocytes for use in the PAT assay. In brief, spleens were homogenized into a single cell suspension by passage through a 100 µm filter followed by lysis of the red blood population using ammonium chloride based red blood cell lysis buffer (Sigma, St. Louis, MO, USA). Intact white blood cells (2×10^8 per condition) were separated from red blood cell debris via centrifugation and subsequently re-suspended in isotonic extraction buffer (50 mM HEPES, pH 7.8, with 1.25 M sucrose, 5 mM EGTA, and 125 mM potassium chloride containing protease inhibitor cocktail (Millipore-Sigma, Burlington, MA, USA) and lysed by sonication. The post-mitochondrial supernatant was obtained via a low-speed centrifugation (12,000× *g*) and was subsequently centrifuged at 100,000× *g* for one hour to obtain the ER microsomal pellet. This pellet was re-suspended in 50 mm MES (pH 6.4) buffer containing 0.05% DDM at a ratio of 10 mg ER microsomes per 1 mL of buffer. Prior to PAT assay, FITC-labeled MGCDRNCK peptide (1 mM, 100× stock) was treated with 10 mM DTT at room temperature for 1 h to reduce disulfide-linked peptide dimers. To initiate reactions, the reduced peptide was added to the aqueous reaction buffer containing the ER microsomes to yield a final concentration of 10 µM peptide in 0.05% DDM, 0.1 mm DTT and 50 mm MES, pH 6.4, and reactions were incubated at 30 °C for 2 to 60 min. After reaction completion, 10 µL of reaction volume was spotted on reverse-phase C18 TLC plates uniplates (Analtech, Newark, DE, USA) per time point and resolved using a 40% acetonitrile mobile phase. Post-run fluorescent peptides were visualized under UV fluorescent light to determine the ratio of palmitoylated to non-palmitoylated peptide. For TLC evaluation of the cytosolic DHHC6/SELENOK complexes, a similar protocol was followed with modifications. As described above, the intermediates generated by incubating cytosolic DHHC6, soluble SELENOK (U92 → A, U92 → C, U92), and NBD-palmitoyl-CoA at pH 7.4 were washed in the same buffer and incubated with the CD36 peptide in 0.05% DDM, 0.1 mm DTT and 50 mm MES, pH 6.4, and reactions carried out at 30 °C for 2 to 15 min. Thin layr chromatography (TLC) was carried out as described above.

3. Results

3.1. SELENOK Deficiency Leads to Decreased Target Peptide Palmitoylation Using an In Vitro Assay

We set out to test the requirement of SELENOK for S-acylation (i.e., palmitoylation) of a target peptide by the DHHC6 in the ER membrane. To this end, we purified ER microsomes from splenocytes of WT or SELENOK KO mice and tested their capacity to palmitoylate a peptide from a known palmitoylation target of DHHC6/SELENOK, CD36 [10]. Using thin layer chromatography to differentiate between the native and S-acylated forms of a FITC-labeled CD36 peptide (MGCDRNCK), we found that ER microsomal preparations from SELENOK KO splenocytes exhibited lower levels of palmitoylation compared to WT controls (Figure 1A). Western blotting confirmed that this was not due to differences in enzyme levels (DHHC6) in the microsomal preparations (Figure 1B). These experiments were repeated using a time course approach and SELENOK deficient ER microsomes were found to generate approximately 50% less S-acylated peptide over time (Figure 2). These results are consistent with in vivo data in WT versus SELENOK KO mice and validated our ability to utilize TLC-based palmitoylation approaches to evaluate molecular features of SELENOK facilitated DHHC6 catalyzed alkylation.

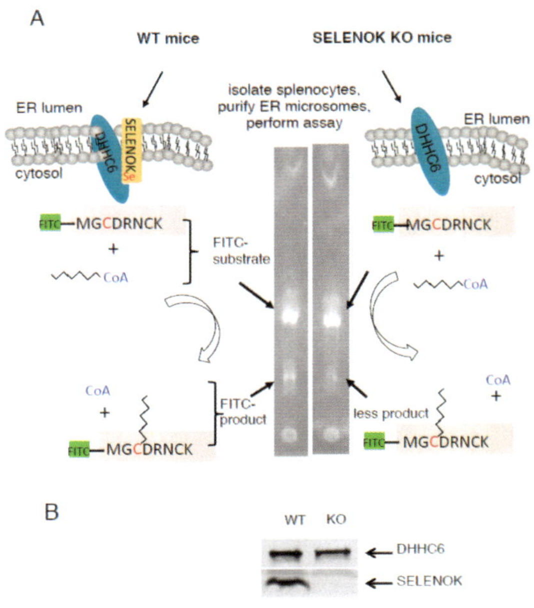

Figure 1. A diagram illustrating protocol for detecting palmitoylation of peptides by murine splenocyte microsomes. (**A**) Splenocytes were isolated from either WT or SELENOK mice, and microsomes were prepared containing ER membranes with or without SELENOK, respectively. Substrates including palmitoyl-CoA and FITC-peptide were added to microsomes for different periods of time after which the reaction mixtures were subjected to reverse-phase TLC. Fluorescent bands corresponding to palmitoylated peptides were identified using UV transillumination. (**B**) For each experiment, equivalent levels of DHHC6 were confirmed using Western blotting.

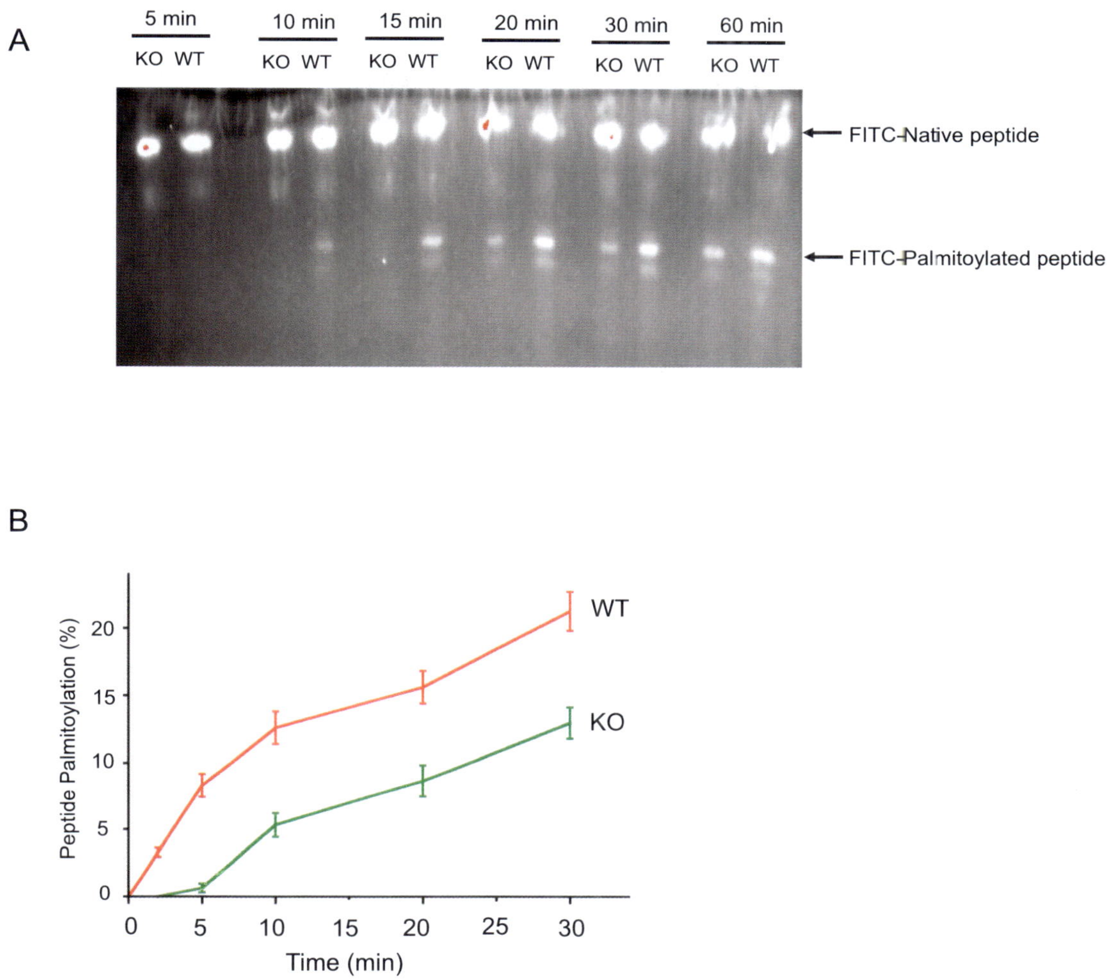

Figure 2. Palmitoylation of target peptides is decreased in SELENOK deficient microsomes. (**A**) A time course for peptide palmitoylation was performed using a TLC-based assay. A representative image for fluorescence imaged with a *uv* transilluminator. Note the imasge was was captured at high exposure to clearly show the palmitoylated peptide bands, which resulted in some red overexposed regions in the native peptide band. (**B**) Three independent experiments were conducted to compare microsomes from WT and SELENOK KO splenocytes. Values at each time point indicate percent of peptide that was palmitoylated = (FITC/(Native + FITC)) × 100. Means ± S.E. are shown.

3.2. The Sec Residue in SELENOK Facilitates S-Acylation of DHHC6

In order to study mechanisms by which SELENOK influences the catalytic activity of DHHC6, we cloned and expressed a soluble version of DHHC6 that contains the SH3 domain to bind to SELENOK and catalytic domain (Figure 3A,B). A flexible linker domain that has been used in previous studies to successfully link protein domains in a similar fashion [20] was used to link these two domains of DHHC6. This cytosolic DHHC6 protein was incubated with variants of full-length SELENOK with different amino acids at the active position of amino acid 92 (U92 → A, U92 → C and U92) that were coupled to StrepTactin™ beads via an N-terminal Strep-II tag. We were able to bind equivalent quantities of cytosolic DHHC6 to all three version of bead-bound SELENOK (Figure 3C).

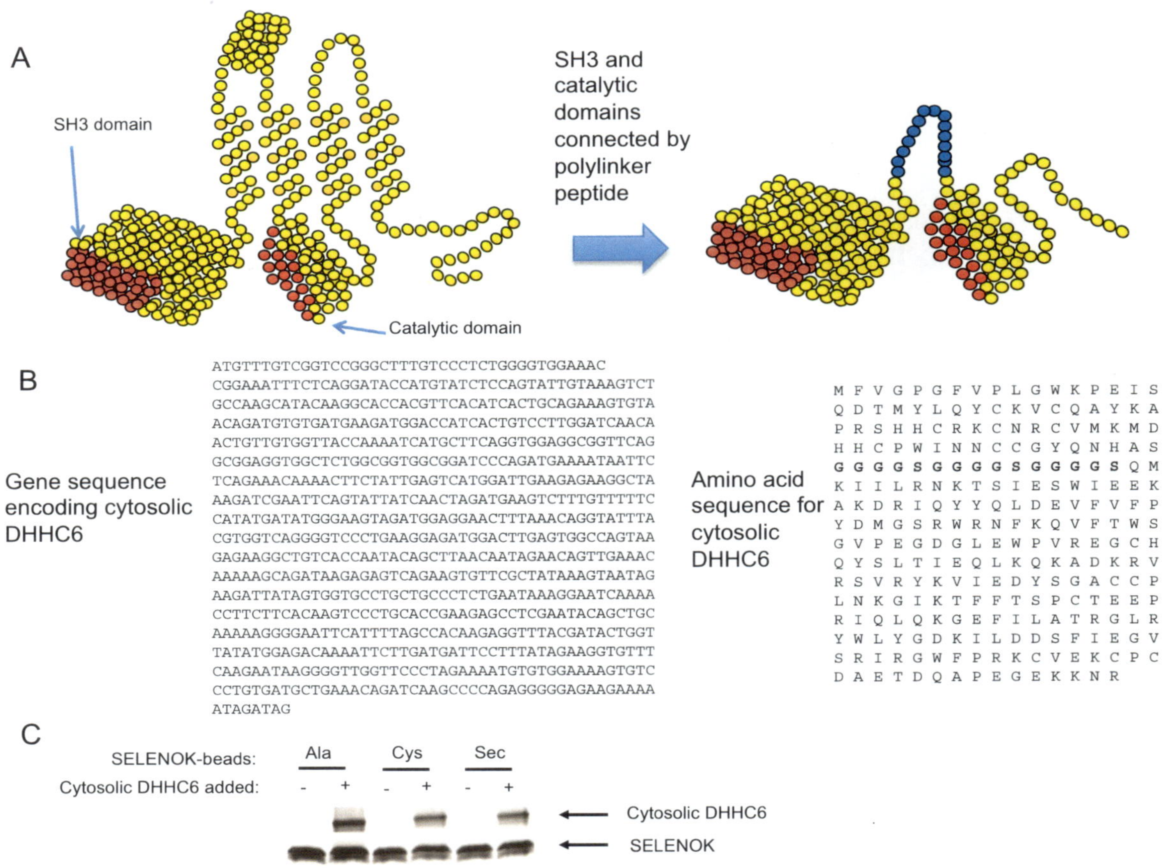

Figure 3. Synthesis of a soluble cytosolic DHHC6 that binds to SELENOK. (**A**) Illustration of full-length DHHC6 with the SH3 and catalytic domains that were used to construct a modified version of DHHC6, which contains both domains connected by a linker domain shown in blue. (**B**) The DNA sequence used to express the cytosolic DHHC6 along with amino acid sequence showing linker region in blue. (**C**) StrepTactin beads were used to pull down 1 μg streptavidin-tagged SELENOK containing either Ala, or Cys, or Sec at amino acid position 92. These beads were divided into two aliquots that were not or were incubated overnight at 4 °C with the cytosolic DHHC6 in a 1:1 molar ratio. Eluted proteins were analyzed by Coomassie blue staining of PAGE, and results show all three versions of SELENOK bound to cytosolic DHHC6. Note that some degradation of the recombinant SELENOK occurred during the overnight incubation giving rise to double bands. Also, these are recombinant proteins and not cell lysates, which leads to no detectable background in lanes corresponding to the "no Cytosolic DHHC6 added" conditions.

These different DHHC6/SELENOK complexes were then incubated with a fluorescent version of palmitoyl-CoA (NBD-palmitoyl-CoA) to allow autoacylation of DHHC6 to occur at different pH. Autoacylation has been shown to exhibit pH dependence, with acylated DHHC enzymes hydrolyzing at low pH (<7.2) but maintaining acylated states at higher pH (between 7.4 and 8.6) [13]. In the case of Erf2/Erf4 autopalmitoylation, the underlying cause for the observed pH dependence was proposed to be the charges on key histidines. Thus, to study the stability of the acylated DHHC6 intermediate, autoacylation of DHHC6 at carried out at pH 6.8 (conducive to hydrolysis), pH 7.4 (low levels of hydrolysis), and pH 8.2 (very low levels of hydrolysis). A fluorescent NBD-palmitoyl-CoA was incubated with the bead-bound DHHC6/SELENOK complexes and the autoacylation of DHHC6 was analyzed by SDS-PAGE. The fluorescent detection of acyl-DHHC6 within the gel showed that Sec-containing SELENOK was most effective at generating or stabilizing acylated DHHC6 (Figure 4A). A fluorescent band corresponding to stable acyl-DHHC6 was detectable at both pH 7.4 and 8.2. As a parallel approach, the gel was stained with Coomassie Blue and this allowed visualization of acylated and non-acylated versions of DHHC6 based on size/mobility differences (Figure 4B). The DHHC6 complexed to Ala-containing SELENOK represents baseline autoacylation of the DHHC protein due to the absence of the important Sec residue at position 92 in SELENOK. Under conditions conducive to hydrolysis of the acylated intermediate (pH 6.8), there was no detection of acyl-DHHC6. Autoacylation of DHHC6 complexed to Ala-containing SELENOK increased under conditions less conducive to hydrolysis (pH 7.4) and was fully acylated under conditions non-conducive to hydrolysis (pH 8.2). Cys-containing SELENOK complexed to DHHC6 generated similar results, suggesting that Cys residue at position 92 did not facilitate acylation of DHHC6 above the baseline autoacylation levels. However, Sec-containing SELENOK complexed to DHHC6 led to stable acyl-DHHC6 under conditions conducive to hydrolysis (pH 6.8), and higher levels of acylation at the less conducive conditions (pH 7.4 and 8.2). These data together with the fluorescent data shown above suggest that Sec at amino acid position 92 in SELENOK stabilizes the acyl-DHHC6 intermediate by protecting the thioester bond of acyl-DHHC6 from hydrolysis that leads to the futile cycle.

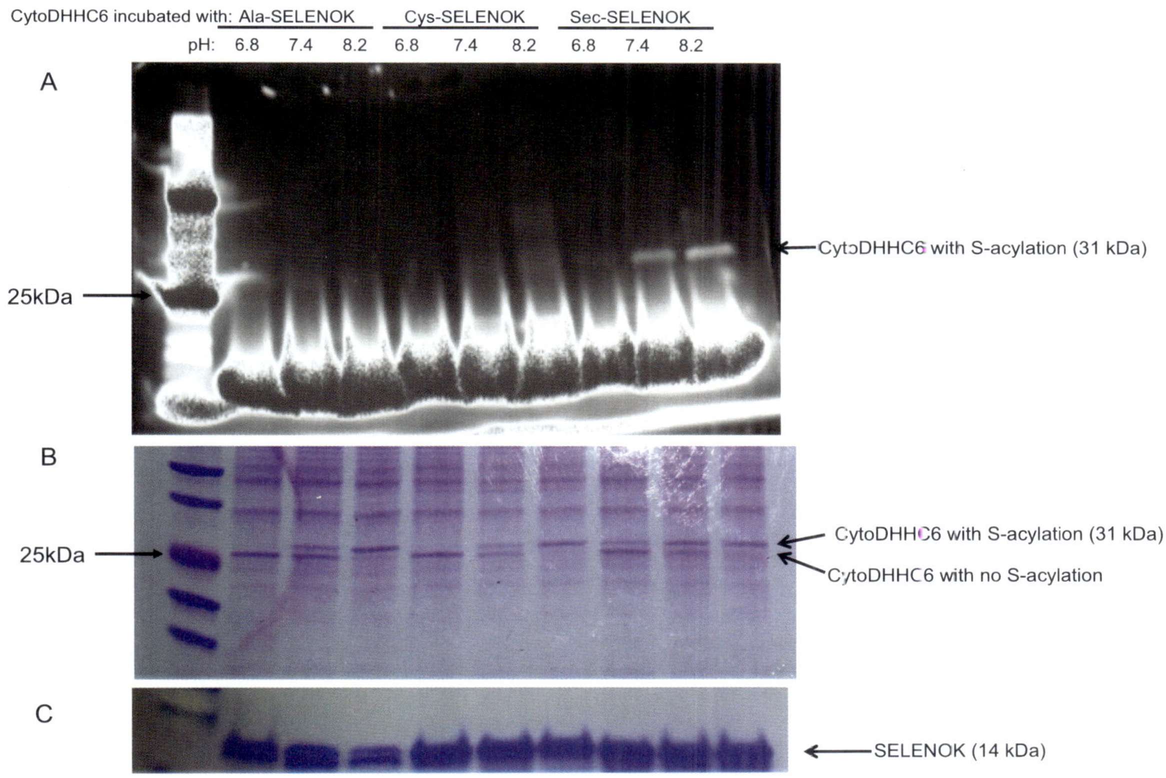

Figure 4. Sec-containing SELENOK stabilizes acyl-DHHC6 intermediate formed during the autopalmitoylation of the enzyme. Cytosolic DHHC6 bound to different versions of SELENOK (U92 $\rightarrow$ A, U92 $\rightarrow$ C, and U92) bound to StrepTactin beads were incubated for 60 min with fluorescent NBD-palmitoyl-CoA in buffer of pH 6.8, 7.4, and 8.2. Beads were then washed, proteins eluted and analyzed by SDS-PAGE. (**A**) The gel was exposed to *uv* using a transilluminator and the acylated DHHC6 visualized at ~31 kDa with highest levels found in the lanes corresponding to Sec-containing SELENOK at pH 7.4 and 8.2. (**B**) Coomassie Blue staining of the gel revealed two bands for DHHC6 ~31 kDa. Based on the pattern within the pH ranges, the upper band corresponds to acylated DHHC6 and the lower band to the nonacylated DHHC6. (**C**) Coomassie Blue staining of the gel in the region of SELENOK (~14 kDa) shows that the protein was eluted from beads at equivalent levels. Note that some degradation of the recombinant SELENOK occurred during the overnight incubation giving rise to double bands.

As another approach to study S-acylation of DHHC6, western blotting was used to analyze the different versions of SELENOK for their ability to facilitate S-acylation of DHHC6. As described above, fluorescent NBD-palmitoyl-CoA was incubated with DHHC6 complexed to different versions of SELENOK (U92 → A, U92 → C, U92) at pH 6.8, 7.4, and 8.2. Similar to the results above, complexing of DHHC6 to Sec-containing SELENOK led to stable acyl-DHHC6 at the conditions conducive to hydrolysis (pH 6.8) with S-acylation increasing under conditions less conducive to hydrolysis (pH 7.4 and 8.2) (Figure 5). As discussed above, Ala-containing SELENOK combined to DHHC6 represents autopalmitoylation of DHHC6 in the absence of functional SELENOK. No stable acyl-DHCC6 intermediate was detected under conditions conducive to hydrolysis (pH 6.8), but acylation of DHHC6 increased when pH was increased. Results for Cys-containing SELENOK were similar to Ala-containing SELENOK, suggesting that Sec residue at position 92 is required for any increase in S-acylation of DHHC6 above baseline levels.

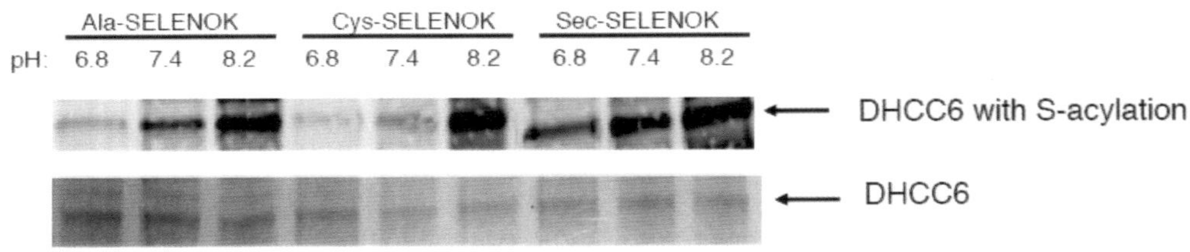

Figure 5. Sec-containing SELENOK is most effective at stabilizing the acyl-DHHC6 intermediate. The autopalmitoylation of cytosolic DHHC6 was performed with different bead-bound versions of SELENOK (U92 → A, U92 → C, and U92) under different pH conditions. Western blotting was performed to detect NBD-palmitate-DHHC6 as a green fluorescent band and the DHHC protein that was detected with anti-DHHC6 and IR-secondary antibodies as a red fluorescent band.

3.3. The Acyl Transfer Function of DHHC6 is Most Efficient with Sec-Containing SELENOK

While the data above suggest the acyl-DHHC6 intermediate is stabilized by binding to Sec-containing SELENOK, this does not demonstrate the ability of DHHC6 to transfer this acyl group to target peptides. Thus, we next incubated the NBD-palmitoyl-DHHC6 intermediates (formed at pH 7.4) with a target peptide corresponding to CD36 for different periods of time. The transfer of the fluorescent NBD-palmitate was analyzed by thin layer chromatography as described above, and results showed that the acyl transfer at 5 and 10 min was most effective for DHHC6 complexed to Sec-containing SELENOK (Figure 6A). This was repeated for 10 and 15 min and again, at 10 min DHHC6 complexed to Sec-containing SELENOK was most effective at transferring the fluorescent palmitate to the target peptide (Figure 6B). By 15 min the levels of acyl-peptide were equivalent for DHHC6 complexed to Ala-, Cys-, and Sec-containing SELENOK. Thus, both stability of the acyl-DHHC6 intermediate and efficiency of transferring the acyl group to target peptides were increased when DHHC6 enzyme was bound to SELENOK that contained Sec at residue 92.

A

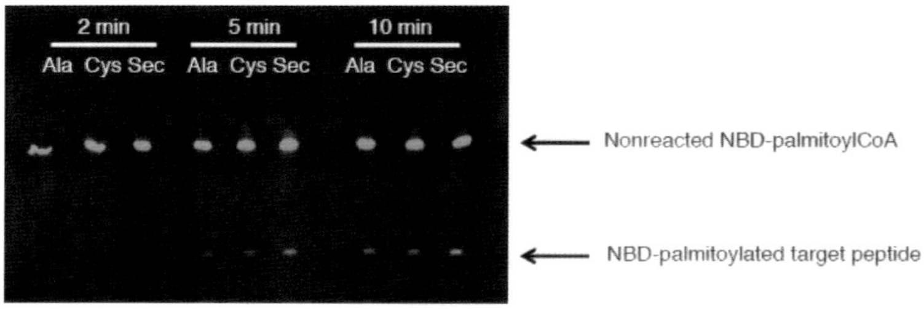

Figure 6. *Cont.*

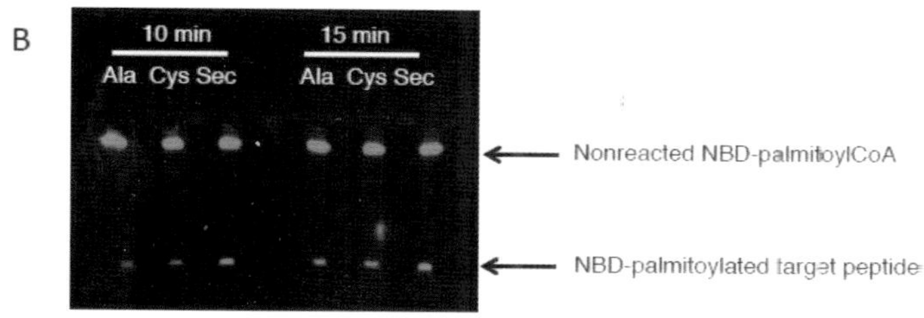

Figure 6. Acyltransferase activity of DHHC6 is most efficient when bound to Sec-containing SELENOK. The NBD-palmitoyl-DHHC6 intermediates formed at pH 7.4 were incubated with CD36 peptide (MGCDRNCK) for different periods of time. Reactions were terminated with SDS on ice and reaction products run on reverse-phase TLC, followed by analysis on a *uv* transilluminator to detect NBD-palmitoyl-peptide. (**A**) The first experiment was run at three time periods of 2, 5, and 10 min. (**B**) The second experiment was run for 10 and 15 min.

4. Discussion

The data presented herein provide insight into how SELENOK bound to DHHC6 may increase the catalytic efficiency of the S-acylation reaction. Our data show that the Sec residue at position 92 of SELENOK is important for stabilizing the autopalmitoylated intermediate, acyl-DHHC6, to prevent hydrolysis of the thioester bond holding the palmitate to the DHHC6 enzyme. This likely increases the time for the enzyme to "find" its target protein within cells to transfer the palmitate group and complete the reaction. Compared to Ala or Cys, Sec at position 92 in SELENOK allows a faster transfer of the palmitate from DHHC6 to Cys residues on target peptides. In fact, SELENOK with Cys at position 92 did not improve stability of the acyl-DHHC6 intermediate above SELENOK with Ala at the same position, particularly at physiological pH (7.4) or pH conducive to hydrolysis (6.8). Also, Cys was similar to Ala at position 92 in SELENOK in terms of ability to promote acyl transfer from acyl-DHHC6 to target peptide. Of course, these results were obtained from cell-free systems that do not inlcude important aspects of DHHC6 catalyzed palmitoylation reactions within cells. For example, a recent study found that DHHC6 may act in concert with DHHC16 to perform its catalytic role in cells [21], and this will need to be considered when studying the influence of SELENOK on DHHC6.

Palmitoylation occurs by a two-step mechanism as best demonstrated in the yeast DHHC enzyme complex, Erf2/Erf4. In *Saccharomyces cerevisiae*, Erf2/Erf4 is a heterodimeric PAT that palmitoylates yeast Ras2 on Cys-318. In the first step, the Erf2 subunit of this PAT complex undergoes autopalmitoylation to create a thioester-linked palmitoyl intermediate. In the second step, this intermediate either undergoes hydrolysis (futile cycle) or carries out the transfer of palmitate from the enzyme cysteine to the cysteine of the Ras substrate [13]. The Erf4 subunit functions to stabilize the Acyl-Erf2 intermediate and to avoid the futile cycle of hydrolysis. Our data suggest SELENOK functions similar to the Erf4 subunit by stabilizing Acyl-DHHC6 and improves the overall transfer of the palmitate to target peptides. Moreover, the Sec residue at position 92 is key for improving intermediate stability and acyl transferase activity. As stated above, Cys at position 92 did not improve acyl-DHHC6 intermediate stability or acyl transferase activity above those levels found with Ala at the same position. Since Ala-containing SELENOK represents a "functionally inactive" form of SELENOK with no redox amino acid (there are no other Cys present in the protein), it appears a Cys residue at position 92 in SELENOK is unable to contribute to DHHC6 catalytic functions. However, there are caveats to these interpretations. First, these data were obtained using a modified, cytosolic form of DHHC6 bound to bead-bound SELENOK. Since the palmitoylation of target proteins by DHCC6/SELENOK in the cell occurs at the surface of the ER membrane, the differences between Sec and Cys in SELENOK may not be fully characterized by in vitro assays. Also, without definitive kinetic data the precise differences in enzymatic activity cannot be determined. Our future research will be aimed at overcoming these two limitations.

These findings highlight the importance that nature has placed on stabilizing the acylated DHHC intermediates formed during palmitoylation reactions. In addition to the Erf2/Erf4 example given above, evidence is emerging that other DHHC enzymes employ different strategies to obtain stable intermediates. For example, DHHC9 contains a key amino acid (Arg148) in the Cys-rich domain that when mutated leads to increased loss of palmitate from its acylated intermediate through hydrolysis, suggesting this residue is important for preventing water mediated nucleophilic attack [22]. The possibility that SELENOK functions to stabilize the acyl-DHHC6 intermediate and prevent hydrolysis before the acyl group can be transferred to a target protein highlights the importance of this step in the palmitoylation reaction that physiologically occurs on the cytosolic side of the ER membrane. Synthesis of SELENOK requires sufficient dietary selenium and dedicated translational machinery to insert the 21st amino acid into position 92 [1,3,18]. Exactly how SELENOK uses its Sec residue to stabilize the acyl-DHHC6 intermediate was not determined in this study. It may involve acyl-transfer equilibrium between the thioester bond in DHHC6 and a selenol ester bond in SELENOK that prevents hydrolysis of thioester bond by transferring the acyl group to Sec as a selenol ester bond and then back to DHHC. In fact, SELENOK has been shown to form dimers and experimental evidence highlights the reactivity of selenoesters with selenocystines, so there is the possibility that complex thioester (in DHHC6) and selenoester (In one or more SELENOKs) bonds are involved in the catalytic mechanism [16,23].

5. Conclusions

Overall, our data suggest increasing the efficiency of DHHC6 catalyzed palmitoylation requires Sec in SELENOK that cannot be replaced by Cys. Without SELENOK present in the immune cells, the stability of the acylated DHHC6 intermediate is compromised leading to reduced palmitoylation of key proteins involved in promoting immune cell functions like proliferation, migration, and cytokine secretion. Thus, these new data provide mechanistic insight into previous findings showing that the SELENOK knockout mice exhibit compromised immunity and our laboratory plans to expand on these cell-free assays as we move forward with further in vitro and in vivo experiments.

Acknowledgments: This research was supported by NIH grant R01AI089999, P20GM103457, and core facilities supported by P30GM114737, P30GM103341, G12RR003061, G12MD007601.

Author Contributions: Gregory J. Fredericks and Peter R. Hoffmann conceived and designed the experiments; Gregory J. Fredericks and FuKun W. Hoffmann and Johann Urschitz performed the experiments; Robert J. Hondal and Sharon Rozovsky designed and generated reagents; Gregory J. Fredericks and Peter R. Hoffmann wrote the paper.

Conflicts of Interest: The authors declare no conflicts of interest.

References

1. Bulteau, A.L.; Chavatte, L. Update on selenoprotein biosynthesis. *Antioxid. Redox Signal.* **2015**, *23*, 775–794. [CrossRef] [PubMed]
2. Snider, G.W.; Ruggles, E.; Khan, N.; Hondal, R.J. Selenocysteine confers resistance to inactivation by oxidation in thioredoxin reductase: Comparison of selenium and sulfur enzymes. *Biochemistry* **2013**, *52*, 5472–5481. [CrossRef] [PubMed]
3. Reich, H.J.; Hondal, R.J. Why nature chose selenium. *ACS Chem. Biol.* **2016**, *11*, 821–841. [CrossRef] [PubMed]
4. Reeves, M.A.; Hoffmann, P.R. The human selenoproteome: Recent insights into functions and regulation. *Cell. Mol. Life Sci.* **2009**, *66*, 2457–2478. [CrossRef] [PubMed]
5. Fredericks, G.J.; Hoffmann, F.W.; Rose, A.H.; Osterheld, H.J.; Hess, F.M.; Mercier, F.; Hoffmann, P.R. Stable expression and function of the inositol 1,4,5-triphosphate receptor requires palmitoylation by a DHHC6/selenoprotein K complex. *Proc. Natl. Acad. Sci. USA* **2014**, *111*, 16478–16483. [CrossRef] [PubMed]
6. Mitchell, D.A.; Vasudevan, A.; Linder, M.E.; Deschenes, R.J. Protein palmitoylation by a family of DHHC protein S-acyltransferases. *J. Lipid Res.* **2006**, *47*, 1118–1127. [CrossRef] [PubMed]

7. Dietrich, L.E.; Ungermann, C. On the mechanism of protein palmitoylation. *EMBO Rep.* **2004**, *5*, 1053–1057. [CrossRef] [PubMed]
8. Verma, S.; Hoffmann, F.W.; Kumar, M.; Huang, Z.; Roe, K.; Nguyen-Wu, E.; Hashimoto, A.S.; Hoffmann, P.R. Selenoprotein K knockout mice exhibit deficient calcium flux in immune cells and impaired immune responses. *J. Immunol.* **2011**, *186*, 2127–2137. [CrossRef] [PubMed]
9. Gottlieb, C.D.; Linder, M.E. Structure and function of dhhc protein S-acyltransferases. *Biochem. Soc. Trans.* **2017**, *45*, 923–928. [CrossRef] [PubMed]
10. Norton, R.L.; Fredericks, G.J.; Huang, Z.; Fay, J.D.; Hoffmann, F.W.; Hoffmann, P.R. Selenoprotein K regulation of palmitoylation and calpain cleavage of ASAP2 is required for efficient fcgammar-mediated phagocytosis. *J. Leukoc. Biol.* **2017**, *101*, 439–448. [CrossRef] [PubMed]
11. Meiler, S.; Baumer, Y.; Huang, Z.; Hoffmann, F.W.; Fredericks, G.J.; Rose, A.H.; Norton, R.L.; Hoffmann, P.R.; Boisvert, W.A. Selenoprotein K is required for palmitoylation of CD36 in macrophages: Implications in foam cell formation and atherogenesis. *J. Leukoc. Biol.* **2013**, *93*, 771–780. [CrossRef] [PubMed]
12. Fredericks, G.J.; Hoffmann, P.R. Selenoprotein K and protein palmitoylation. *Antioxid. Redox Signal.* **2015**, *23*, 854–862. [CrossRef] [PubMed]
13. Jennings, B.C.; Linder, M.E. DHHC protein S-acyltransferases use similar ping-pong kinetic mechanisms but display different acyl-coa specificities. *J. Biol. Chem.* **2012**, *287*, 7236–7245. [CrossRef] [PubMed]
14. Mitchell, D.A.; Mitchell, G.; Ling, Y.; Budde, C.; Deschenes, R.J. Mutational analysis of saccharomyces cerevisiae Erf2 reveals a two-step reaction mechanism for protein palmitoylation by DHHC enzymes. *J. Biol. Chem.* **2010**, *285*, 38104–38114. [CrossRef] [PubMed]
15. Mitchell, D.A.; Hamel, L.D.; Ishizuka, K.; Mitchell, G.; Schaefer, L.M.; Deschenes, R.J. The Erf4 subunit of the yeast Ras palmitoyl acyltransferase is required for stability of the Acyl-Erf2 intermediate and palmitoyl transfer to a Ras2 substrate. *J. Biol. Chem.* **2012**, *287*, 34337–34348. [CrossRef] [PubMed]
16. Swarthout, J.T.; Lobo, S.; Farh, L.; Croke, M.R.; Greentree, W.K.; Deschenes, R.J.; Linder, M.E. DHHC9 and GCP16 constitute a human protein fatty acyltransferase with specificity for H- and N-Ras. *J. Biol. Chem.* **2005**, *280*, 31141–31148. [CrossRef] [PubMed]
17. Liu, J.; Zhang, Z.; Rozovsky, S. Selenoprotein K form an intermolecular diselenide bond with unusually high redox potential. *FEBS Lett.* **2014**, *588*, 3311–3321. [CrossRef] [PubMed]
18. Zhang, Z.; Liu, J.; Rozovsky, S. Preparation of selenocysteine-containing forms of human selenok and selenos. *Methods Mol. Biol.* **2018**, *1661*, 241–263. [PubMed]
19. Huang, Z.; Hoffmann, F.W.; Fay, J.D.; Hashimoto, A.C.; Chapagain, M.L.; Kaufusi, P.H.; Hoffmann, P.R. Stimulation of unprimed macrophages with immune complexes triggers a low output of nitric oxide by calcium-dependent neuronal nitric-oxide synthase. *J. Biol. Chem.* **2012**, *287*, 4492–4502. [CrossRef] [PubMed]
20. Chen, X.; Zaro, J.L.; Shen, W.C. Fusion protein linkers: Property, design and functionality. *Adv. Drug Deliv. Rev.* **2013**, *65*, 1357–1369. [CrossRef] [PubMed]
21. Abrami, L.; Dallavilla, T.; Sandoz, P.A.; Demir, M.; Kunz, B.; Savoglidis, G.; Hatzimanikatis, V.; Van Der Goot, F.G. Identification and dynamics of the human ZDHHC16-ZDHHC6 palmitoylation cascade. *Elife* **2017**, *6*, e27826. [CrossRef] [PubMed]
22. Mitchell, D.A.; Hamel, L.D.; Reddy, K.D.; Farh, L.; Rettew, L.M.; Sanchez, P.R.; Deschenes, R.J. Mutations in the X-linked intellectual disability gene, zDHHC9, alter autopalmitoylation activity by distinct mechanisms. *J. Biol. Chem.* **2014**, *289*, 18582–18592. [CrossRef] [PubMed]
23. Mitchell, N.J.; Malins, L.R.; Liu, X.; Thompson, R.E.; Chan, B.; Radom, L.; Payne, R.J. Rapid additive-free selenocystine-selenoester peptide ligation. *J. Am. Chem. Soc.* **2015**, *137*, 14011–14014. [CrossRef] [PubMed]

2

Transcription Factor ETS-1 and Reactive Oxygen Species: Role in Vascular and Renal Injury

Yan-Ting Shiu [1] and Edgar A. Jaimes [2,3,*]

1 Division of Nephrology and Hypertension, University of Utah, Salt Lake City, UT 84112, USA; Y.Shiu@hsc.utah.edu
2 Renal Service, Memorial Sloan Kettering Cancer Center, New York, NY 10065, USA
3 Renal Division, Weill Cornell Medical College, New York, NY 10065, USA
* Correspondence: jaimese@mskcc.org

Abstract: The E26 avian erythroblastosis virus transcription factor-1 (ETS-1) is a member of the ETS family and regulates the expression of a variety of genes including growth factors, chemokines and adhesion molecules. Although ETS-1 was discovered as an oncogene, several lines of research show that it is up-regulated by angiotensin II (Ang II) both in the vasculature and the glomerulus. While reactive oxygen species (ROS) are required for Ang II-induced ETS-1 expression, ETS-1 also regulates the expression of p47*phox*, which is one of the subunits of nicotinamide adenine dinucleotide phosphate (NADPH) oxidase and a major source of ROS in the kidney and vasculature. Thus, there appears to be a positive feedback between ETS-1 and ROS. ETS-1 is also upregulated in the kidneys of rats with salt-sensitive hypertension and plays a major role in the development of end-organ injury in this animal model. Activation of the renin angiotensin system is required for the increased ETS-1 expression in these rats, and blockade of ETS-1 or haplodeficiency reduces the severity of kidney injury in these rats. In summary, ETS-1 plays a major role in the development of vascular and renal injury and is a potential target for the development of novel therapeutic strategies to ameliorate end-organ injury in hypertension.

Keywords: ETS-1; reactive oxygen species; vascular injury; renal injury

---

1. Introduction

Originally discovered as an oncogene, ETS-1 is now known to regulate several important biological processes in various normal cell types beyond tumors, including the regulation of immune cell functions. ETS-1 is the founding member of the ETS family, the members of which share a unique DNA binding domain called the ETS domain. The name "ETS" originates from a sequence that was discovered in 1983 in the E26 avian erythroblastosis virus, where it forms a transforming gene together with Δ*gag* and *c-myb*, which encodes a 135-kDa gag-myb-ets fusion protein [1–3]. This newly discovered sequence was called the E26 transformation-specific sequence. In human, currently the ETS family consists of 28 members, which are classified into 4 distinct classes based on the in vitro derived binding site (Class I, II, III, IV) and 12 subfamilies based on ETS domain sequence homology (ETS, ERG, PEA3, ETV, TCF, GABP, ELF1, SPI1, TEL, ERF, SPDEF, and ESE) [4,5]. ETS-1 is the first discovered in the ETS family and belongs to Class I and the ETS subfamily.

In humans, the ETS-1 gene is located on chromosome 11 (11q24.3). The human TATA-less ETS-1 gene contains 8 exons, designated as exon A (first exon) followed by exons III–IX (last seven exons) [6]. Its product is the major isoform of ETS-1, which has 441 amino acids and is referred to as p54. The p54 isoform can be divided into 6 domains (Figure 1) (adapted from [7,8]). The A and B domains are regulatory units. In particular, the B domain (between amino acids 54 and 135) is the "pointed domain", which is characterized by a sterile alpha motif (SAM) and is the second most common domain present in ETS proteins. The C domain (between amino acids 135 and 243) is the transactivation domain and contains a high content of acidic residues. The D domain (between amino acids 243 and 331) comprises two regulatory units. While its *N*-terminal unit contains several calcium-responsive phosphorylation sites, its C-terminal unit is part of an autoinhibitory module that also includes the F domain. The key functional unit of this autoinhibitory module has three inhibitory helices, which are HI-1 and HI-2 in the D domain and H4 in the F domain. The E domain (between amino acids 331 and 415) is the DNA binding ETS domain and is present in all ETS proteins. It is composed of 85 amino acids and characterized by a winged helix-turn-helix (wHTH) motif that specifically recognizes DNA sequences containing a GGAA/T core element. This domain comprises three α-helices and four β-strands that are arranged as H1-S1-S2-H2-H3-S3-S4. The autoinhibitory module's helices block the ETS domain's DNA binding activity by interacting with the H1-helix within the ETS domain, rendering the ETS domain in a closed confirmation and cannot bind DNA.

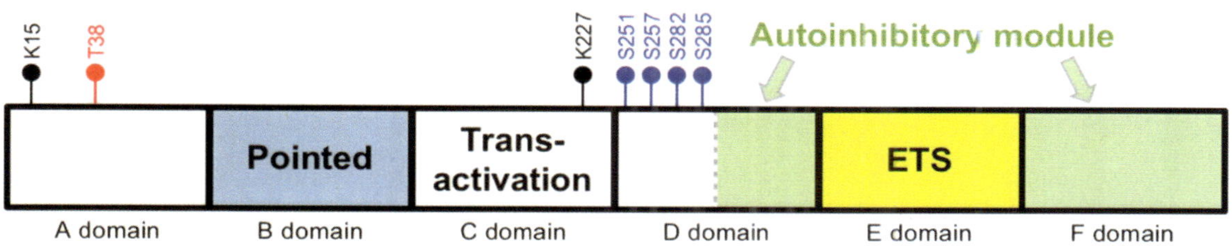

Figure 1. Domains of the most abundant isoform of ETS-1. Black circles are the lysine (K) sumoylation sites. Blue circles are the Ca^{2+}-dependent serine (S) phosphorylation sites. The red circle is the Ras-dependent threonine (T) phosphorylation site. Note that the schematic domain lengths are not proportional to the numbers of amino acids within each domain.

2. Regulation

The transcriptional activity of ETS-1 can be modulated through posttranslational modifications (including phosphorylation, ubiquitinylation, acetylation and sumoylation), other transcription factors, and its nuclear transportation.

2.1. Posttranslational Modifications

Phosphorylation of threonine 38 (Thr38) in the A domain by the mitogen-activated kinases extracellular signal regulated kinases 1 and 2 (ERK1/2) in the Ras-Raf-MAPK pathway increases the transcriptional activity of ETS-1 to promote DNA transcription [9–11]. The adjacent B domain (the pointed domain) serves as a docking site for ERK2. Phosphorylation of ETS-1 at Thr38 enhances the association of ETS-1 with two transcriptional co-activating proteins p300 and cAMP response element-binding protein (CREB) binding protein (CBP), resulting in an increase in the transactivational activity of their target genes [12,13]. The C-domain (the transactivation domain) is necessary for the interaction of ETS-1 with CBP/p300. Finally, it has been shown that in response to transforming growth factor (TGF)-β signaling, ETS-1 becomes acetylated and dissociated from the CBP/p300 complexes [14].

On the other hand, phosphorylation of serine residues in the D domain by calmodulin-dependent kinase II (CaMKII) inhibits DNA binding [15]. This inhibition is mediated by two mechanisms. First, serine phosphorylation in the D domain's *N*-terminal unit increases the inhibitory effect of its C-terminal unit by stabilizing the inhibitory structure mentioned above. Second, serine phosphorylation of ETS-1 enhances its association with an E3 ubiquitin ligase, the ring finger and WD repeat domain 2 protein (RFWD2), which leads to its ubiquitination and subsequent degradation through the ubiquitin–proteasome pathway [16,17]. The exact lysine residue(s) of ETS-1 involved in ubiquitination are not yet known. Finally, mutation of the sumoylation sites in ETS-1 (K15 and K227) lead to increased transcriptional activity by ETS-1, suggesting that sumoylation of ETS-1 inhibits in its activity in transactivating genes [17,18].

2.2. By Transcription Factors

ETS-1 activity is further regulated through direct interactions with other transcription factors. As mentioned above, the autoinhibitory module binds to the ETS domain and the inhibitory structure is reinforced by serine phosphorylation. However, the autoinhibitory module of ETS-1 has been shown to interact with runt-related transcription factor 1 (Runx1, also termed acute myelogenous leukemia 1 (AML1) or core-binding factor α2 (CBFα2)), paired box protein Pax-5 (Pax5), transcription factor E3 (TFE3), and upstream stimulatory factor 1 (USF 1) to relieve autoinhibition [19–24]. It is important to note that, when two ETS DNA binding sites are present in the correct orientation and spacing, the autoinhibitory module of an ETS-1 protein can interact with the adjacent ETS-1 to relieve autoinhibitory function [25].

2.3. By Nuclear Transport

Another important mechanism by which the function of ETS proteins can be regulated is through nuclear transport. A specific region in the ETS-1 protein (between amino acids 369 and 388) called the nuclear localization sequence facilitates its movement from the cytoplasm into the nucleus, which is required for its function as a transcription factor [26].

2.4. Regulation of Its Expression

The expression of ETS-1 is affected by a wide spectrum of factors. Here we focus on angiotensin II (Ang II), which is a critical mediator of renal injury and vascular inflammation. In the context of kidney fibrosis, we have demonstrated that Ang II-induced expression of ETS-1 in mesangial cells was mediated by ROS [27]. In the vasculature, Ang II induced the expression of ETS-1 in cultured rat aortic smooth muscle cells, which was mediated by the $G_{q/11}$-Src-Ras pathway [28]. More about the induction of ETS-1 by Ang II and the functional consequences are presented below.

3. Effects of Angiotensin II on ETS-1 Expression and the Functional Consequences in the Vasculature and Kidney

3.1. In Vitro Studies

Angiotensin (Ang) II is a well-known mediator in the development of hypertension, atherosclerosis and renal injury [29]. Multiple studies support a role for NADPH oxidase-derived reactive oxygen species (ROS) as intermediaries of several effects of Ang II [30], including promoting lipoprotein oxidation, vascular smooth muscle hypertrophy, mesangial cell hypertrophy, extracellular matrix formation and endothelial injury [31,32] (Figure 2).

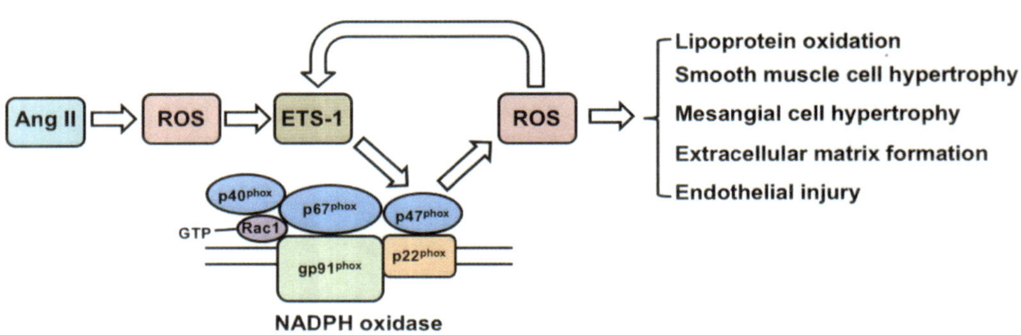

Figure 2. Regulation of ETS-1 by angiotensin II and the functional consequences. Ang II: Angiotensin II; ROS: reactive oxygen species; NADPH: nicotinamide adenine dinucleotide phosphate.

In vascular smooth muscle cells, ETS-1 is induced in response to a variety of inflammatory stimuli, including Ang II [33–35]. Furthermore, Ang-II induced production of the chemokine monocyte chemoattractant protein-1, the vascular cell adhesion molecule-1, and plasminogen activator inhibitor-1 in the vascular wall cells was mediated by ETS-1 [36]. In mesangial cells, Ang II increases the expression of ETS-1 via increased generation of ROS. In these cells, ETS-1 activates the production of fibronectin by directly binding an activating its promoter [37]. Thus, Ang-II induced ETS-1 in vascular smooth muscle cells and mesangial cells are of functional consequences.

In vitro studies have also demonstrated that ETS-1 is a downstream transcriptional effector of ROS. In several ovarian cancer cell lines, the expression of ETS-1 is induced by H_2O_2 [38]. In these cells, the induction of ETS-1 is associated with binding of the transcription factor Nrf2 to an antioxidant response element within the *ETS-1* gene promoter. ETS-1 can also collaborate with the transcription factor activator protein-1 to regulate gene expression of the matrix metalloproteinase-1 in response to H_2O_2 in a fibrosarcoma cell line [39]. On the other hand, ETS-1 regulates the expression of p47*phox*, which is one of the subunits of NADPH oxidase and a major source of ROS in the kidney and vasculature [40]. Taken together, these studies support a dual role of ETS-1 as a downstream mediator of ROS, as well as an upstream regulator of ROS via regulating the expression of genes that are involved in the ROS generation (Figure 2).

As we and others have shown, the production of ROS is a critical determinant in Ang II-induced vascular remodeling that is independent of changes in blood pressure [32,41,42]. ROS also play a major role as mediators of extracellular matrix deposition, mesangial cell proliferation and hypertrophy in the kidney in response to Ang II [32]. In glomerular mesangial cells, we have shown that Ang II-induced ETS-1 expression is prevented by ROS inhibition, suggesting that ROS are necessary for ETS-1 expression [27]. We also showed that ETS-1 is one of the transcription factors that transactivate the expression of fibronectin induced by Ang II. This transactivation occurs through the interaction of ETS-1 with CREB and p300. In addition, we showed that the phosphorylation of ETS-1 induced by Ang II involves both ERK-MAPK and PI3K/Akt pathways [37].

3.2. *In Vivo Studies*

The renal expression of ETS-1 is augmented in a variety of models of renal injury. In the anti-Thy model of glomerulonephritis, the expression of ETS-1 is increased in the glomerular mesangium and to a lesser degree in podocytes and glomerular endothelium [43]. In a model of acute renal failure, the tubular expression of ETS-1 is increased and associated with increased expression of cyclin D, suggesting that ETS-1 participates in the control of tubular regeneration in acute renal failure [44]. In rats with anti-glomerular basement induced glomerulonephritis, there is also increased expression of ETS-1 in the glomeruli and in the interstitium [45].

In vivo studies have also determined that Ang II increases renal ETS-1 expression. We have found that the infusion of Ang II results in a 3-fold increase in ETS-1 mRNA expression and a 4-fold increase in ETS-1 protein expression as compared with control mice [46] (Figure 3). By immunofluorescence, we determined that the increase in ETS-1 expression was mostly in the glomeruli. In these mice, blockade of ETS-1 utilizing a dominant negative peptide (ETS-DN) reduced proteinuria, mesangial expansion and expression of α-smooth muscle actin, a well-validated marker of renal fibrosis [46]. Blockade of ETS-1 also reduced the mRNA and protein expression of the growth factors TGF-β and CTGF, as well as cell proliferation and macrophage infiltration [46]. The infusion of Ang II resulted in increased expression of NOX4 and nitrotyrosine, which were also reduced by ETS blockade. These findings demonstrate that the inductive effects of Ang II on renal fibrosis, inflammation and increased oxidative stress are at least in part mediated by ETS-1. Importantly, ETS-1 blockade did not have a significant effect on blood pressure in mice infused with Ang II.

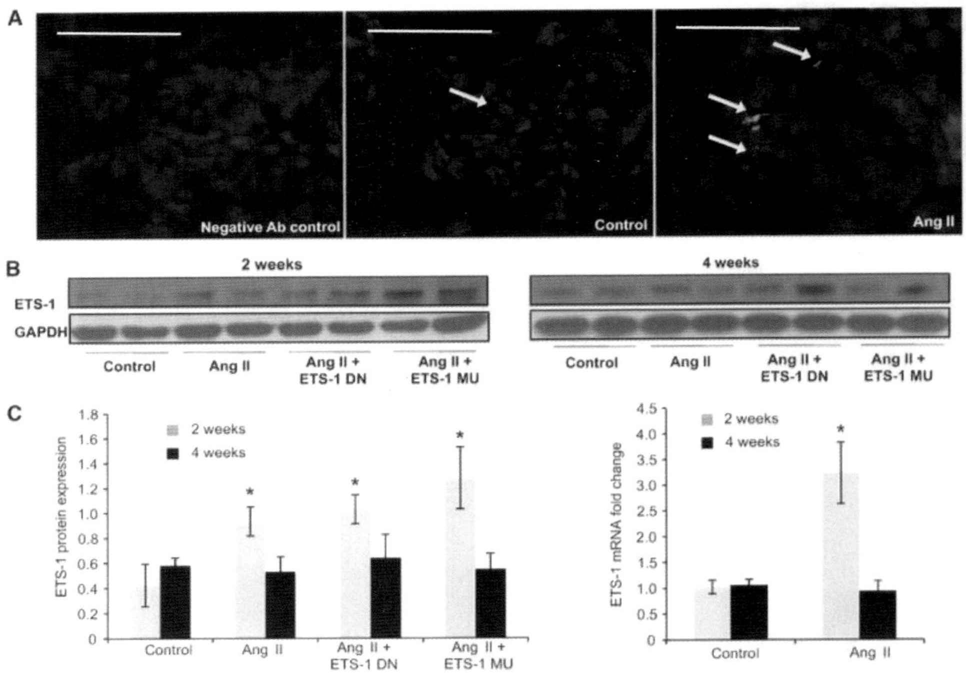

Figure 3. Angiotensin II (Ang II) increases cortical ETS-1 expression. (**A**) Representative confocal photomicrographs showing low basal expression of ETS-1 (green) in control kidney cortex, which is predominantly glomerular and increased by Ang II. (Bar = 50 μm); (**B**) The renal cortical ETS-1 protein expression increases after 2 weeks of Ang II as assessed by Western blot ($n = 6$, * $p < 0.05$ vs. control) and returns to baseline after 4 weeks of Ang II. The expression of ETS-1 was not significantly modified by treatment with either ETS-1 dominant-negative (ETS-1 DN) or ETS-1 mutant (ETS-1 MU) peptide; (**C**) Densitometric analysis for ETS-1 showing significant increases in ETS-1 protein expression after 2 but not after 4 weeks of Ang II. Neither ETS-1 DN nor ETS-1 MU modified ETS-1 protein expression. Data expressed as mean ± SEM are normalized to GAPDH (* $p < 0.05$ vs. control; $n = 6$). The infusion of Ang II for 2 weeks resulted in increases in cortical ETS-1 mRNA expression as assessed by real-time reverse transcriptase polymerase chain reaction ($n = 6$; * $p < 0.05$ vs. control) and returns to baseline levels after 4 weeks of Ang II. GAPDH: glyceraldehyde 3-phosphate dehydrogenase. (Right panel).

Others have demonstrated that in response to systemic Ang II infusion, ETS-1 is induced in vascular smooth muscle cells and endothelial cells of the mouse thoracic aorta [36]. Furthermore, Ang II-induced arterial wall thickening, perivascular fibrosis, cardiac hypertrophy and recruitment of T cells and macrophages to the vessel wall were significantly diminished in *ETS-1*$^{-/-}$ mice as compared with control mice. Ang II-induced cyclin-dependent kinase inhibitor p21CIP, plasminogen activator inhibitor-1, and monocyte chemoattractant protein-1 were also reduced in the aorta of ETS-1$^{-/-}$ mice compared with wild-type controls [36].

In addition, Ang II-induced production of H_2O_2 and superoxide anion (O_2^-) was blunted in vascular smooth muscle cells from *ETS-1*$^{-/-}$ mice. In primary human aortic smooth muscle cells, Ang II-induced ROS production and the induction of the NADPH oxidase subunit p47phox were inhibited by small interfering RNA of ETS-1. In addition, blockade of ETS-1 with ETS-DN reduced Ang II–induced ROS production and medial hypertrophy in the mouse thoracic aorta [47].

4. ETS-1 in Neointima Formation

The formation of neointimal hyperplasia is a common response to vascular injury. It is the result of migration and proliferation of vascular smooth muscle cells into the intimal layer and is the major cause of restenosis after percutaneous coronary intervention such as balloon angioplasty and stenting [48]. Using a rat carotid artery balloon injury model, we found that mRNA expression of ETS-1 was increased rapidly (within 2 h) in injured carotid arteries and we confirmed increased nuclear expression of ETS-1 within 24 h postinjury [48]. Importantly, we found that blockade of ETS-1 with ETS-1 DN effectively inhibited neointima formation in this model (Figure 4). We also demonstrated that ETS-1 mediated the formation of arterial neointima in this model by regulating the activation of proinflammatory cytokines and adhesion molecules, including IL-6, monocyte chemoattractant protein 1 (MCP-1), P-selectin, and E-selectin [48]. Neointima formation can also occur in the vein, such as in an arteriovenous fistula (created by a direct anastomosis between an artery and a vein) or an arteriovenous graft that is used as hemodialysis vascular access. Using a mouse model of carotid-jugular fistula, we found that the mRNA expression of ETS-1 was increased in the venous limb of the fistula, and we confirmed increased expression of ETS-1 predominantly in the neointima and overlying endothelium [49]. Furthermore, blockade of ETS-1 with ETS-1 DN inhibited the formation of neointima in the mouse carotid-jugular fistula, as well as reduced the expression of nitric oxide synthase 2, NOX2, NOX4, E-selectin, and MCP-1 [49]. While we also found an increased protein and nuclear expression of ETS-1 in the neointima of a porcine carotid-jugular graft model, we did not find an increase of ETS-1 at the mRNA level [49].

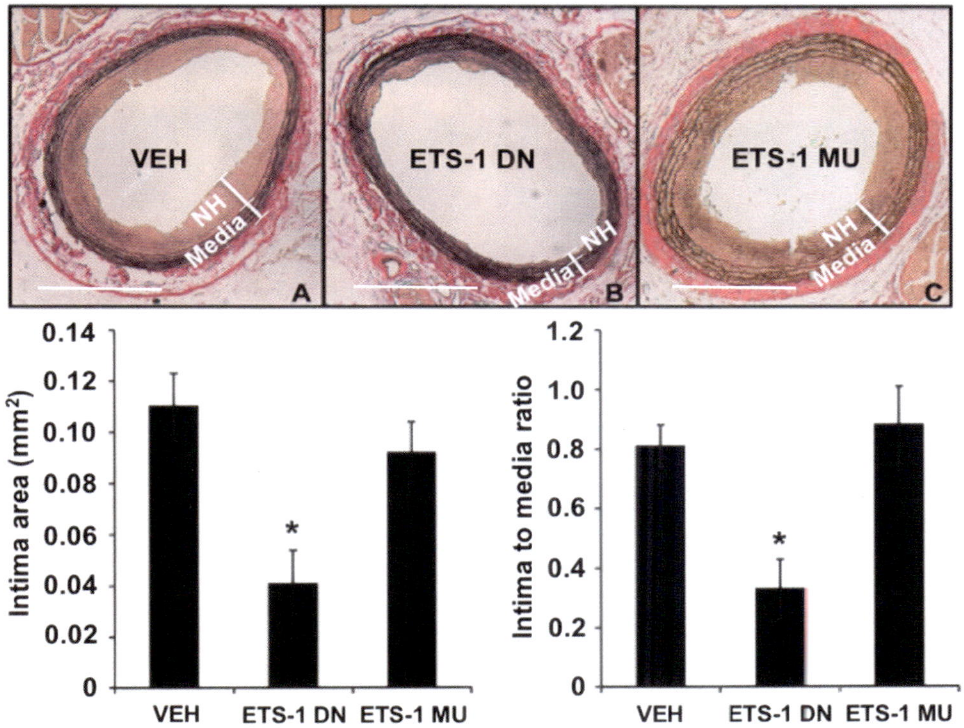

Figure 4. A single injection of ETS-1 DN (10 mg/kg) inhibited the formation of neointimal hyperplasia (NH) in injured rat carotid arteries. Top, elastic Van Gieson-stained tissue sections of carotid arteries from rats treated with (**A**) saline vehicle (VEH); (**B**) ETS-1 DN; or (**C**) ETS-1 mutant (MU) 14 days after balloon injury. Bottom, composite data are shown as mean ± SEM ($n = 6$ per group). * $p < 0.05$ compared to the VEH group. (Bar = 50 µm).

5. ETS-1 in Salt-Sensitive Hypertension

Salt-sensitive (SS) hypertension affects over 50% of the general population [50] and is associated with a high risk for hypertensive end-organ damage including atherosclerosis, left ventricular hypertrophy and chronic kidney disease [51]. As we have previously shown, SS hypertension is characterized by reduced cardiovascular and renal NO bioavailability [51]. The renin angiotensin system (RAS) has been recognized as an endocrine, paracrine, autocrine and intracrine system [52–54]. Although all organs have elements of the RAS, the kidney is unique in that it has every component of the RAS [55]. Importantly the tissue concentration of Ang II in the kidneys are several fold higher than can be explained by Ang II delivery from arterial blood flow [56]. Dahl salt-sensitive rats (DS rats) are a well-established model of salt-sensitive hypertension that develop hypertension when fed a high salt diet [57]. Although these rats have low levels of circulating RAS several studies have shown improvement of cardiac and renal function when treated with an angiotensin-converting enzyme (ACE) inhibitor or angiotensin II receptor blockers (ARB) [58–63], suggesting local activation of RAS. Although these rats have suppressed plasma renin when placed on a high salt diet the kidney levels of angiotensinogen are markedly increased indicating a paradoxical augmentation of intrarenal angiotensinogen that appears to be mediated dependent on the generation of reactive oxygen species [64–66].

We have demonstrated increased glomerular expression of ETS-1 in hypertensive Dahl salt-sensitive rats [67]. These rats had a significant increase in the phosphorylated ETS-1 level without a change in the total ETS-1 level. Phosphorylated ETS-1 was primarily located in the glomeruli and predominantly expressed in the glomerular epithelium and to a lesser degree in the glomerular endothelium (Figure 5).

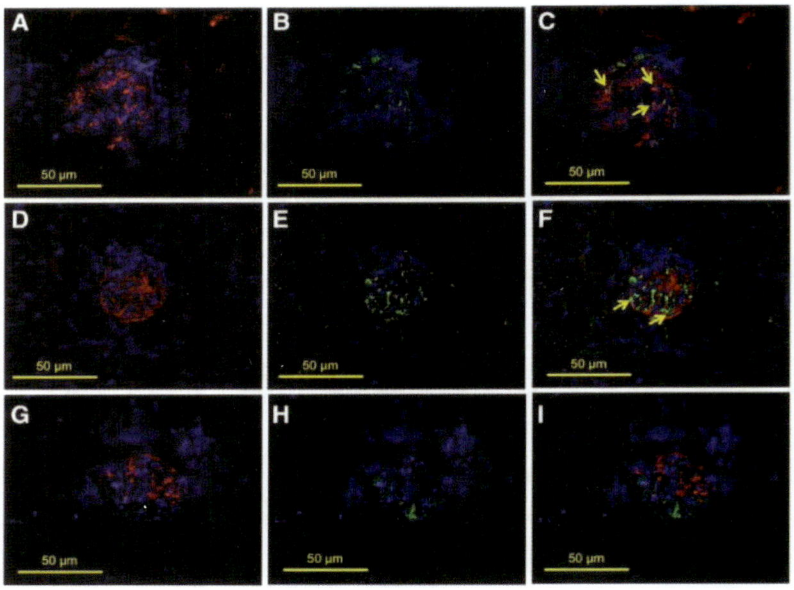

Figure 5. Glomerular expression of transcription factor avian erythroblastosis virus E26 oncogen homolog-1 (ETS-1) in hypertensive Dahl salt-sensitive (DS) rats. Colocalization studies were performed to characterize the expression of ETS-1 in the glomerular endothelium (CD31), podocytes (synaptopodin), or mesangium (desmin). (**A–C**) show positive stain for CD31 (**A**, red), ETS-1 (**B**, green), and some areas in which there is colocalization of CD31 and ETS-1 indicating endothelial expression of ETS-1 (**C**, arrows); (**D–F**) show positive stain for synaptopodin (**D**, red), ETS-1 (**E**, green), and areas in which there is colocalization of ETS-1 and synaptopodin indicating expression of ETS-1 in podocytes (**F**, arrows); (**G–I**) show positive stain for desmin (**G**, red), ETS-1 (**H**, green); no clear evidence of colocalization of ETS-1 and desmin was observed (**I**), suggesting lack of expression of ETS-1 in mesangial areas (×40 magnification).

Studies have demonstrated that Dahl salt-sensitive rats, when fed a high salt diet and made hypertensive, have increased local activation of the RAS, characterized by sustained levels of Ang II, increased levels of angiotensinogen and increased expression of the AT1 receptor [64]. In addition, as others and we have shown, salt-sensitive hypertension is associated with reduced NO bioavailability and increased ROS production [51,68–70]. In support of the role for increased RAS activation in salt-sensitive hypertension, AT1 receptor blockade ameliorates cardiac and/or renal dysfunction in these rats, suggesting an important role for RAS in the development of end-organ injury in salt-sensitive hypertension [65,66]. We observed an increased level of phosphorylated ETS-1 in hypertensive DS rats, and this increase was significantly reduced by RAS blockade with ARB, suggesting that increased RAS activation mediates increased ETS-1 phosphorylation in hypertensive DS rats [67]. To determine the role of ETS-1 in the pathogenesis of renal injury in salt-sensitive hypertension, we used a dominant negative ETS-1 peptide that competes for DNA binding with ETS-1 but does not initiate gene transcription. We observed that ETS-1 blockade reduced ETS-1 phosphorylation, which is consistent with a positive feedback of ETS-1 on its own activation.

ETS-1 blockade alone resulted in significant reductions in glomerular injury score, fibronectin expression, proteinuria and macrophage infiltration but had no significant effect on interstitial fibrosis. RAS blockade alone also reduced glomerular injury score, proteinuria and macrophage infiltration but had no significant effect on fibronectin production or fibrosis. In contrast, concomitant ETS-1 and RAS blockade had additive effects on all parameters examined. In addition, we observed that ETS-1 blockade resulted in a significant reduction in the urinary excretion of TGF-β, suggesting that ETS-1 may be a direct regulator of TGF-β in hypertensive DS rats. In contrast, RAS blockade did not modify the urinary excretion of TGF-β, indicating that other pathways independent of RAS participate in the production of TGF-β in hypertensive DS rats. Both ETS-1 blockade alone and RAS blockade alone had very small effects on blood pressure as measured by radio-telemetry. However, rats with combined ETS-1 and RAS blockade had blood pressures that were similar to those from rats on a normal salt diet, indicating that ETS-1 may also be playing a role in blood pressure regulation either directly or indirectly. These findings also suggest that the additional beneficial effects of concomitant ETS-1 and RAS blockade are in large part due to their effects on blood pressure [67].

To better understand the interaction between RAS and ETS-1, we measured the expression of some of main components of RAS in the different experimental groups. We and others have previously shown that hypertensive DS rats had significant increases in the urinary excretion of angiotensinogen and intrarenal concentration of Ang II, which are indicative of increased RAS activation. Both ETS-1 blockade alone as well as RAS blockade alone induced significant reductions in the urinary excretion of angiotensinogen and tissue levels of Ang II. Concomitant ETS-1 and RAS blockade further reduced the urinary excretion of angiotensinogen. These findings suggest that ETS-1 also plays a role in the regulation of the RAS, through the mechanisms are unclear.

In our recent studies, when placed on high salt diet, DS rats with only one functioning ETS-1 gene had lower glomerular injury score, less albuminuria, lower serum creatinine and less kidney fibrosis when compared to wild type controls [71]. Moreover, transplant of a kidney from rats with only one copy of the ETS-1 gene into salt resistant rats (DR) resulted in less glomerular injury and proteinuria as compared to rats transplanted with a kidney receiving a transplant from a DS rat. These results demonstrate that reduced renal expression of ETS-1 prevents hypertension-associated kidney injury in SS rats [71].

6. Conclusions

In conclusion, multiple sources of experimental evidence demonstrate a role of ETS-1 in vascular and renal injury. ETS-1 is upregulated by Ang II and regulates the expression of cytokines, growth factors and adhesion molecules. Reactive oxygen species are required for ETS-1 expression in response to Ang II but at the same time ETS-1 regulates the activity of NADPH oxidase in the vasculature. ETS-1 is upregulated the vasculature following injury and drives the formation of neointima. ETS-1 is also upregulated in salt-sensitive hypertension, where it plays an important role in the development of end-organ injury. The current evidence suggests that ETS-1 could be a potential therapeutic target for the treatment or prevention of end-organ injury in hypertension since beneficial RAS and ETS-1 blockade have additive beneficial effects on the severity of injury suggesting that ETS-1 can also be upregulated independently of RAS activation.

Funding: This research was funded by U.S. Department of Veterans Affairs: I01BX001073 (EAJ) and a National Institutes of Health R01DK100505 grant (YTS).

Acknowledgments: The authors thank Daniel B. Pike for assistance in preparing this manuscript.

Conflicts of Interest: The authors declare no conflicts of interest.

References

1. Leprince, D.; Gegonne, A.; Coll, J.; de Taisne, C.; Schneeberger, A.; Lagrou, C.; Stehelin, D. A putative second cell-derived oncogene of the avian leukaemia retrovirus E26. *Nature* **1983**, *306*, 395–397. [CrossRef] [PubMed]
2. Nunn, M.F.; Seeburg, P.H.; Moscovici, C.; Duesberg, P.H. Tripartite structure of the avian erythroblastosis virus E26 transforming gene. *Nature* **1983**, *306*, 391–395. [CrossRef] [PubMed]
3. Watson, D.K.; McWilliams-Smith, M.J.; Nunn, M.F.; Duesberg, P.H.; O'Brien, S.J.; Papas, T.S. The ets sequence from the transforming gene of avian erythroblastosis virus, E26, has unique domains on human chromosomes 11 and 21: Both loci are transcriptionally active. *Proc. Natl. Acad. Sci. USA* **1985**, *82*, 7294–7298. [CrossRef] [PubMed]
4. Hollenhorst, P.C.; McIntosh, L.P.; Graves, B.J. Genomic and biochemical insights into the specificity of ETS transcription factors. *Ann. Rev. Biochem.* **2011**, *80*, 437–471. [CrossRef] [PubMed]
5. Findlay, V.J.; LaRue, A.C.; Turner, D.P.; Watson, P.M.; Watson, D.K. Understanding the role of ETS-mediated gene regulation in complex biological processes. *Adv. Cancer Res.* **2013**, *119*, 1–61. [PubMed]
6. Iotsova, V.; Crepieux, P.; Montpellier, C.; Laudet, V.; Stehelin, D. TATA-less promoters of some Ets-family genes are efficiently repressed by wild-type p53. *Oncogene* **1996**, *13*, 2331–2337. [PubMed]
7. Garrett-Sinha, L.A. Review of Ets1 structure, function, and roles in immunity. *Cell. Mol. Life Sci.* **2013**, *70*, 3375–3390. [CrossRef] [PubMed]
8. Dittmer, J. The biology of the Ets1 proto-oncogene. *Mol. Cancer* **2003**, *2*, 29. [CrossRef] [PubMed]
9. Yang, B.S.; Hauser, C.A.; Henkel, G.; Colman, M.S.; Van Beveren, C.; Stacey, K.J.; Hume, D.A.; Maki, R.A.; Ostrowski, M.C. Ras-mediated phosphorylation of a conserved threonine residue enhances the transactivation activities of c-Ets1 and c-Ets2. *Mol. Cell. Biol.* **1996**, *16*, 538–547. [CrossRef] [PubMed]
10. Slupsky, C.M.; Gentile, L.N.; Donaldson, L.W.; Mackereth, C.D.; Seidel, J.J.; Graves, B.J.; McIntosh, L.P. Structure of the Ets-1 pointed domain and mitogen-activated protein kinase phosphorylation site. *Proc. Natl. Acad. Sci. USA* **1998**, *95*, 12129–12134. [CrossRef] [PubMed]
11. Wasylyk, B.; Hagman, J.; Gutierrez-Hartmann, A. Ets transcription factors: Nuclear effectors of the Ras-MAP-kinase signaling pathway. *Trends Biochem. Sci.* **1998**, *23*, 213–216. [CrossRef]
12. Foulds, C.E.; Nelson, M.L.; Blaszczak, A.G.; Graves, B.J. Ras/mitogen-activated protein kinase signaling activates Ets-1 and Ets-2 by CBP/p300 recruitment. *Mol. Cell. Biol.* **2004**, *24*, 10954–10964. [CrossRef] [PubMed]
13. Nelson, M.L.; Kang, H.S.; Lee, G.M.; Blaszczak, A.G.; Lau, D.K.; McIntosh, L.P.; Graves, B.J. Ras signaling requires dynamic properties of Ets1 for phosphorylation-enhanced binding to coactivator CBP. *Proc. Natl. Acad. Sci. USA* **2010**, *107*, 10026–10031. [CrossRef] [PubMed]
14. Czuwara-Ladykowska, J.; Sementchenko, V.I.; Watson, D.K.; Trojanowska, M. Ets1 is an effector of the transforming growth factor beta (TGF-beta) signaling pathway and an antagonist of the profibrotic effects of TGF-beta. *J. Biol. Chem.* **2002**, *277*, 20399–20408. [CrossRef] [PubMed]
15. Cowley, D.O.; Graves, B.J. Phosphorylation represses Ets-1 DNA binding by reinforcing autoinhibition. *Genes Dev.* **2000**, *14*, 366–376. [PubMed]
16. Nishida, T.; Terashima, M.; Fukami, K.; Yamada, Y. PIASy controls ubiquitination-dependent proteasomal degradation of Ets-1. *Biochem. J.* **2007**, *405*, 481–488. [CrossRef] [PubMed]
17. Ji, Z.; Degerny, C.; Vintonenko, N.; Deheuninck, J.; Foveau, B.; Leroy, C.; Coll, J.; Tulasne, D.; Baert, J.L.; Fafeur, V. Regulation of the Ets-1 transcription factor by sumoylation and ubiquitinylation. *Oncogene* **2007**, *26*, 395–406. [CrossRef] [PubMed]
18. Nishida, T.; Terashima, M.; Fukami, K. PIASy-mediated repression of the Ets-1 is independent of its sumoylation. *Biochem. Biophys. Res. Commun.* **2006**, *345*, 1536–1546. [CrossRef] [PubMed]

19. Sieweke, M.H.; Tekotte, H.; Jarosch, U.; Graf, T. Cooperative interaction of Ets-1 with USF-1 required for HIV-1 enhancer activity in T cells. *EMBO J.* **1998**, *17*, 1728–1739. [CrossRef] [PubMed]
20. Garvie, C.W.; Hagman, J.; Wolberger, C. Structural studies of Ets-1/Pax5 complex formation on DNA. *Mol. Cell.* **2001**, *8*, 1267–1276. [CrossRef]
21. Tian, G.; Erman, B.; Ishii, H.; Gangopadhyay, S.S.; Sen, R. Transcriptional activation by ETS and leucine zipper-containing basic helix-loop-helix proteins. *Mol. Cell. Biol.* **1999**, *19*, 2946–2957. [CrossRef] [PubMed]
22. Kim, W.Y.; Sieweke, M.; Ogawa, E.; Wee, H.J.; Englmeier, U.; Graf, T.; Ito, Y. Mutual activation of Ets-1 and AML1 DNA binding by direct interaction of their autoinhibitory domains. *EMBO J.* **1999**, *18*, 1609–1620. [CrossRef] [PubMed]
23. Goetz, T.L.; Gu, T.L.; Speck, N.A.; Graves, B.J. Auto-inhibition of Ets-1 is counteracted by DNA binding cooperativity with core-binding factor alpha2. *Mol. Cell. Biol.* **2000**, *20*, 81–90. [CrossRef] [PubMed]
24. Fitzsimmons, D.; Lukin, K.; Lutz, R.; Garvie, C.W.; Wolberger, C.; Hagman, J. Highly cooperative recruitment of Ets-1 and release of autoinhibition by Pax5. *J. Mol. Biol.* **2009**, *392*, 452–464. [CrossRef] [PubMed]
25. Baillat, D.; Begue, A.; Stehelin, D.; Aumercier, M. ETS-1 transcription factor binds cooperatively to the palindromic head to head ETS-binding sites of the stromelysin-1 promoter by counteracting autoinhibition. *J. Biol. Chem.* **2002**, *277*, 29386–29398. [CrossRef] [PubMed]
26. Boulukos, K.E.; Pognonec, P.; Rabault, B.; Begue, A.; Ghysdael, J. Definition of an Ets1 protein domain required for nuclear localization in cells and DNA-binding activity in vitro. *Mol. Cell. Biol.* **1989**, *9*, 5718–5721. [CrossRef] [PubMed]
27. Pearse, D.D.; Tian, R.X.; Nigro, J.; Iorgulescu, J.B.; Puzis, L.; Jaimes, E.A. Angiotensin II increases the expression of the transcription factor ETS-1 in mesangial cells. *Am J. Physiol. Ren. Physiol.* **2008**, *294*, F1094–F1100. [CrossRef] [PubMed]
28. Abe, K.; Nakashima, H.; Ishida, M.; Miho, N.; Sawano, M.; Soe, N.N.; Kurabayashi, M.; Chayama, K.; Yoshizumi, M.; Ishida, T. Angiotensin II-induced osteopontin expression in vascular smooth muscle cells involves Gq/11, Ras, ERK, Src and Ets-1. *Hypertens. Res.* **2008**, *31*, 987–998. [CrossRef] [PubMed]
29. Dzau, V.J. Theodore Cooper Lecture: Tissue angiotensin and pathobiology of vascular disease: A unifying hypothesis. *Hypertension* **2001**, *37*, 1047–1052. [CrossRef] [PubMed]
30. Taniyama, Y.; Hitomi, H.; Shah, A.; Alexander, R.W.; Griendling, K.K. Mechanisms of reactive oxygen species-dependent downregulation of insulin receptor substrate-1 by angiotensin II. *Arterioscler. Thromb. Vasc. Biol.* **2005**, *25*, 1142–1147. [CrossRef] [PubMed]
31. Nedeljkovic, Z.S.; Gokce, N.; Loscalzo, J. Mechanisms of oxidative stress and vascular dysfunction. *Postgrad. Med. J.* **2003**, *79*, 195–199. [CrossRef] [PubMed]
32. Jaimes, E.A.; Galceran, J.M.; Raij, L. Angiotensin II induces superoxide anion production by mesangial cells. *Kidney Int.* **1998**, *54*, 775–784. [CrossRef] [PubMed]
33. Goetze, S.; Kintscher, U.; Kaneshiro, K.; Meehan, W.P.; Collins, A.; Fleck, E.; Hsueh, W.A.; Law, R.E. TNFalpha induces expression of transcription factors c-fos, Egr-1, and Ets-1 in vascular lesions through extracellular signal-regulated kinases 1/2. *Atherosclerosis* **2001**, *159*, 93–101. [CrossRef]
34. Hultgardh-Nilsson, A.; Cercek, B.; Wang, J.W.; Naito, S.; Lovdahl, C.; Sharifi, B.; Forrester, J.S.; Fagin, J.A. Regulated expression of the ETS-1 transcription factor in vascular smooth muscle cells in vivo and in vitro. *Circ. Res.* **1996**, *78*, 589–595. [CrossRef] [PubMed]
35. Naito, S.; Shimizu, S.; Maeda, S.; Wang, J.; Paul, R.; Fagin, J.A. Ets-1 is an early response gene activated by ET-1 and PDGF-BB in vascular smooth muscle cells. *Am. J. Physiol.* **1998**, *274*, C472–C480. [CrossRef] [PubMed]
36. Zhan, Y.; Brown, C.; Maynard, E.; Anshelevich, A.; Ni, W.; Ho, I.C.; Oettgen, P. Ets-1 is a critical regulator of Ang II-mediated vascular inflammation and remodeling. *J. Clin. Investig.* **2005**, *115*, 2508–2516. [CrossRef] [PubMed]
37. Hua, P.; Feng, W.; Rezonzew, G.; Chumley, P.; Jaimes, E.A. The transcription factor ETS-1 regulates angiotensin II-stimulated fibronectin production in mesangial cells. *Am. J. Physiol. Ren. Physiol.* **2012**, *302*, F1418–F1429. [CrossRef] [PubMed]
38. Wilson, L.A.; Gemin, A.; Espiritu, R.; Singh, G. ETS-1 is transcriptionally up-regulated by H_2O_2 via an antioxidant response element. *FASEB J.* **2005**, *19*, 2085–2087. [CrossRef] [PubMed]

39. Nelson, K.K.; Subbaram, S.; Connor, K.M.; Dasgupta, J.; Ha, X.F.; Meng, T.C.; Tonks, N.K.; Melendez, J.A. Redox-dependent matrix metalloproteinase-1 expression is regulated by JNK through Ets and AP-1 promoter motifs. *J. Biol. Chem.* **2006**, *281*, 14100–14110. [CrossRef] [PubMed]
40. Landmesser, U.; Cai, H.; Dikalov, S.; McCann, L.; Hwang, J.; Jo, H.; Holland, S.M.; Harrison, D.G. Role of p47(phox) in vascular oxidative stress and hypertension caused by angiotensin II. *Hypertension* **2002**, *40*, 511–515. [CrossRef] [PubMed]
41. Jaimes, E.A.; Tian, R.X.; Pearse, D.; Raij, L. Up-regulation of glomerular COX-2 by angiotensin II: Role of reactive oxygen species. *Kidney Int.* **2005**, *68*, 2143–2153. [CrossRef] [PubMed]
42. Zhou, M.S.; Jaimes, E.A.; Raij, L. Vascular but not cardiac remodeling is associated with superoxide production in angiotensin II hypertension. *J. Hypertens.* **2005**, *23*, 1737–1743. [CrossRef] [PubMed]
43. Raffetseder, U.; Wernert, N.; Ostendorf, T.; van Roeyen, C.; Rauen, T.; Behrens, P.; Floege, J.; Mertens, P.R. Mesangial cell expression of proto-oncogene Ets-1 during progression of mesangioproliferative glomerulonephritis. *Kidney Int.* **2004**, *66*, 622–632. [CrossRef] [PubMed]
44. Tanaka, H.; Terada, Y.; Kobayashi, T.; Okado, T.; Inoshita, S.; Kuwahara, M.; Seth, A.; Sato, Y.; Sasaki, S. Expression and function of Ets-1 during experimental acute renal failure in rats. *J. Am. Soc. Nephrol.* **2004**, *15*, 3083–3092. [CrossRef] [PubMed]
45. Naito, T.; Razzaque, M.S.; Nazneen, A.; Liu, D.; Nihei, H.; Koji, T.; Taguchi, T. Renal expression of the Ets-1 proto-oncogene during progression of rat crescentic glomerulonephritis. *J. Am. Soc. Nephrol.* **2000**, *11*, 2243–2255. [PubMed]
46. Feng, W.; Chumley, P.; Hua, P.; Rezonzew, G.; Jaimes, D.; Duckworth, M.W.; Xing, D.; Jaimes, E.A. Role of the transcription factor erythroblastosis virus E26 oncogen homolog-1 (ETS-1) as mediator of the renal proinflammatory and profibrotic effects of angiotensin II. *Hypertension* **2012**, *60*, 1226–1233. [CrossRef] [PubMed]
47. Ni, W.; Zhan, Y.; He, H.; Maynard, E.; Balschi, J.A.; Oettgen, P. Ets-1 is a critical transcriptional regulator of reactive oxygen species and p47(phox) gene expression in response to angiotensin II. *Circ. Res.* **2007**, *101*, 985–994. [CrossRef] [PubMed]
48. Feng, W.; Xing, D.; Hua, P.; Zhang, Y.; Chen, Y.F.; Oparil, S.; Jaimes, E.A. The transcription factor ETS-1 mediates proinflammatory responses and neointima formation in carotid artery endoluminal vascular injury. *Hypertension* **2010**, *55*, 1381–1388. [CrossRef] [PubMed]
49. Feng, W.; Chumley, P.; Allon, M.; George, J.; Scott, D.W.; Patel, R.P.; Litovsky, S.; Jaimes, E.A. The transcription factor E26 transformation-specific sequence-1 mediates neointima formation in arteriovenous fistula. *J. Am. Soc. Nephrol.* **2014**, *25*, 475–487. [CrossRef] [PubMed]
50. Weinberger, M.H.; Miller, J.Z.; Luft, F.C.; Grim, C.E.; Fineberg, N.S. Definitions and characteristics of sodium sensitivity and blood pressure resistance. *Hypertension* **1986**, *8*, II127–II134. [CrossRef] [PubMed]
51. Zhou, M.S.; Adam, A.G.; Jaimes, E.A.; Raij, L. In salt-sensitive hypertension, increased superoxide production is linked to functional upregulation of angiotensin II. *Hypertension* **2003**, *42*, 945–951. [CrossRef] [PubMed]
52. Navar, L.G.; Harrison-Bernard, L.M.; Nishiyama, A.; Kobori, H. Regulation of intrarenal angiotensin II in hypertension. *Hypertension* **2002**, *39*, 316–322. [CrossRef] [PubMed]
53. Re, R.N. Intracellular renin and the nature of intracrine enzymes. *Hypertension* **2003**, *42*, 117–122. [CrossRef] [PubMed]
54. Kobori, H.; Ozawa, Y.; Suzaki, Y.; Prieto-Carrasquero, M.C.; Nishiyama, A.; Shoji, T.; Cohen, E.P.; Navar, L.G. Young Scholars Award Lecture: Intratubular angiotensinogen in hypertension and kidney diseases. *Am. J. Hypertens.* **2006**, *19*, 541–550. [CrossRef] [PubMed]
55. Kobori, H.; Nangaku, M.; Navar, L.G.; Nishiyama, A. The intrarenal renin-angiotensin system: From physiology to the pathobiology of hypertension and kidney disease. *Pharmacol. Rev.* **2007**, *59*, 251–287. [CrossRef] [PubMed]
56. Ingert, C.; Grima, M.; Coquard, C.; Barthelmebs, M.; Imbs, J.L. Contribution of angiotensin II internalization to intrarenal angiotensin II levels in rats. *Am. J. Physiol. Renal Physiol.* **2002**, *283*, F1003–F1010. [CrossRef] [PubMed]
57. Iwai, J.; Dahl, L.K.; Knudsen, K.D. Genetic influence on the renin-angiotensin system: Low renin activities in hypertension-prone rats. *Circ. Res.* **1973**, *32*, 678–684. [CrossRef] [PubMed]

58. Hayakawa, H.; Coffee, K.; Raij, L. Endothelial dysfunction and cardiorenal injury in experimental salt-sensitive hypertension: Effects of antihypertensive therapy. *Circulation* **1997**, *96*, 2407–2413. [CrossRef] [PubMed]
59. Kodama, K.; Adachi, H.; Sonoda, J. Beneficial effects of long-term enalapril treatment and low-salt intake on survival rate of dahl salt-sensitive rats with established hypertension. *J. Pharmacol. Exp. Ther.* **1997**, *283*, 625–629. [PubMed]
60. Otsuka, F.; Yamauchi, T.; Kataoka, H.; Mimura, Y.; Ogura, T.; Makino, H. Effects of chronic inhibition of ACE and AT1 receptors on glomerular injury in dahl salt-sensitive rats. *Am. J. Physiol.* **1998**, *274*, R1797–R1806. [CrossRef] [PubMed]
61. Hayashida, W.; Kihara, Y.; Yasaka, A.; Inagaki, K.; Iwanaga, Y.; Sasayama, S. Stage-specific differential activation of mitogen-activated protein kinases in hypertrophied and failing rat hearts. *J. Mol. Cell. Cardiol.* **2001**, *33*, 733–744. [CrossRef] [PubMed]
62. Sakata, Y.; Masuyama, T.; Yamamoto, K.; Doi, R.; Mano, T.; Kuzuya, T.; Miwa, T.; Takeda, H.; Hori, M. Renin angiotensin system-dependent hypertrophy as a contributor to heart failure in hypertensive rats: Different characteristics from renin angiotensin system-independent hypertrophy. *J Am. Coll. Cardiol.* **2001**, *37*, 293–299. [CrossRef]
63. Nishikimi, T.; Mori, Y.; Kobayashi, N.; Tadokoro, K.; Wang, X.; Akimoto, K.; Yoshihara, F.; Kangawa, K.; Matsuoka, H. Renoprotective effect of chronic adrenomedullin infusion in Dahl salt-sensitive rats. *Hypertension* **2002**, *39*, 1077–1082. [CrossRef] [PubMed]
64. Kobori, H.; Nishiyama, A.; Abe, Y.; Navar, L.G. Enhancement of intrarenal angiotensinogen in Dahl salt-sensitive rats on high salt diet. *Hypertension* **2003**, *41*, 592–597. [CrossRef] [PubMed]
65. Nishiyama, A.; Yoshizumi, M.; Rahman, M.; Kobori, H.; Seth, D.M.; Miyatake, A.; Zhang, G.X.; Yao, L.; Hitomi, H.; Shokoji, T.; et al. Effects of AT1 receptor blockade on renal injury and mitogen-activated protein activity in Dahl salt-sensitive rats. *Kidney Int.* **2004**, *65*, 972–981. [CrossRef] [PubMed]
66. Onozato, M.L.; Tojo, A.; Kobayashi, N.; Goto, A.; Matsuoka, H.; Fujita. T. Dual blockade of aldosterone and angiotensin II additively suppresses TGF-beta and NADPH oxidase in the hypertensive kidney. *Nephrol. Dial. Transplant.* **2007**, *22*, 1314–1322. [CrossRef] [PubMed]
67. Feng, W.; Chumley, P.; Prieto, M.C.; Miyada, K.; Seth, D.M.; Fatima, H.; Hua, P.; Rezonzew, G.; Sanders, P.W.; Jaimes, E.A. Transcription factor avian erythroblastosis virus E26 oncogen homolog-1 is a novel mediator of renal injury in salt-sensitive hypertension. *Hypertension* **2015**, *65*, 813–820. [CrossRef] [PubMed]
68. Zhou, M.S.; Hernandez Schulman, I.; Pagano, P.J.; Jaimes, E.A.; Raij, L. Reduced NAD(P)H oxidase in low renin hypertension: Link among angiotensin II, atherogenesis, and blood pressure. *Hypertension* **2006**, *47*, 81–86. [CrossRef] [PubMed]
69. Elbashir, S.M.; Harborth, J.; Weber, K.; Tuschl, T. Analysis of gene function in somatic mammalian cells using small interfering RNAs. *Methods* **2002**, *26*, 199–213. [CrossRef]
70. Meng, S.; Roberts, L.J., 2nd; Cason, G.W.; Curry, T.S.; Manning, R.D., Jr. Superoxide dismutase and oxidative stress in Dahl salt-sensitive and -resistant rats. *Am. J. Physiol. Regul. Integr. Comp. Physiol.* **2002**, *283*, R732–R738. [CrossRef] [PubMed]
71. Feng, W.; Chen, B.; Xing, D.; Li, X.; Fatima, H.; Jaimes, E.A.; Sanders, P.W. Haploinsufficiency of the Transcription Factor Ets-1 Is Renoprotective in Dahl Salt-Sensitive Rats. *J. Am. Soc. Nephrol.* **2017**, *28*, 3239–3250. [CrossRef] [PubMed]

3

A Possible Role for Singlet Oxygen in the Degradation of Various Antioxidants

Athinoula L. Petrou [1,*], Petros L. Petrou [2], Theodoros Ntanos [1] and Antonis Liapis [1]

1 Laboratory of Inorganic Chemistry, Department of Chemistry, National and Kapodistrian University of Athens, Panepistimiopolis, 15771 Athens, Greece; theontanos@hotmail.com (T.N.); a-liapis@hotmail.com (A.L.)
2 Private practice in Cardiology, 6–8 Acheans Street, Nicosia 1101, Cyprus; lambrosp@spidernet.com.cy
* Correspondence: athpetrou@chem.uoa.gr

Abstract: The thermodynamic parameters E_{act}, $\Delta H^{\neq}$, $\Delta S^{\neq}$, and $\Delta G^{\neq}$ for various processes involving antioxidants were calculated using literature kinetic data (k, T). The $\Delta G^{\neq}$ values of the antioxidants' processes vary in the range 91.27–116.46 $kJmol^{-1}$ at 310 K. The similarity of the $\Delta G^{\neq}$ values (for all of the antioxidants studied) is supported to be an indication that a common mechanism in the above antioxidant processes may be taking place. A value of about 10–30 $kJmol^{-1}$ is the activation energy for the diffusion of reactants depending on the reaction and the medium. The energy 92 $kJmol^{-1}$ is needed for the excitation of O_2 from the ground to the first excited state ($^1\Delta_g$, singlet oxygen). We suggest the same role of the oxidative stress and specifically of singlet oxygen to the processes of antioxidants as in the processes of proteinaceous diseases. We therefore suggest a competition between the various antioxidants and the proteins of proteinaceous diseases in capturing singlet oxygen's empty π^* orbital. The concentration of the antioxidants could be a crucial factor for the competition. Also, the structures of the antioxidant molecules play a significant role since the various structures have a different number of regions of high electron density.

Keywords: antioxidants; oxidative stress; singlet oxygen; free energy of activation; enthalpy of activation; entropy of activation; activation energy

1. Introduction

In a recent article of ours [1], we have presented a possible role of oxidative stress and singlet oxygen in diverse diseases. In that article we have presented the calculated values of the free energies of activation of various reactions of proteins of proteinaceous diseases. From the values of the $\Delta Gs^{\neq}$, we came to the conclusion that the rate determining steps of the various reactions that were studied could be the formation of singlet oxygen from ground state oxygen and the diffusion of the various reactants, proteins, DNA, in general biomolecules.

Having presented the above (possible) role of singlet oxygen (a major component of oxidative stress) in the pathogenesis of neurodegenerative and other disorders, we concluded that antioxidant administration or donation of reagents bearing regions of high electron density (bases) may be useful in the prevention and treatment of neurodegenerative diseases and the other disorders that were studied. In the last paragraph of [1] entitled "future strategies", we have explained our goal for our studies that were to be followed.

There we stated that to achieve the delay of disease progression, the candidate antioxidant or base must be supplied as early as possible, in order to prevent irreversible neuronal loss. The antioxidant or base should also be tailored to the region of generation of O_2 ($^1\Delta_g$), i.e., to neurons rich in lipids and/or metal ions. A critical property of the chosen antioxidant or basic properties-bearing reagent is to be able to penetrate the blood–brain barrier after systemic administration in order to reach a critical therapeutic level within the CNS (Central Nervous System). The antioxidants should be ones that could prevent lipid, protein and DNA peroxidation, and thus prevent production of the $^1O_2$ ($^1\Delta_g$). They could also be able to capture singlet oxygen's empty π^* orbital [1]. Suitable bases should also be ones that could donate a pair of electrons in the empty π^* orbital of the produced O_2 ($^1\Delta_g$), in order to prevent its reaction with protein, lipid, DNA, etc. The antioxidants and bases (reagents bearing regions of high electron density) should react with the O_2 ($^1\Delta_g$), faster than lipids, proteins, DNA, etc. Thus, the $\Delta Gs^{\neq}$ of their reactions should be smaller than the $\Delta Gs^{\neq}$ that are presented in [1]. This means that the rate constants of the reactions should be greater than the ones reported in Supplementary Table S1 of [1].

In this paper, we present the results of our calculations on the activation parameters of reactions of various antioxidants with oxygen under various temperatures of treatment and we show that there is a possibility the reactive species in these oxidations to be the singlet oxygen species due to the values of the $\Delta Gs^{\neq}$. So, we suggest the same mechanism, that is, the formation of singlet oxygen and its reaction with the antioxidants. Concluding, we suggest that a competition might exist between antioxidants and the proteins of proteinaceous diseases in capturing the singlet oxygen's empty π^* orbital.

Oxidative Stress, Reactive Oxygen Species (ROS), Proteinaceous diseases and the proteins related to them: Aβ-amyloid (Alzheimer's disease, AD), Tau proteins [Alzheimer's disease and Parkinson's disease], α-Synuclein (Parkinson's disease), Prion: PrP (Prion Proteins), Amylin or islet amyloid polypeptide (IAPP) (type II diabetes), α-Crystallins (Cataracts) are briefly presented in [1].

1.1. Antioxidants

Living organisms have complex systems of antioxidants in body tissues, in order to balance their oxidative state. These antioxidants are produced internally (endogenous) or are taken with diet (exogenous):

(a) Endogenous antioxidants—the ones which are produced by the body. Examples are: superoxide dismutase, catalase, glutathione peroxidase, and glutathione.
(b) Exogenous antioxidants—the ones which come from the diet. Examples are: vitamin C, carotenoids, polyphenols, sulforafanes, curcumin, anthocyanins, etc.

Many antioxidant-based clinical trials and therapeutic interventions have been disappointing in their therapeutic benefit [2]. It has been reported [3–5] that while numerous evidence points to increased levels of oxidative stress playing a causal role in a number of neurodegenerative conditions, the understanding of the specific role of oxidative stress in the genesis and/or propagation of neurodegenerative diseases is poorly defined. Even more challenging to the "oxidative stress theory of neurodegeneration" is the fact that many antioxidant-based clinical trials [3,4] and therapeutic interventions have been largely disappointing in their therapeutic benefit [2]. Based on our research work, we attribute the above finding to (a) the antioxidants that were tried might not be able to pass through the Blood Brain Barrier (BBB); (b) their structure might not be the suitable one to capture the empty π^* orbital of O_2 ($^1\Delta_g$) bearing very few regions of high electron density that (c) their in vitro concentration might not be high enough in order to compete with the large amount of proteins present. We explain a, b, c, in more detail, below.

1.2. The Electronic Structure and the Energy above Ground State of Two Excited States of Oxygen. The First Excited State, the Singlet Oxygen State

The two outer electrons of molecular oxygen are located at the antibonding π^* orbitals. In the ground state the two π^* electrons occupy the equivalent in energy π^*_{2py}, π^*_{2pz} orbitals (see below), whereas in the first excited state, the $^1\Delta_g$, they occupy one of these orbitals, leaving the second one empty. The highest occupied molecular orbitals (HOMO) of the ground state ($^3\Sigma_g{}^-$), the first excited state ($^1\Delta_g$) and the second excited state ($^1\Sigma_g{}^+$) of the oxygen molecule are [6]:

$\pi^* \underline{\uparrow}\ \ \underline{\uparrow}\ \pi^*$	$\pi^* \underline{\uparrow\downarrow}\ \underline{\ \ }\ \pi^*$	$\pi^* \underline{\uparrow}\ \ \underline{\downarrow}\ \pi^*$
Ground state	First excited state	Second excited state
$2S + 1 = 3$	$2S + 1 = 1$	$2S + 1 = 1$
${}^3\Sigma_g{}^-$	${}^1\Delta_g$, 92 $kJmol^{-1}$ above ground state	${}^1\Sigma_g{}^+$, 155 $kJmol^{-1}$ above ground state

Thus, the first excited state, the ${}^1\Delta_g$ state, which is energetically 92 $kJmol^{-1}$ above the ground state, bears an empty π^* orbital where it can accommodate a pair of electrons. This availability of accepting a pair of electrons in the empty π^* orbital, gives to singlet oxygen strong acidic properties. So, singlet oxygen having this ability can behave like a strong electrophile reacting with reagents bearing regions of high electron density, causing oxidative damage to them. These reagents may be biomolecules [1] or components of foods that are bearing antioxidant qualities [7]. Guanine, in the molecule of DNA, nitrogen and oxygen in proteinic molecules, nitrogen, and oxygen in amino acids, etc., can act as bases accommodating their pair of electrons in the singlet oxygen's empty π^* orbital [1]. Also antioxidants bearing electron densities like beta-carotene's and lycopene's conjugated double bonds, astaxanthin's polyene chain, and terminal rings, sulforafane's O, N, S lone pairs of electrons etc. can accommodate them in the empty π^* orbital of singlet oxygen, provided that their geometry and energy suits to the π^* orbital's geometry and energy (see below).

The general reactions taking place could be presented by the Equations:

$$O_2\left({}^1\Delta_g\right) + \text{biomolecule(s) bearing regions of high electron density} \rightleftarrows \\ [\text{adduct } (O_2/\text{biomolecule(s)})]^{\neq} \rightleftarrows \text{oxidation products of biomolecule(s)}$$

$$O_2\left({}^1\Delta_g\right) + \text{antioxidant} \rightleftarrows [\text{adduct } (O_2/\text{antioxidant})]^{\neq} \rightleftarrows \text{oxidation products of antioxidants}$$

Singlet oxygen quenching [8] may be both physical and chemical quenching. Physical quenching leads to the deactivation of singlet oxygen by going to the ground triplet oxygen state. This can be achieved by energy transfer or charge transfer. There is no consumption of oxygen and no product formation. Singlet oxygen quenching by energy transfer takes place when the energy level of a quencher is very near or below that of singlet oxygen. Singlet oxygen quenchers by energy transfer are carotenoids with 9 or more conjugated double bonds. Tocopherols, curcumin, carotenoids, urate, phenolics, and ascorbate can quench singlet oxygen and the singlet oxygen quenching activity of carotenoids depends on the number of conjugated double bonds in their structure and the nature of substituents in the β-ionone ring. When a quencher bears high reduction potential and low triplet energy, it quenches singlet oxygen by a charge transfer mechanism. Quenchers of this type are amines, phenols (including tocopherols), iodide, sulfides, and azides, which all have many electrons. By donating an electron to singlet oxygen, the quencher forms a singlet state charge transfer complex and then by intersystem crossing changes the complex to the triplet state. Chemical quenching of singlet oxygen is a reaction involving the oxidation of a quencher. β-carotene, ascorbic acid, amino acids (such as histidine, cysteine, tryptophan, and methionine), peptides, tocopherols, and phenolics are chemical quenchers and they are all oxidized by singlet oxygen [9–12].

It should also be mentioned that many of the antioxidants that are discussed in this article quench singlet oxygen via both ways, physical as well as chemical quenching, and the physical quenching will not necessarily lead to destruction of the antioxidants. For example, carotenoids quench singlet oxygen mainly via energy transfer to generate the carotenoid triplet excited state, and this can then simply lose its energy as heat to decay back to the ground state. Tocopherols have also been shown to both chemically and physically quench singlet oxygen and astaxanthin is a very fast quencher of singlet oxygen.

Singlet Oxygen has also been extensively studied in relation to the photodynamic field [13–17].

1.3. Diffusion—Controlled Reactions, Activation Energy of Diffusion

Diffusion-controlled reactions (in solution) are reactions in which every collision of the reacting molecules leads to products. Their rates are only limited by the activation energy of diffusion that has values ranging from 10 to 30 kJmol^{-1} and are dependent on the nature of the solvent [18–20].

1.4. Food Antioxidants

In the following presentation, the term "antioxidant" refers mainly to compounds in foods, such as anthocyanins, carotenoids, polyphenols, sulforafane, vitamins, etc. Also, in the description of the various antioxidants that follows, we will explain which regions of high electron density, or which pairs of electrons in their molecular structure can be accommodated to singlet oxygen's empty π^* orbital. We must note here that not only lone pairs must be available in the various compounds-candidates for reaction with singlet oxygen's empty π^* orbital, but also the energy of their molecular orbitals should suit the energy of the singlet oxygen's (LUMO) orbitals. Overlapping between orbitals takes place provided that the energy and geometry of the orbitals suit. In Figure 1, structures of the antioxidants studied in the articles reviewed and others are presented.

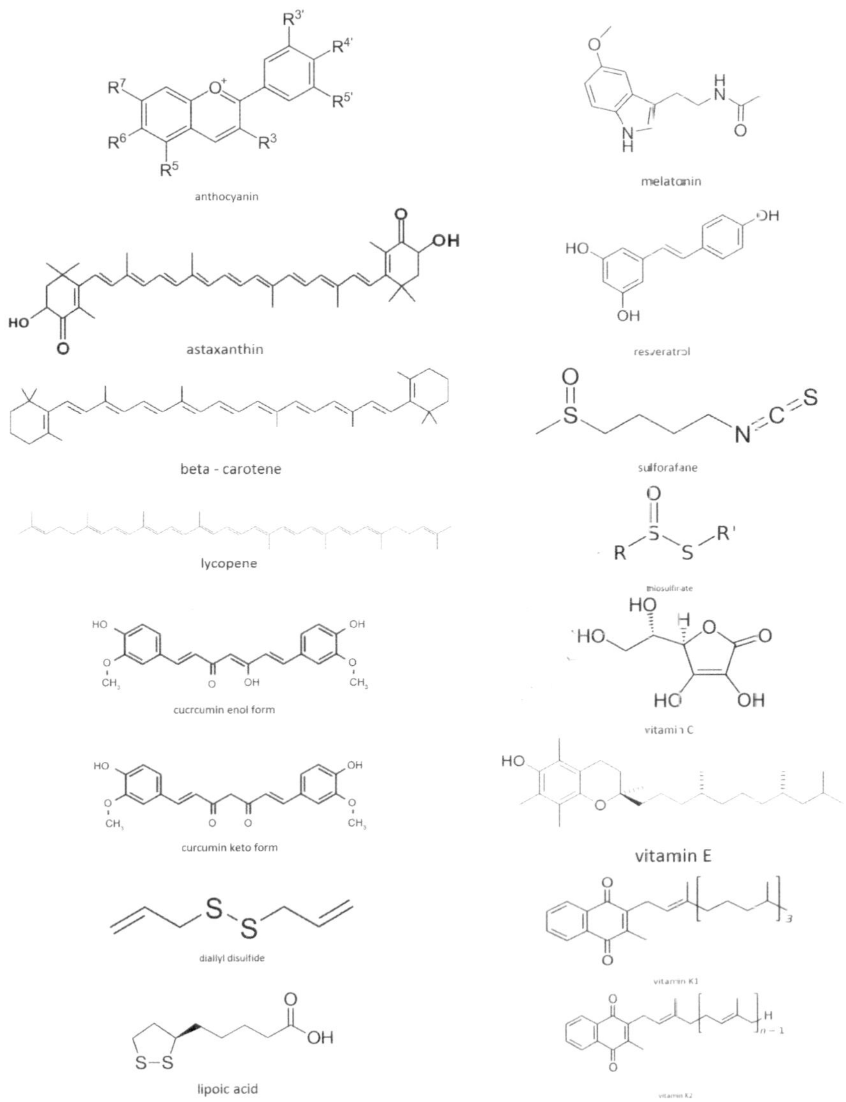

Figure 1. *Cont.*

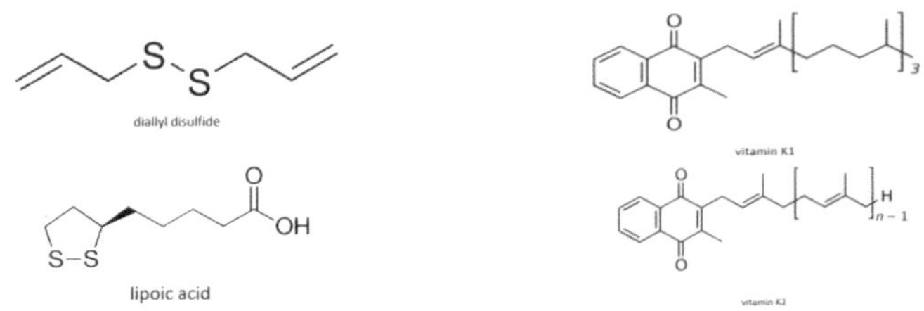

Figure 1. Chemical Structures of various antioxidants.

1.5. Oxidative Stress, Singlet Oxygen and Antioxidants—The Goal of Our Research (Meta-Analysis and Review of Literature Data)

We have already presented evidence, using the Free Energy of activation values, that oxidative stress and specifically singlet oxygen play a significant role in neurodegenerative diseases, in cataract formation, in diabetes, and in carcinogenesis [1]. The brain is especially vulnerable to oxidative stress damage because of its high rate of oxygen consumption, its abundant lipid content, and the relative paucity of antioxidant enzymes as compared with other organs [1].

Reactive oxygen and nitrogen species, such as super oxide anion, hydrogen peroxide, hydroxyl radical, and nitric oxide (O_2^{-}•, H_2O_2, •OH, $OONO^-$), and their biological metabolites also play an important role in carcinogenesis. The presence of free radicals in a biosystem could lead to mutation, transformation, and ultimately cancer [1 and refs therein].

Since oxidative stress, as it was outlined in [1] plays a crucial role in the above mentioned disorders (neurodegenerative disorders, diabetes, cataract, cancer) we searched for the Free Energies of activation that are needed in the biological (human) systems in order for the above various (proteinaceous) disorders to be initiated. A search in the literature led us to realize that the calculation of $\Delta G^{\neq}$ [$\Delta G^{\neq} = \Delta H^{\neq} - T \cdot \Delta S^{\neq}$] of the various processes would give us reasonable results. Having done this, we came to the conclusion that the processes that we have studied, which lead to the above disorders, all have $\Delta G^{\neq}$ values that vary between 92.8 and 127 $kJmol^{-1}$ at 310 K [1]. Knowing that ~ 92 $kJmol^{-1}$ is the energy needed for the production of singlet oxygen ([1] and refs therein), and that the activation energy of diffusion has values ranging from 10 to 30 $kJmol^{-1}$, we were guided to propose a possible mechanism for the pathway(s) that leads to the studied disorders. The Free Energies of activation that were calculated using the data of the papers cited were similar. This similarity led us to conclude that a common mechanism is possibly taking place. The possible mechanism has been presented [1]. Having presented the above (possible) role of singlet oxygen (a major component of oxidative stress) in the pathogenesis of neurodegenerative and other disorders, we concluded that antioxidant administration or donation of reagents bearing regions of high electron density (bases) may be useful in the prevention and treatment of neurodegenerative diseases and the other disorders that were studied.

In this paper, we present the results of our calculations on the activation parameters of reactions of various antioxidants with oxygen under various temperatures of treatment and we show, based on the $\Delta G^{\neq}$ values, that the reactive species in these oxidations might also be the singlet oxygen species, $^1\Delta_g$. Suggesting a mechanism for the reaction: antioxidant + O_2, we propose the same rate determining step, that is, the formation of singlet oxygen that then reacts with the antioxidant. 92 $kJmol^{-1}$ is the energy needed for the production of $^1\Delta_g$ and 10–30 $kJmol^{-1}$ is the diffusion of the reactants' activation energy. Having found similar values of $\Delta Gs^{\neq}$ for the reactions: antioxidants + O_2 and proteins + O_2 or biomolecules + O_2 we suggest that a competition exists between antioxidants and the proteins of proteinaceous diseases or biomolecules in general in capturing the singlet oxygen's empty π^* orbital. In Figure 2, we present schematically the calculated values of $\Delta Gs^{\neq}$.

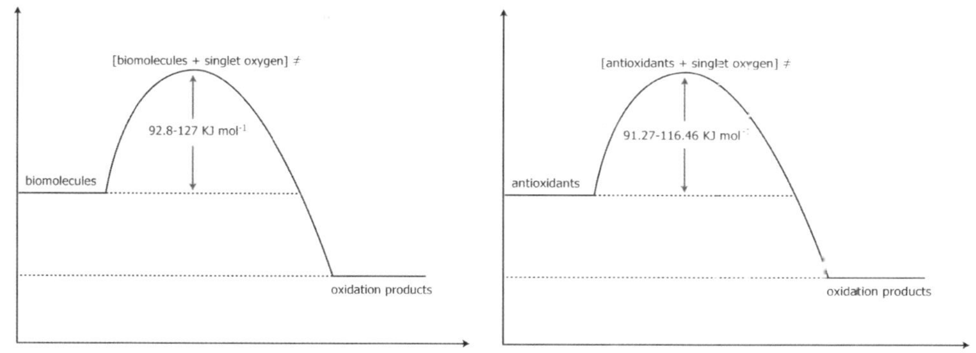

(a) (b)

Figure 2. Free energies of activation for the reactions: (**a**) biomolecules + singlet oxygen and (**b**) antioxidants + singlet oxygen.

We also, in this paper, present and describe the characteristics of the structures of the various antioxidants that make them strong competitors with proteins, DNA, biomolecules in general that are candidates for capturing the singlet oxygen's empty π^* orbital.

The results of our calculations are presented in Table 1.

2. Method of Calculations

The Eyring-Polanyi or activated complex theory relation—Free energy of activation. For the calculation of the thermodynamic parameters of activation of the various processes that were studied and are presented in this article, we have applied the kinetic equations Arrhenius and Eyring-Polanyi according to the activated complex theory to the literature data (k, T) for the various antioxidant processess. The Arrhenius equation, the calculation of E_{act} from a plot of it, the Eyring-Polanyi equation, the calculation of $\Delta H^{\neq}$ and $\Delta S^{\neq}$ from a plot of it, and the calculation of $\Delta G^{\neq}$ from the thermodynamic relation $\Delta G^{\neq} = \Delta H^{\neq} - T\Delta S^{\neq}$ are in detail presented in [1].

So, this paper is a meta-analysis and review of literature data that refer to antioxidant reactions with oxygen at various conditions (various temperatures, various pH, in the presence of light or without the presence of light, etc.).

The $\Delta S^{\neq}$ values for all of the antioxidants' reactions with oxygen are found to be negative, implying that the reacting species ($^3O_2$) becomes more organised at the activated step, ($^1O_2$) justifying our mechanism (see below) [18,20–22].

3. Results

Application of the Arrhenius and the Eyring-Polanyi Equations to Cases Related to Thermal and with Oxygen Treatment of Various Food Antioxidants

We have applied the Arrhenius and the Eyring-Polanyi equations to literature data (k, T) that are related to thermal and with oxygen treatment of various food antioxidants and we have calculated the parameters E_{act}, $\Delta H^{\neq}$, $\Delta S^{\neq}$, and $\Delta G^{\neq}$. It has been shown that similar processes have similar $\Delta G^{\neq}$ values (at the same temperatures), but may differ in the enthalpic and the entropic contributions [18–22]. We will present and compare the calculated activation parameters ($\Delta H^{\neq}$, $\Delta S^{\neq}$, $\Delta G^{\neq}$, along with the E_{act}) for the cases related to treatment of various food antioxidants (Table 1).

4. Discussion

From Table 1, it is shown that the values of E_{act} lie between 4.13 and 100.48 $kJmol^{-1}$. The $\Delta H^{\neq}$ values range between 1.13 and 97.75 $kJmol^{-1}$. The $\Delta S^{\neq}$ has values ranging between −318.66 and −46.68 $JK^{-1}\ mol^{-1}$.

The $\Delta G^{\neq}$ values range between 91.27 and 116.46 $kJmol^{-1}$ at 310 K for all of the cases of the food antioxidants studied.

From the above ranges it is concluded that independently of the nature of the antioxidant (anthocyanin, beta-carotene, curcumin, lycopene, polyphenols, sulforafane, vitamin C, etc.) or the kind of process that is taking place, (thermal treatment, pH effect, with presence or without the presence of light, oxygen reaction, etc.), the values of E_{act}, $\Delta H^{\neq}$ and $\Delta S^{\neq}$ cover a broad range, whereas the $\Delta G^{\neq}$ values cover a narrow range. In this narrow range a value of 10–30 $kJmol^{-1}$ is needed for the diffusion of the reactants, depending on the reaction and the medium. So, it remains a value of 92 $kJmol^{-1}$. This value of 92 $kJmol^{-1}$ is equal to the energy needed for the oxygen molecule, O_2, to go from the ground state to the first excited state, the $^1\Delta_g$ state, the singlet oxygen state (see above Section 1.2).

Concluding, we can say that, independently of the nature of the antioxidant and of the process that is taking place, the Free Energy of activation is actually equal to the energy that is needed for the production of singlet oxygen from ground state oxygen, [rate determining step (rds), excitation energy], to which the amount of the activation energy for the diffusion of the reactants is added. This fact raises some questions that need to be answered (see below, Section 4.3).

In the following analysis, we will, in short, present the various antioxidants, explaining specifically their ability, due to their structure, of capturing the singlet oxygen's empty π^* orbital.

Before analyzing the various cases of antioxidants, we present the thermal injury due to normal body temperature [23]. After completing the analysis of all the cases of antioxidants that were studied, we present a case of oxygen-free reaction of diallyl disulfide for comparison with the reaction of diallyl disulfide in the presence of oxygen. We show that without the presence of O_2, that is, without the formation of $^1\Delta_g$ the Free Energy of activation differs considerably from the values that were found with the antioxidants (diallyl disulfide) in the presence of O2 [135.81 $kJmol^{-1}$ at 310 K vs. 101.21 $kJmol^{-1}$ and 91.27 $kJmol^{-1}$ at 310 K (case j), Table 1].

4.1. Analytically the Various Cases that were Studied Are:

4.1.1. Destructive Processes due to Normal Body Temperature

Case a: Thermal injury due to normal body temperature [23]

In this work, the authors report that at physiologic temperature, 37 °C, over 0.2% of cells are irreversibly lost from the proliferating population each hour as a result of heat injury [23]. The very important question raised by the authors is whether any of the destructive processes takes place at rates that are significant when compared to the lifespans of the cells and the various organisms. If so, then the heat destruction due to the physiologic temperatures must be considered as a critical factor determining the aging of organisms. The authors have found evidence that in the case of hamster cells in vitro this is true [23]. According to the authors the exact nature of the thermal destruction due to physiologic temperatures was not known (at 1973), but "*it probably involves the denaturation of certain proteins and nucleic acids. In simplest terms, thermal injury is a result of a number of molecular events, each of which is activated by the thermal free-energy pool* [23]". The rate determining step (rds) has a rate constant which is the k of the slowest and critical reaction, if reactions of various rates are involved. The authors having found E_{act} = 8.0 electron volts/cell reported that this is equivalent to the rupture of only 30–40 hydrogen bonds/cell. They report $\Delta G^{\neq}$, the free energy of activation as being 1.2 eV/cell. They also report $\Delta S^{\neq}$ = 507 entropy units (eu). The above values are very high for most of the chemical reactions, but are typical of the denaturation of proteins, because of the required rupture of many hydrogen bonds [23]. This rupture of hydrogen bonds must be related to the rds since it leads to positive $\Delta S^{\neq}$ (increase of degrees of freedom). In the cases that will follow, of the reactions of antioxidants, the $\Delta S^{\neq}$ are negative suggesting loss of entropy, that is, increased organisation (decrease of degrees of freedom, decrease of the number of free species.). This will be explained by the mechanism for the rest of the cases, which will be presented, that is, the capture of the singlet oxygen's empty π^* orbital by the antioxidants' lone pairs of electrons or regions of high electron density (unsaturated bonds) etc. If heat injury at 37 °C in mammalian cells in vitro proceeds at the rate indicated by the authors' experiments, we could wonder about the accumulation of irreversible thermal lesions in long-lived cells in vivo. The authors are questioning whether this might be a major factor in the functional decline of the aging organisms.

Our calculations according to the authors' results give $\Delta G^{\neq}$ = 112.8 (92 + 20.8) $kJmol^{-1}$ at 310 K. We suggest a mechanism according to which singlet oxygen's empty π^* orbital is captured by the lone pairs of electrons of the –O and/or –N groups that participated in the hydrogen bonding. The hydrogen bonds were destroyed, as the authors suggest, by heat. The process is composite due to high values of $\Delta H^{\neq}$ (766.89 $kJmol^{-1}$) and $\Delta S^{\neq}$ (2110.41 $JK^{-1}mol^{-1}$) (Table 1). Thus the $\Delta S^{\neq}$ of the composite process is a sum of a negative value due to the reaction of singlet oxygen with proteins ($^1\Delta_g$ + proteins) and a very positive value ($\Delta S^0 > 0$) due to the disruption of the hydrogen bonds that preceded. We thus suggest the establishment of pre-equilibria (prior to the rds) that have high positive values of ΔH^0 and ΔS^0. The 112.8 $kJmol^{-1}$ at 310 K value shows that the denaturation of proteins and nucleic acids may be indeed a reaction with singlet oxygen's empty π^* orbital.

4.1.2. Anthocyanins (Also Anthocyans)

Food plants that are rich in anthocyanins have a purple, red, blue, or black colour. Also, some of the colors of autumn leaves are due to the presence of anthocyanins [24,25]. Anthocyanins play an antioxidant role against reactive oxygen species (ROS) caused by abiotic stresses, such as overexposure to UV-light [26] and extreme temperatures [27,28].

The aromatic rings in the molecular structure of anthocyanins can offer electron density to the empty π^* orbital of singlet oxygen. Also the positively charged oxygen atom can accept electron density from the occupied π^* orbital of $^1\Delta_g$ (singlet oxygen), the HOMO.

Case b: Degradation kinetics of anthocyanins [29]

The authors report on a study about the determination of the degradation kinetic parameters for blackberry anthocyanins in both juice and concentrate during heating and storage at various temperatures [29].

The activation energy value for the degradation of blackberry anthocyanins during heating was found to be 58.95 $kJmol^{-1}$ for the (blackberry) juice. During storage anthocyanin in the blackberry juice concentrate degraded more rapidly than that in blackberry juice with the activation energies being 65.06 $kJmol^{-1}$ and 75.5 $kJmol^{-1}$, respectively. Factors influencing the anthocyanin stability include pH, oxygen, enzymes, light, ascorbic acid, sulfur dioxide or sulphite salts, sugars, metal ions, and copigments [30]. Heat treatment is one of the most important factors that affect the stability of anthocyanins.

Our calculated values of E_{act}, $\Delta H^{\neq}$, $\Delta S^{\neq}$ are presented in Table 1.

$\Delta G^{\neq}$ = 109.33 $kJmol^{-1}$ at 310 K. We suggest reaction of anthocyanins with oxygen and occupancy of singlet oxygen's empty π^* orbital by anthocyanins' regions of high electron density. That explains the negative $\Delta S^{\neq}$ and the numerical value (92 + 17) $kJmol^{-1}$ of $\Delta G^{\neq}$

Case c: Degradation kinetics of anthocyanins [31]

Anthocyanin stability was tested for seven food products: blood orange juice, two blackberry juices with high and low content of suspended insoluble solids (SIS), and four roselle extracts. The highest content of anthocyanins was found in the blackberry juice. Anthocyanins in blood orange juice degraded with the highest rate constant followed by the blackberry juices and the roselle extracts. Activation energies were found to be 66 $kJmol^{-1}$ for blood orange and 37 $kJmol^{-1}$ for blackberry. For roselle extracts, the activation energies were 47–61 $kJmol^{-1}$. Slight protection for the anthocyanins was provided by a high SIS content for the blackberry juices. Besides their health effects [32], beneficial effects for human diseases have also been referred [33]. The reduction of risks of coronary heart disease, cancer and stroke have been reported [34]. The sensitivity of anthocyanins in the various food products may be depended on the chemical composition, the dissolved oxygen concentration and the chemical structure of anthocyanin.

Our calculations gave: $\Delta G^{\neq}$ 106.75 (= 92 + 14.75) $kJmol^{-1}$ at 310 K and 108.47 (= 92 + 16.47) $kJmol^{-1}$ at 310 K (case c, Table 1). Reaction of anthocyanin with oxygen takes place and occupancy of singlet oxygen's empty π^* orbital by regions of high electron density of anthocyanins. That is why $\Delta S^{\neq}$ is negative and $\Delta G^{\neq}$ is the sum of 92 $kJmol^{-1}$ + the diffusion activation energy.

4.1.3. Carotenoids or Tetraterpenoids

They are categorized as xanthophylls, which contain oxygen and carotenes that are purely hydrocarbons, not containing oxygen. Carotenoids that contain unsubstituted beta-ionone rings and other carotenoids, such as beta-carotene, alpha-carotene, beta-cryptoxanthin, and gamma-carotene, can act as antioxidants.

Carotenoids contain polyene chain, long conjugated double bonds, which carry out antioxidant activities by quenching singlet oxygen and scavenging radicals to terminate chain reactions in the cell membrane.

So, the biological benefits of carotenoids may be due to their antioxidant properties attributed to their physical and chemical interactions with cell membranes. Their highly unsaturated chemical structure makes them very susceptible to thermal degradation and oxidation.

Tomato carotenoids: Tomato carotenoids act as antioxidants to help protect cells and include carotenes and xanthophylls. The provitamin A carotenes are converted to vitamin A inside the body and are important in the eyes (visual cycle). Other carotenoids in tomatoes can also accumulate in the eyes and help to filter damaging rays of light.

Xanthophylls: The main xanthophylls in tomatoes are lutein and zeaxanthin and are yellow pigments. They contain oxygen atoms besides carbon and hydrogen atoms (see above carotenes). Vitamin A, lutein, and zeaxanthin are very important to the health of the eyes.

Lutein: Lutein is a xanthophyll and one of the 600 known naturally occurring carotenoids.

Zeaxanthin: Zeaxanthin is one of the two primary xanthophyll carotenoids that are contained within the retina of the eye. Within the central macula zeaxanthin is the dominant component, whereas in the peripheral retina, lutein predominates.

Beta-carotene: β-carotene being highly conjugated is a colored red-orange pigment abundant in plants and fruits. As a hydrocarbon lacking functional groups, it is very lipophilic. Among the carotenes, β-carotene is distinguished by having beta-rings at both ends of the molecule. β-carotene is the most common form of carotene in plants. In nature, β-carotene is a precursor (inactive form) to vitamin A via the action of beta-carotene 15, 15′-monooxygenase [35].

Pairs of electrons or electron density in the molecular structure of beta-carotene that can be accommodated to singlet oxygen's empty π^* orbital: the conjugated bonds of the polyene chain are regions of high electron density, and thus they can react with singlet oxygen's empty π^* orbital. They can also trap radicals in the cell membrane. However, as stated above, carotenoids quench singlet oxygen mainly via energy transfer.

Lycopene: Lycopene is a phytochemical, a bright red carotene, insoluble in water, which is found in tomatoes and other red fruits and vegetables. Parsley and asparagus contain also lycopene [36] though they are not red as the chlorophyll present in these foods masks the presence of the lycopene. Although chemically lycopene is a carotene, it has no the vitamin A activity [37]. Lycopene may help to prevent breast and prostate cancer.

The eleven conjugated double bonds are responsible for lycopene's deep red color and its antioxidant activity in vitro.

Pairs of electrons or electron density regions in the molecular structure of lycopene that can be accommodated to singlet oxygen's empty π^* orbital: lycopene being a polyunsaturated hydrocarbon bears regions of high electron density, the conjugated double bonds, and thus they can be accommodated in the empty π^* orbital. The polyene chain in lycopene can also trap radicals in the cell membrane.

Case d: Antioxidant activity and carotenoids content [38]

Carrot has the highest carotene content among foods [38]. The authors studied the influence of air drying temperature on antioxidant activity and carotenoids content to establish the degradation kinetics. The activation energy value that was found and reported is 23.7 $kJmol^{-1}$. The authors concluded that the drying process significantly decreased the carrot antioxidant activity. Our calculations based on the authors' results are presented in Table 1. $\Delta G^{\neq}$ = 114.31 $kJmol^{-1}$ at 310 K. Again, singlet oxygen's empty π^* orbital reacts with carotenoids' regions of high electron density.

Case e: Degradation of carotenoid antioxidants [39]

Bioavailability of lycopene is believed to be increased by processing, such as cooking or chopping, because of the breaking down the cell walls, increasing the accessibility of carotenoids [39]. Processing also converts some of the trans-isomers of lycopene to the more bioavailable cis-isomers. Heat and light induces lycopene oxidation and isomerization. The all-trans form isomerises to the cis-form. The aim of the authors' study was to determine the effect of temperature and time on the degradation kinetics of lycopene and beta-carotene content in tomato paste produced from Roma (i) and Ajindi-Kerewa (ii) tomato cultivars [39]. The activation energies of lycopene degradation obtained from the Arrhenius plots are 8.65 $kJmol^{-1}$ [(ii) cultivar lycopene] and 4.63 $kJmol^{-1}$ [(i) cultivar lycopene]. While the activation energies of lycopene degradation in (ii) tomatoes are twice that in (i) those of beta-carotene degradation are almost the same in the two cultivars: 4.81 $kJmol^{-1}$ [(ii) cultivar beta-carotene] and 4.14 $kJmol^{-1}$ [(i) cultivar beta-carotene].

Our calculations give for [(ii) cultivar lycopene], $\Delta G^{\neq}$ = 101.11 $kJmol^{-1}$, at 310 K. For [(i) cultivar lycopene $\Delta G^{\neq}$ = 99.48 $kJmol^{-1}$ at 310 K.

The [(ii) cultivar beta-carotene] gives $\Delta G^{\neq}$ = 100.44 $kJmol^{-1}$ at 310 K.

The [(i) cultivar beta-carotene] gives $\Delta G^{\neq}$ = 99.41 $kJmol^{-1}$ at 310 K.

The $\Delta G^{\neq}$ values are almost similar. We suggest similar mechanisms for the two cultivars, the mechanism that we have already suggested for carotenoids and anthocyanins [see also below Section 4.2 mechanism of the studied antioxidants' reactions with oxygen].

Case f: Beta-carotene degradation [40]

The authors' results indicate that at high concentrations oxygen diffusion becomes a limiting factor in agreement with our mechanism, according to which the studied reaction is the reaction of the antioxidant (beta-carotene) with oxygen. The highly unsaturated chemical structure of carotenoids makes them very susceptible to thermal degradation and oxidation in agreement with our mechanism (Section 4.2), according to which the empty π^* orbital of $^1\Delta g$ accommodates electron density from the highly unsaturated chemical structure of carotenoids.

First order kinetics is expected if beta-carotene and oxygen are the only reactants and if a large excess of oxygen is present [40]. Presumably, the carotene is uniformly dispersed in the fatty acid layer through which oxygen has to diffuse before the oxidation can occur. This work propose E_{act} = 22.8 Kcal mol^{-1} that is, 95.4 $kJmol^{-1}$. Our calculations gave E_{act} = 95.73 $kJmol^{-1}$ and $\Delta G^{\neq}$ = 107.37 $kJmol^{-1}$ at 310 K. Again we suggest the mechanism of Section 4.2.

Curcumin: Curcumin is a chemical produced by some plants.

Curcumin contains a molecular structure in the presence of hydroxyl and keto moieties on the enol and keto form of the molecule which are responsible for the high antioxidant properties. The unsaturated bonds of the chain trap radicals in the cell membrane, while the terminal rings of curcumin could scavenge radicals at the outer and inner parts of the cell membrane.

Case g: Stability of curcumin during storage [41]

Limited information is available concerning curcumin stability in microencapsulated turmeric oleoresin. There exists a need to investigate the storage stability of this curcumin in inclusion complex that contributes to unique yellow colour of turmeric oleoresin. Activation energy in the presence of light was 23.88 $kJmol^{-1}$ and in the dark was 13.65 $kJmol^{-1}$. Relatively low activation energy obtained in the authors' study for both with or without light indicates that degradation will continue at a measurable rate at low temperatures, for instance, during storage, leading to a limited shelf life.

Our calculations give: E_{act} = 24.213 $kJmol^{-1}$ and $\Delta G^{\neq}$ = 94.912 $kJmol^{-1}$ at 310 K for the reactions taking place in the presence of light.

Our calculations give: E_{act} = 11.803 $kJmol^{-1}$, $\Delta G^{\neq}$ = 99.32 $kJmol^{-1}$ at 310 K for the reactions taking place without the presence of light. We suggest the mechanism of Section 4.2.

According to our results, the degradation in the presence of light ($\Delta G^{\neq}$ = 94.912 $kJmol^{-1}$ at 310 K) is faster than without the presence of light ($\Delta G^{\neq}$ = 99.32 $kJmol^{-1}$ at 310 K).

According to the authors' results, in the dark the degradation is faster (23.88 $kJmol^{-1}$ in the presence of light and in the dark 13.65 $kJmol^{-1}$). This finding cannot be correct and it justifies our suggestion of using $\Delta G^{\neq}$ instead of E_{act}.

4.1.4. Polyphenols also Polyhydroxyphenols

Polyphenols are molecules with large conjugated systems of π electron configurations bearing aromatic rings. They are reactive towards oxidation possessing a significant binding affinity for proteins, leading to the formation of soluble and insoluble protein-polyphenol complexes [42].

Polyphenols, which often have antioxidant properties in vitro, are not necessarily antioxidants in vivo, due to extensive metabolism [43]. The catechol group, which acts as an electron acceptor, is responsible for the antioxidant activity [44] in many polyphenols.

There are many different structures of phenolic compounds and this makes it difficult to come to broad conclusions about their specific health effects.

Although in vitro experiments show that polyphenols are good antioxidants, the antioxidant actions in vivo are shown to be probably minor or absent [45] [see in Section 4.1 our comments for case h]. By still undefined mechanisms, flavonoids and other polyphenols may reduce the risk of cancer and cardiovascular disease [46]. Polyphenols in vivo are poorly (less than 5%) conserved with most of the absorbed existing as chemically modified metabolites [47]. The increase in antioxidant capacity of blood observed after the consumption of foods rich in polyphenols has been proposed not to be caused by the polyphenols themselves, but most probably by increased levels of uric acid as derived from the metabolism of flavonoids [47,48]. Generally, foods contain complex mixtures of polyphenols [49]. Some polyphenols interfere with the absorption of essential nutrients, especially iron and other metal ions, and so they are considered antinutrients. They also bind to digestive enzymes and other proteins, particularly in ruminants [50] behaving as antinutrients.

Pairs of electrons in the molecular structure of polyphenols that can be accommodated to singlet oxygen's empty π^* orbital are the oxygen lone pairs the phenyl rings' electron densities and the unsaturated double bonds' electron densities wherever they exist.

Case h: Thermal degradation of polyphenols [51]

In this study, the authors examined the thermal degradation of the semi-solid residue (grape marc) with high content of antioxidants and its filtered extract [51].

Degradation kinetics was studied in terms of total phenol content, antioxidant activity, and anthocyanin content. The activation energy for the grape marc is slightly higher than that for the filtered extract. Due to their diverse structure, different polyphenols are found in the distinct parts of the grape skin and seed. Some of them are free and can be found in vacuoles, while others are associated to cell wall compounds or to polysaccharide structures in the skin cells [51].

Thermal treatments on enhanced polyphenol extraction degrade active compounds. The E_{act} for grape marc was found to be 55.980 $kJmol^{-1}$ and for filtered extract 53.196 $kJmol^{-1}$.

Our calculations give for grape marc $\Delta G^{\neq} = 94.86$ kJmol^{-1} at 310 K and for filtered extract $\Delta G^{\neq} = 94.46$ kJmol^{-1} at 310 K. These values suggest that the mechanism that we propose is valid for the cases of polyphenols as well. However, in vivo the situation may be different due to the extensive metabolism [43].

Sulforafane (SF): Sulforafane is an organosulfur compound. It is found in cruciferous vegetables.

SF is of interest since it primarily modulates the activities of phase II enzymes that convert carcinogens to inactivate metabolites, thereby preventing them from interacting with DNA [52]. SF can also inhibit histone deacetylase activity in human colorectal and prostate cancer cells, leading to cancer prevention [53,54].

Regions of high electron density in the molecular structure of SF that can be accommodated to singlet oxygen's empty π^* orbital are the unsaturated bonds. The atoms S, N, O bear lone pairs of electrons, which can also be accommodated to singlet oxygen's empty π^* orbital.

Case i: Degradation kinetics of sulforaphane [55]

It has been proved that SF lowers the risks of various cancers, such as breast cancer, lung cancer, colorectal cancer, prostate cancer and/or bladder cancer [55]. SF is not a stable compound, and its stability is affected by pH, temperature, heating time, oxygen, and possibly by some food components [55].

This work [55] deals with thermal degradation kinetics of SF in broccoli extract at selected temperatures and pH values [55]. The authors' results indicated that SF is unstable at high temperatures and is more heat-stable in acidic food products. The $\Delta G^{\neq}$ values, as calculated by us, based on the results of work [55], are almost the same for the various values of pH, SF being though more stable in acidic pHs (higher values of $\Delta Gs^{\neq}$ implying lower values of rate constants k and thus lower degradation rates meaning more stable SF).

Our calculations based on the authors' results give (Table 1) for pH = 2.2, $\Delta G^{\neq} = 114.95$ kJmol^{-1} at 310 K. For pH = 3.0, $\Delta G^{\neq} = 115.08$ kJmol^{-1} at 310 K, for pH = 4.0 $\Delta G^{\neq} = 112.32$ kJmol^{-1} at 310 K, for pH = 5.0 $\Delta G^{\neq} = 110.2$ kJmol^{-1} at 310 K and for pH = 6.0 $\Delta G^{\neq} = 108.9$ kJmol^{-1} at 310 K.

The above values suggest that the mechanism that we propose (Section 4.2) is valid for the case of SF as well.

Diallyl disulphide: Diallyl disulfide is derived from garlic and a few other plants of the genus Allium [56]. Diallyl disulfide, diallyl trisulfide and diallyl tetrasulfide are principal components of the distilled oil of garlic which is insoluble in water yellow liquid. Upon crushing garlic and other plants of the Alliaceae family, allicin is released, the decomposition of which produces diallyl disulfide. Diallyl disulfide is responsible for the many of the health benefits of garlic.

Diallyl disulfide increases the production of the enzyme glutathione S-transferase which acts as a detoxicator of the cells. Garlic protects nerve cells from oxidative stress in vitro [57–64].

By causing detoxification in the liver, diallyl disulfide can offer protection of liver during the chemotherapy [65,66].

The organosulfur compounds that are released from Alliaceae plant cells possess antimicrobial, insecticidal and larvicidal properties [67]. The inhibition of the growth of molds and bacteria by garlic oil is due to diallyl disulfide. It also acts against helicobacter pylori allicin acting more efficiently [68,69]. Due to its antimicrobial effects diallyl disulfide together with tobramycin is used in preparations, which are used for the (selective) decontamination of the organs before surgical operations. Such preparations prevent endotoxemia in heart valve operations [70].

Diallyl disulfide is responsible for garlic's action in preventing the colorectal cancer [71]. Diallyl disulfide affects cancer cells more than normal cells [72]. Garlic may protect from the development of cardiovascular diseases. Oxidative stress may be a reason for some of these diseases, such as atherosclerosis or coronary heart disease. Diallyl disulfide reduces oxidative stress by participating in the detoxification of the cell along with some other mechanisms [73]. Diallyl disulfide can also lead to a short-term lowering of blood pressure [74] by activating the TRPA1 ion channel.

In a review article titled "Herbal medicine for the treatment of cardiovascular disease (clinical consideration)" [75], the authors refer to the important qualities of garlic. Also, the effect of a garlic oil preparation on serum lipoproteins and cholesterol metabolism was reported [76]. Promise for improving some cardiovascular risk factors by garlic's properties is referred in [77]. There are also reports with title "Garlic prevents plaque" [78] and "garlic prevents blood clots" [79].

Pairs of electrons in the molecular structure of diallyl disulphide that can be accommodated to singlet oxygen's empty π^* orbital are the sulfur lone pairs and the double bonds' electron density.

Thiosulfinate: Thiosulfinate is a functional group consisting of the linkage R-S(O)-S-R (R are organic substituents).

Pairs of electrons in the molecular structure of thiosulfinate that can be accommodated to singlet oxygen's empty π^* orbital are O and S lone pairs of electrons.

Case j: Antioxidant activity and degradation of thiosulfinates of garlic [80]

In the work [80], the rate constants for loss of thiosulfinate and for loss of antioxidant activity were found to increase with blanching temperature. The activation energies were 7.67 $kJmol^{-1}$ and 89.75 $kJmol^{-1}$, respectively. The antioxidant activity was correlated with thiosulfinates and the antioxidant activity, along with the thiosulfinate contents were decreased with increasing blanching time. Banerjee et al. [81] support that thiosulfinates not only have antioxidant activity, but also can stimulate the synthesis of glutathione, which is an important antioxidant. Heat treatment of garlic affects the antioxidant activity of thiosulfinate because of the inactivation of alliinase, which is responsible for the formation of these compounds through interaction with alliin [82]. The antioxidant activity may be associated with the presence of phenolic compounds such as flavonoids and mericitin [83].

Antioxidant Activity: a loss of antioxidant activity was observed over time during blanching. This results from the damage to the plant tissue by heating, which leads to the exposure of antioxidant compounds [84]. Yin and Cheng [85] reported that the activity of organosulfur compounds is lowered by high temperatures due to inactivation by heat of alliinase, the enzyme that is responsible for the formation of thiosulfinates [86]. This confirms the high loss of these compounds in the presented study. It was suggested that the antioxidant activity was due to thiosulfinates and to other compounds such as the phenolics, which were not evaluated in the study.

Our calculations gave for antioxidant activity $\Delta G^{\neq} = 101.21$ $kJmol^{-1}$ at 310 K, and for loss of thiosulfinates $\Delta G^{\neq} = 91.27$ $kJmol^{-1}$ at 310 K. The value of $\Delta G^{\neq}$ for loss of thiosulfinates could suggest that there is no need for diffusion for this process to take place, something that is expected. It could also mean that singlet oxygen is not involved here.

The calculated values suggest that the proposed mechanism (Section 4.2) is valid for the case of the antioxidant activity and thiosulfinate degradation of garlic as well.

Vitamin C: Vitamin C (Ascorbic acid) is a water soluble monosaccharide. During primate evolution, one of the enzymes needed to synthesize ascorbic acid (enzyme gulonolactone oxidase) has been lost by mutation. Humans and apes must obtain it from the diet since it is a vitamin [87]. Most other animals being able to produce it in their bodies do not require it in their diets [88]. It is essential for collagen, carnitine, and neurotransmitters biosynthesis [89]. By reaction with glutathione, it remains in its reduced form. Ascorbic acid, being a redox catalyst, can reduce and thus neutralise, reactive oxygen species (ROS) such as hydrogen peroxide [90] (antioxidant action).

Pairs of electrons in the molecular structure of vitamin C that can be accommodated to singlet oxygen's empty π^* orbital are the lone pairs of oxygen atoms. Regions of high electron density are also the double bonds.

Case k: Vitamin C degradation [91]

Various vitamin C tablet samples were examined e.g., standard ascorbic acid solution (Merck), vitamin C 200 mg tablets, Ascovit 100 mg tablets with orange taste and vitamin C nose drops 10%.

The variations of vitamin C concentration were studied as a function of light exposition at various temperatures. The values of E_{act} that were found are: standard ascorbic acid solution.

(Merck) 8.73 kcalmol^{-1} (36.53 kJmol^{-1}), 200 mg tablet 6.65 kcalmol^{-1} (27.82 kJmol^{-1}), Ascovit 100 mg tablet 2.62 kcalmol^{-1} (10.96 kJmol^{-1}), Vitamin C nose drops 8.39 kcalmol^{-1} (35.10 kJmol^{-1}).

The calculated by us values of $\Delta G^{\neq}$ are: standard ascorbic acid solution (Merck) $\Delta G^{\neq}$ = 97.79 kJmol^{-1} at 310 K, 200 mg tablet $\Delta G^{\neq}$ = 93.6 kJmol^{-1} at 310 K, Ascovit 100 mg tablet $\Delta G^{\neq}$ = 94.26 kJmol^{-1} at 310 K, Vitamin C nose drops $\Delta G^{\neq}$ = 95.73 kJmol^{-1} at 310 K.

Thus, the $\Delta G^{\neq}$ values for the various samples were very similar and very close to the value of 92 kJmol^{-1}, that is, close to the energy that is needed for the excitation of ground state oxygen to the first excited state, the singlet oxygen state.

Case l: Temperature and high pressure effect on lycopene and vitamin C [92]

The aim of the study was to determine the kinetics of vitamin C and lycopene degradation of watermelon juice under various temperatures and high pressures [92]. According to the authors in the conditions of processing (thermal and high pressure), lycopene is found to be more stable than vitamin C. Thermal treatment resulted in faster degradation rates of the two components compared to the high pressure treatment. It has been found that there is a relation between lycopene consumption with diet and lower incidence in prostate and oral cancers. It may also lower the risks of cardiovascular disease [92]. Vitamin C is unstable towards oxygen, heat, light, and metal catalysts. Lycopene changes during processing and storage. It undergoes oxidation and isomerization from all-trans to mono-cis or poly-cis forms [92]. In fruits and vegetables the all-trans isomer is the most predominant and is also the most thermodynamically stable form [92]. The thermal degradation of vitamin C is faster than that of lycopene. So, the E_{act} value for the thermal degradation of vitamin C of watermelon juice was found to be 18.37 kcalmol^{-1} (76.86 kJmol^{-1}) whereas the corresponding value of lycopene of watermelon juice was found to be 23.35 kcal mol^{-1} (97.7 kJmol^{-1}).

Our calculations give for E_{act} of vitamin C degradation 76.92 kJmol^{-1} and for $\Delta G^{\neq}$ = 105.528 kJmol^{-1} at 310 K. The E_{act} of lycopene degradation is found to be 97.21 kJmol^{-1}, and the $\Delta G^{\neq}$= 116.46 kJmol^{-1} at 310 K.

The above presented values suggest that the proposed mechanism (Section 4.2) is valid also for the case of lycopene and vitamin C.

Case m: Oxidation of vitamin C [93]

Vitamin C is important in the functioning of the brain. Fruits and vegetables like oranges, berries, potatoes, greens, and tomatoes are the main sources of vitamin C for humans. The oxidation of vitamin C occurs very quickly in a basic environment at high temperatures. The amount of vitamin C is significantly reduced if it is stored at room temperature [93]. The results of the authors' research indicate that between 40 and 80 °C the kinetics of the oxidation of ascorbic acid, vitamin C, is a first order reaction and the activation energy for this reaction was found to be 20.73 kJmol^{-1}. Our calculations, according to the authors' results, gave the following values: E_{act} = 41.65 kJmol^{-1} and $\Delta G^{\neq}$ = 108.47 kJmol^{-1} at 310 K.

Again the proposed mechanism (Section 4.2) is valid also for the case of vitamin C oxidation.

Cysteine: Cysteine is a semi-essential proteinogenic amino acid. The thiol (–SH) side chain in cysteine often participates in enzymatic reactions. It is oxidized to give the disulfide (–S–S–) derivative cystine, which plays an important structural role in many proteins.

Cysteine has antioxidant properties due to the ability of thiols to undergo redox reactions. Cysteine's antioxidant properties are expressed in the tripeptide glutathione, which occurs in humans as well as other organisms. Glutathione is biosynthesized from its constituent amino acids, cysteine, glycine, and glutamic acid. Cysteine is an important source of sulfide in human metabolism.

Pairs of electrons in the molecular structure of cysteine that can be accommodated to singlet oxygen's empty π^* orbital are lone pairs on O, N and S atoms.

4.1.5. Fumaric Acid or Trans-Butenedioic Acid

Fumaric acid activates the Nrf2 antioxidant response pathway, the primary cellular defense against the cytotoxic effects of oxidative stress [94].

Pairs of electrons in the molecular structure of fumaric acid that can be accommodated to singlet oxygen's empty π^* orbital are the O lone pairs and the conjugated double bonds' electron density.

Case n: Effect of antioxidants [vitamin C, cysteine, fumaric acid] on the stability of an HTK (histidine-tryptophane-α-ketoglutaric acid) solution [95]

The study aimed at determining the stability of an HTK (histidine-tryptophane-α-ketoglutaric acid, solutions in transplantology) solution using the changes of the histidine content i.e., the stability of the amino acid as affected by various antioxidants (vitamin C, cysteine, fumaric acid). When solutions containing histidine are stored, the process of the compound's oxidation takes place, according to the authors, who support that the reaction consists mainly of the addition of the free radical to the aromatic ring. The authors state, that this is a relatively quick reaction as the resulting free radical adducts are stabilized by the resonance action of the aromatic ring [95]. The study shows that vitamin C is the most effective antioxidant.

E_{act} reported by the authors: HTK 23.945 cal mol^{-1} (100.186 Jmol^{-1}). Our calculations gave for $\Delta G^{\neq}$ = 113.92 kJmol^{-1} at 310 K. So, we believe that the units of the results for all cases in [95] are not calmol^{-1} but kcalmol^{-1}.

HTK + cysteine, E_{act} = 21.980 cal mol^{-1} (91.96 Jmol^{-1}). Our calculations gave for $\Delta G^{\neq}$ = 114.96 kJmol^{-1} at 310 K.

HTK + vitamin C, E_{act} = 23.453cal mol^{-1} (98.127 Jmol^{-1}). Our calculations gave for $\Delta G^{\neq}$ = 115.61 kJmol^{-1} at 310 K.

HTK + fumaric acid, E_{act} = 21.440 cal mol^{-1} (89.70 Jmol^{-1}). Our calculations gave for $\Delta G^{\neq}$ = 114.87 kJmol^{-1} at 310 K.

Vitamin C is proved to be a more effective antioxidant since $\Delta G^{\neq}$ is the highest, and thus the rate constant (of oxidation) is the lowest, and so the degradation (oxidation) is the slowest.

The proposed mechanism (Section 4.2) is, according to the above results, valid also for the cases of the antioxidants vitamin C, cysteine and fumaric acid.

Walnut oil: Walnut oil is oil extracted from walnuts Juglans regia (Persian walnuts). Walnuts are rich in phytonutrients being excellent sources of phosphorous, selenium, magnesium, iron, zinc, and calcium. Walnuts and/or walnut oil provide big levels of Vitamins B_1, B_2, and B_3, along with Vitamin E and niacin.

Niacin, known also as nicotinic acid, together with nicotinamide, it makes up the group known as vitamin B_3 complex.

The oil provides polyunsaturated fatty acids, monounsaturated fatty acids, and saturated fatty acids. Unlike most nuts that are high in monounsaturated fatty acids, walnut oil is composed largely of polyunsaturated fatty acids, particularly alpha-linolenic acid and linoleic acid, and it does contain oleic acid [96]. It does not contain cholesterol.

Walnut oil is edible, and, like all nut seed and vegetable oils will undergo rancidification accelerated by heat, light and oxygen.

Pairs of electrons in walnut oil constituents that can be accommodated to singlet oxygen's empty π^* orbital are the oxygen, nitrogen and sulfur lone pairs and the aromatic rings' and double bonds' electron densities.

Case o: Kinetic parameters of walnut oil [97]

Rancimat was one of the tests that were developed for testing the resistance to oxidation of fats. Being easy for use and due to its repeatability has become a popular method that is used up to now [98,99]. Rancimat test allows for estimating the induction period (IP) or the oxidative stability index (OSI), which is the period before oil rapid oxidation. The oxidation reaction rate constants

(k) of walnut oil at various temperatures were determined. The presence of double bonds increases the oxidation rate [100]. This is explained by the mechanism that we propose as follows: the double bonds' electron densities react with the empty π^* orbital of singlet oxygen. The activation energy E_{act} of walnut crude oil was determined to be 80.327 $kJmol^{-1}$. The amount of polyunsaturated fatty acids (linoleic, linolenic, and oleic acids) in vegetable oils has decisive role in their oxidative stability so that by increasing the polyunsaturated fatty acids, the oil oxidative stability is reduced [101]. According to our mechanism (Section 4.2), the polyunsaturated acids react with singlet oxygen's empty π^* orbital through the electron densities of the unsaturated bonds. The presence of polyunsaturated fatty acids in vegetable oils affect their activation energies. In general, it has been reported that high levels of polyunsaturated acids (linoleic acid and linolenic) reduce the activation energy, (increase of decomposition rate due to unsaturated bonds that react with the empty π^*). The value of enthalpy and entropy of activation of walnuts crude oil was found by the authors to be $\Delta H^{\neq} = 77.27$ $kJmol^{-1}$ and $\Delta S^{\neq} = -55.76$ $JK^{-1}mol^{-1}$, respectively. The $E_{act} = 80.32$ $kJmol^{-1}$, the $\Delta G^{\neq} = 94.56$ $kJmol^{-1}$ at 310 K calculated by us according to the $\Delta H^{\neq}$ and $\Delta S^{\neq}$ reported by the authors.

Our calculations gave: $E_{act} = 10.04$ $kJmol^{-1}$, $\Delta H^{\neq} = 6.99$ $kJmol^{-1}$, $\Delta S^{\neq} = -307.8$ $JK^{-1}mol^{-1}$, $\Delta G^{\neq} = 102.4$ $kJmol^{-1}$ at 310 K.

The differences in the calculated values of the thermodynamic parameters are due to the different units of the rate constants that were expressed by the authors in the unit "per hour". They should be expressed "per second" since the Planck's constant is expressed in Joule.sec. The Planck's constant is involved in the Eyring equation.

4.1.6. Oxygen-Free Reaction of Diallyl Disulfide

Case p: Kinetics and mechanism of diallyl disulfide thermal decomposition [102]

The work deals with diallyl disulfide pyrolysis, that is, reaction under oxygen-free conditions. Diallyl disulfide is present in garlic oil and posseses anticarcinogenic properties [103,104].

In this work [102] the experimental system was evacuated, that is, the experiments were designed in such a way that, there was no reaction with oxygen. This means that our mechanism that are valid in the presence of O_2 cannot be applied in this case where the mechanism must be different and the thermodynamic parameters would have different values. Especially the $\Delta G^{\neq}$ does not correspond to reaction with singlet oxygen. The $\Delta G^{\neq}$ value is different from the values for the other cases (a–o) reported in this paper which are: (a) similar; (b) they have values equal to 92 $kJmol^{-1}$ + E_{act} for diffusion. The $\Delta G^{\neq}$ for this case p is 135.81 $kJmol^{-1}$ at 310 K, completely different from the values for all of the cases of the food antioxidants that were studied that range between 91.27 and 116.46 $kJmol^{-1}$ at 310 K.

Analytically our calculations based on the authors' results give: $E_{act} = 123.32$ $kJmol^{-1}$, $\Delta H^{\neq} = 119.60$ $kJmol^{-1}$, $\Delta S^{\neq} = -52.30$ $JK^{-1}mol^{-1}$, $\Delta G^{\neq} = 135.81$ $kJmol^{-1}$ at 310 K, a completely different from the other cases value.

In addition to the above case p we searched for more cases of reactions of antioxidants under oxygen-free conditions in order to add weight to the conclusion that singlet oxygen is involved in the degradation process. The following cases (a), (b), (c) lead to the conclusion that the $\Delta G^{\neq}$ becomes higher under oxygen-free conditions:

(a) The kinetics of quercetin (a plant polyphenol from the flavonoid group) oxidation in the absence of air [105]. The authors state that: "The results, ... show clearly that the absence, ... or at least substantial reduction, of oxygen content markedly slows down quercetin oxidation." This means that quercetin oxidation becomes slower, that is, the $\Delta G^{\neq}$ value becomes higher.

(b) "Circulating air increased the rate of lycopene degradation" [106]. This suggests that the absence of oxygen decreased the degradation, which means that increased the $\Delta G^{\neq}$ value.

(c) "Oxygen-free conditions reduce lycopene losses significantly" [107]. This means that without the presence of oxygen lycopene is degraded more slowly meaning that the $\Delta G^{\neq}$ value is higher.

Conclusion: Except for the case (a), for which we found positive $\Delta S^{\neq}$ and we suggest a composite mechanism, all other values of $\Delta S^{\neq}$ are negative which agrees with the mechanism that we propose, according to which the lone pairs of electrons or the electron densities of the antioxidants are accommodated at the singlet oxygen's empty π^* orbital. This procedure happening at the rate determining step leads to a higher organization in the transition state than in the reactants, that is, leads to less degrees of freedom, since the two species become one.

Other important Antioxidants for which we had no available data for our calculations are:

Astaxanthin ($C_{40}H_{52}O_4$) is an antioxidant that crosses the blood brain barrier. It has been reported by Naguib et al. [108] that astaxanthin has higher antioxidant activity compared to various carotenoids such as α-carotene, lutein, lycopene and β-carotene. Actually antioxidant activity of astaxanthin was 10 times more than zeaxanthin, lutein, canthaxanthin, β-carotene and 100 times higher than α-tocopherol [109].

Astaxanthin contains a molecular structure in the presence of hydroxyl and keto moieties on each ionone ring, which are responsible for the high antioxidant properties [108,110]. The polyene chain in astaxanthin traps radicals in the cell membrane, while the terminal ring of astaxanthin could scavenge radicals at the outer and inner parts of the cell membrane. So, astaxanthin's molecular structure enables it to stay both in and outside the cell membrane. Vitamin C and β-carotene can be positioned inside the lipid bilayer so astaxanthin gives better protection than the above two antioxidants.

Astaxanthin can be found in high concentrations within the retina. It has been reported that astaxanthin, along with the similar fat-soluble carotenoids lutein and zeaxanthin, may help in absorbing some of the blue light and near-UV rays that the retinas are exposed to daily. There are studies suggesting that aside from cataracts and macular degeneration astaxanthin benefits include cardiovascular health, brain aging, cancer, diabetes, as well as other diseases and conditions [111].

Coenzyme Q-10 is produced naturally in our body. It crosses the blood brain barrier. It is used for cell growth and to protect cells from damage that could lead to cancer.

The oxidized molecule that has three isoprenoid units is called Q3.

CoQ10 contains a molecular structure in the presence of keto moieties on ring, which are responsible for the high antioxidant properties. The polyene chain in CoQ10 traps radicals in the cell membrane, while the terminal ring of CoQ10 could scavenge radicals at the outer and inner parts of cell membrane.

Glutathione (GSH) is an important antioxidant in some bacteria and archaea, in fungi, plants, and animals. Glutathione prevents damage to important cellular components that are caused by reactive oxygen species, such as free radicals, heavy metals, peroxides, and lipid peroxides [112]. Glutathione, serving as an electron donor reduces disulfide bonds of proteins to cysteines. During this process, glutathione is oxidized to glutathione disulfide (GSSG/L-(–)-glutathione). Oxidized glutathione can be reduced back by NADPH (an electron donor) and glutathione reductase [113]. A measure of cellular oxidative stress is often used the ratio of reduced to oxidized glutathione within cells [114,115].

Glutathione is one of the most important antioxidants in cells due to its high concentration and its central role in maintaining the cell's redox state [116].

Pairs of electrons in the molecular structure of glutathione that can be accommodated to singlet oxygen's empty π^* orbital are the lone pairs of O, N, S, the double bonds' electron density. Also, the positively charged nitrogen atom can accept electron density from the occupied π^* orbital of $^1\Delta_g$ (singlet oxygen), the HOMO.

Lipoic acid (LA), also known as α-lipoic acid (ALA) and thioctic acid is an organosulfur compound derived from octanoic acid. LA contains two sulfur atoms connected by a disulfide bond and is thus considered to be oxidized.

Lipoic acid is an antioxidant. Although the body can synthesize LA, it can also be absorbed from the diet. Maximum blood levels of LA are achieved 30–60 min after dietary supplementation, and it is thought to be largely metabolized in the liver [117]. In Germany, LA is approved as a drug for the treatment of diabetic neuropathy since 1966 [118].

Pairs of electrons in the molecular structure of lipoic acid that can be accommodated to singlet oxygen's empty π^* orbital are the lone pairs of O and S, and the double bond's electron density.

Melatonin, N-acetyl-5-methoxy, tryptamine, is a hormone that is produced by the pineal gland in animals and regulates sleep and wakefulness [119]. In animals, melatonin is involved in the synchronization of the circadian rhythms including sleep-wake timing, seasonal reproduction, blood pressure regulation, and many others [120]. It also functions as synchronizer of the biological clock. In animals, many of its biological effects are due to its role as an antioxidant [121]. It plays a particular role in the protection of nuclear and mitochondrial DNA [122].

Melatonin is a powerful wide-spectrum antioxidant [123,124] that easily cross the blood-brain-barrier [121,125,126] and cell membranes. This antioxidant is a direct scavenger of radical oxygen and nitrogen species, including OH•, O_2^-•, and NO• [127,128]. Melatonin, once oxidized, upon reacting with free radicals cannot be reduced to its former state because it forms several stable end-products. For this reason it has been referred to as a terminal (or suicidal) antioxidant [129]. It has been proven that melatonin is twice as active as vitamin E, and is believed to be the most effective lipophilic antioxidant [130]. A very important characteristic of melatonin is that its metabolites are also scavengers in what is referred to as the cascade reaction [123]. When melatonin is compared to synthetic, mitochondrial-targeted antioxidants (MitoQ and MitoE), it is proved to be a comparable protector against mitochondrial oxidative stress [131].

Pairs of electrons in the molecular structure of melatonin that can be accommodated to singlet oxygen's empty π^* orbital are the lone pairs of O and N, and the electron densities of the rings and of the double C=O bond.

Vitamin E is the name for eight related fat-soluble vitamins tocopherols and tocotrienols, with antioxidant properties [132,133]. The body preferentially absorbs and metabolises the form α-tocopherol [134] which has the highest bioavailability. Its action is protecting membranes from oxidation by reacting with lipid radicals that are produced in the lipid peroxidation chain reaction [132,135]. During lipid peroxidation, singlet oxygen is produced [1]. Vitamin E removes the free radicals and stops the propagation reaction. The result of this reaction is oxidized by singlet oxygen α-tocopheroxyl radicals that can be recycled back to the active reduced form through reduction by other antioxidants, such as ascorbate, retinol or ubiquinol [136]. It has been suggested that the most important function of α-tocopherol is as a signaling molecule having no significant role in antioxidant metabolism [137,138].

Tocotrienols are a rarer form of Vitamin E. It crosses the blood brain barrier. Tocotrienols may be important in protecting neurons from damage [139].

Pairs of electrons in the molecular structure of vitamin E that can be accommodated to singlet oxygen's empty π^* orbital are the oxygen lone pairs and the phenyl ring's electron density. According to its structure, vitamin E may not be a significant antioxidant since there are not many regions of high electron density to capture singlet oxygen's empty π^* orbital (see below "mechanism of action" of the studied antioxidants).

Vitamin K_2 has recently been revealed as an important nutrient in protecting against heart disease [140]. It achieves this by guiding the body to add the calcium in the bones and teeth and not in the arteries and soft tissue. The structures of both vitamins K_1 and K_2 show why K_2 can act as an antioxidant, whereas K_1 not as a good one.

Regions of high electron density are the double bonded oxygens that bear pairs of electrons that can be accommodated in the singlet oxygen's empty π^* orbital. This also applies for the chain double bonds that exist in K_2 but not in K_1. The molecular structure bears the presence of keto moieties on the ring, which are responsible for high antioxidant properties. The polyene chain in vitamin K_2 traps radicals in the cell membrane, while the terminal ring of vitamin K_2 could scavenge radicals at the outer and inner parts of cell membrane.

4.2. Mechanism of the Studied Antioxidants' Reactions with Oxygen

The results of our calculations that are presented in Table 1 suggest that for all of the cases (a–o), the free energy of activation could be the sum of the 92 $kJmol^{-1}$ and the E_{act} of diffusion of the reactants. As in the already studied reactions of proteins of proteinaceous diseases the free energy of activation reveals that the rds is the production of singlet oxygen which then reacts with proteins, DNA, biomolecules etc. In the present work again the rds is found to be the formation of singlet oxygen which then reacts with the antioxidants. Examining the structures of the various antioxidants, we can conclude that this might be the case: the various antioxidants, like the proteins of proteinaceous diseases, bear regions of high electron density (basic properties), and thus they can react with the empty π^* orbital of singlet oxygen (strong acidic properties). So, there is a possibility of the two following reactions taking place in the two different systems: (a) Proteins, DNA, biomolecules + singlet oxygen's empty π^* orbital, and (b) antioxidants + singlet oxygen's empty π^* orbital. For these two cases the rates of the reactions are:

For both cases: Vrds = k $[O_2]$ = cT exp − (92/RT). $[O_2]$, Rds reaction: $^3\Sigma_g \quad O_2 \rightarrow {}^1\Delta g\ O_2$

(a) For the reactions of biomolecules with the produced at the rds singlet oxygen:

$V_{(\text{biomolecules+singlet oxygen's empty } \pi^* \text{ orbital})} = k_{(b+so)}\ [^1O_2]\ [\text{biomolecules}] = c.\ T.\ \exp\ (-\Delta G^{\neq}{}_{(b+so)}/RT)$ $[^1O_2]$ [biomolecules], where $^1O_2$ is the singlet oxygen, (b + so): (biomolecules + singlet oxygen).

(b) For the reactions of antioxidants with the produced at the rds singlet oxygen:

$V_{(\text{antioxidants+singlet oxygen's empty } \pi^* \text{ orbital})} = k_{(a+so)}\ [^1O_2]\ [\text{antioxidants}] = c.\ T.\ \exp\ (-\Delta G^{\neq}{}_{(a+so)}/RT)$ $[^1O_2]$ [antioxidants], where $^1O_2$ is the singlet oxygen, (a + so): (antioxidants + singlet oxygen).

The values of $\Delta G^{\neq}{}_{(b+so)}$ and $\Delta G^{\neq}{}_{(a+so)}$ are almost similar (see Figure 1) the $\Delta G^{\neq}{}_{(a+so)}$ being slightly smaller which implies slightly higher rate of reaction if the concentrations [biomolecules] and [antioxidants] and $k_{(b+so)}$ and $k_{(a+so)}$ were the same. Assuming that the $k_{(b+so)}$ and $k_{(a+so)}$ are very big and similar since they correspond to reactions of an excited state, $^1\Delta_g$ (with acidic properties) and molecules bearing basic properties then the decisive role that is played by the relation of the concentrations of [biomolecules] and of [antioxidants]. Unfortunately the [biomolecules] is a lot higher than the [antioxidants]. Thus, the rate of reaction of biomolecules is a lot higher than the rate of the reaction of antioxidants. In most of the antioxidants, there are more than one sites of attack by singlet oxygen because they bear many regions that can react, for example, many double bonds, many lone pairs of electrons due to the presence of oxygen(s), nitrogen(s), or sulfur atoms etc. This multiplies the "concentration" of the antioxidants (statistical kinetics). However, the same applies for the "concentration" of the biomolecules (proteins, DNA, etc.): it is multiplied because of the existence of many regions of high electron density due to many lone pairs of electrons in the many oxygen, nitrogen, and sulfur atoms in their molecules. Concluding, the solution is to increase the "concentration" of the antioxidants in order to create:

$$V_{(\text{biomolecules+singlet oxygen's empty } \pi^* \text{ orbital})} < V_{(\text{antioxidants+singlet oxygen's empty } \pi^* \text{ orbital})}$$

and thus the antioxidants to win the competition with proteins, DNA, etc., in capturing singlet oxygen's empty π^* orbital.

Table 1. Kinetic data (k, T) and calculated thermodynamic parameters (E_{act}, $\Delta H^{\neq}$, $\Delta S^{\neq}$, $\Delta G^{\neq}$) for reactions of various antioxidants.

	$T^{(i)}$ (K)	$\ln k^{(i)}$	$E_{act}^{(ii)}$ $kJmol^{-1}$	$\Delta H^{\neq (iii)}$ $kJ^{-1}mol^{-1}$	$\Delta S^{\neq (iii)}$ $JK^{-1}mol^{-1}$	$\Delta G^{\neq (iii)}$ $kJmol^{-1}$
Case a Thermal injury due to normal body temperature [23]						
	314	−10.360	769.52$^{(iii)}$	766.89	2110.41	112.8 at 310 K
	315	−9.8338				
	316	−8.4168				
	317	−7.4544				
	318	−6.6079				
	319	−6.0185				
Case b Degradation kinetics of anthocyanins [29] [blackberry juice and concentrate]						
	333	−11.3732	58.90$^{(iii)}$	56.01	−172.01	109.33 at 310 K
	343	−10.7245	58.95$^{(b)}$			
	353	−10.0979				
	363	−9.6309				
Case c Degradation kinetics of anthocyanins [31] [Guatemala roselle]						
	308	−12.0491	39.27$^{(iii)}$	36.46	−226.7	106.75 at 310 K
	340.5	−10.5013				
	371.5	−9.4347				
Case c Degradation kinetics of anthocyanins [31] [BRJ]						
	308	−12.7647	49.17$^{(iii)}$	46.37	−200.31	108.47 at 310 K
	340.5	−10.7615				
	371.5	−9.4962				
Case d Antioxidant activity and carotenoids content [38]						
	323	−14.5426	23.34$^{(iii)}$	20.53	−302.48	114.31 at 310 K
	333	−14.2012	23.7$^{(d)}$			
	353	−13.7892				
Case e Degradation of carotenoid antioxidants [39] (i) cultivar lycopene						
	333	−9.0420	4.62$^{(iii)}$	1.62	−315.66	99.48 at 310 K
	353	−8.8620	4.63$^{(e)}$			
	373	−8.8049				
	393	−8.7829				
(i) cultivar beta-carotene						
	333	−9.0006	4.13$^{(iii)}$	1.13	−317.03	99.41 at 310 K
	353	−8.898	4.14$^{(e)}$			
	373	−8.8274				
	393	−8.7721				
(ii) cultivar lycopene						
	333	−9.5911	8.64$^{(iii)}$	5.64	−307.97	101.11 at 310 K
	353	−9.2616	8.65$^{(e)}$			
	373	−9.2103				
	393	−9.0852				
(ii) cultivar Beta-carotene						
	333	−9.4129	4.81$^{(iii)}$	1.81	−318.17	100.44 at 310 K
	353	−9.2271	4.81$^{(e)}$			
	373	−9.1616				
	393	−9.1458				
Case f Beta-carotene degradation [40]						
	333	−9.6938	95.73$^{(iii)}$	92.88	−46.782	107.37 at 310 K
	343	−8.4143	95.4$^{(f)}$			
	353	−7.7402				
Case g Stability of curcumin during storage [41] With the presence of light						
	278	−8.4068	24.213$^{(iii)}$	21.752	−235.8	94.912 at 310 K
	306	−7.3488	23.88$^{(g)}$			
	318	−7.1247				
Case g Stability of curcumin during storage [41] Without the presence of light						
	278	−9.4980	11.803$^{(iii)}$	9.342	−290.3	99.32 at 310 K
	306	−9.3534	13.65$^{(g)}$			
	318	−8.74034				

Table 1. *Cont.*

	T[i] (K)	lnk[i]	E_{act}[ii] $kJmol^{-1}$	Δ H≠[iii] $kJ^{-1}mol^{-1}$	Δ S≠[iii] $JK^{-1}mol^{-1}$	Δ G≠[iii] $kJmol^{-1}$
Case h, Thermal degradation of polyphenols [51] [grape marc]						
	353	−7.1185	5.67[iii]	2.45	−298.1	94.86 at 310 K
	373	−6.8831	55.98[h]			
	423	−6.7709				
Case h, Thermal degradation of polyphenols [51] [filtered extract]						
	353	−6.7709	9.03[iii]	5.80	−285.9	94.46 at 310 K
	373	−6.5583	53.196[h]			
	423	−6.2520				
Case i Degradation kinetics of sulforaphane [55]						
pH = 2.2	333	−12.7939	85.36[iii]	82.48	−103.66	114.95 at 310 K
	348	−11.1844				
	355	−10.8479				
	363	−10.2289				
pH = 3.0	333	−12.7939	93.17[iii]	90.29	−79.97	115.08at310 K
	348	−11.0021				
	355	−10.5966				
	363	−10.0213				
pH = 4	333	−12.1007	79.69[iii]	76.80	−114.58	112.32 at 310k
	348	−10.4913				
	355	−10.1548				
	363	−9.7493				
pH = 5	333	−11.4076	71.87[iii]	68.98	−132.98	110.2 at 310 K
	348	−10.1548				
	355	−9.7493				
	363	−9.2675				
pH = 6	333	−11.0021	69.61[iii]	66.73	−136.01	108.9 at 310 K
	348	−9.6584				
	355	−9.3281				
	363	−8.9437				
Case j Antioxidant activity and thiosulfinate degradation of garlic [80]						
Antioxidant activity	353	−5.5090	89.76[iii]	86.74	−46.68	101.21 at 310 K
	363	−4.7736	89.75[j]			
	373	−3.8672				
Case j Antioxidant activity and thiosulfinate degradation of garlic [80]						
Degradation of thiosulfinates	353	−5.5684	7.565[iii]	4.55	−279.7	91.27 at 310 K
	363	−5.5090	7.67[j]			
	373	−5.4299				
Case k, Vitamin C degradation, [91]						
Standard ascorbic acid solution (Merck)	303	−8.7916	36.65[iii]	34.09	−205.47	97.79 at 310 K
	313	−8.3266	36.53[k]			
Vitamin C 200 mg tablet	303	−7.0845	27.64[iii]	25.08	−221.03	93.6 at 310 K
	313	−6.7338	27.82[k]			
Ascovit 100 mg tablet	303	−7.1915	11.02[iii]	8.46	−276.8	94.26 at 310 K
	313	−7.0516	10.96[k]			
Vitamin C nose drops	303	−7.9778	34.89[iii]	32.33	−204.53	95.73 at 310 K
	313	−7.5351	35.10[k]			
Case l, Temperature and high pressure stability of vitamin C [92] [watermelon]						
	343	−8.4300	76.92[iii]	73.98	−101.76	105.528 at 310 K
	353	−8.1404	76.86[l]			
	363	−6.9349				
Case l, Temperature and high pressure stability of lycopene [92] [watermelon]						
	343	−11.911	97.21[iii]	94.27	−71.56	116.46 at 310 K
	353	−11.423	97.7[l]			
	363	−10.024				

Table 1. *Cont.*

	$T^{(i)}$ (K)	$\ln k^{(i)}$	$E_{act}{}^{(ii)}$ $kJmol^{-1}$	$\Delta H^{\neq(iii)}$ $kJ^{-1}mol^{-1}$	$\Delta S^{\neq(iii)}$ $JK^{-1}mol^{-1}$	$\Delta G^{\neq(iii)}$ $kJmol^{-1}$
Case m, Oxidation of vitamin C [93]						
	313	−12.8992	41.65$^{(iii)}$	38.89	−224.4	108.47 at 310 K
	323	−11.5297	20.73$^{(m)}$			
	333	−11.1765				
	343	−10.9159				
	353	−10.9823				
Case n, Effect of antioxidants [vitamin C, cysteine, fumaric acid] on the stability of an HTK solution [95] HTK						
	323	−13.1563	100.48$^{(iii)}$	97.75	−52.15	113.92 at 310k
	333	−12.032	100.186$^{(n)}$			
HTK + cysteine	323	−13.6903	92.31$^{(iii)}$	89.58	−81.87	114.96 at 310 K
	333	−12.6576	91.96$^{(n)}$			
HTK + vitamin C	323	−13.8494	98.20$^{(iii)}$	95.47	−64.98	115.61 at 310 K
	333	−12.7508	98.127$^{(n)}$			
HTK + fumaric acid	323	−13.6903	89.94$^{(iii)}$	87.21	−89.22	114.87 at 310 K
	333	−12.6841	89.70$^{(n)}$			
Case o, Kinetic parameters of walnut oil [97]						
	353	−9.7921	10.04$^{(iii)}$	6.99	−307.8	102.4 at 310 K 94.56 at 310 K calculated by us according to the $\Delta H^{\neq}$, and $\Delta S^{\neq}$ of work [133]
	363	−9.7042	80.32$^{(o)}$	77.27$^{(o)}$	−55.76$^{(o)}$	
	373	−9.6146				
	383	−9.5239				
Oxygen-free conditions Case p kinetics and mechanism of diallyl disulfide thermal decomposition [102]						
	433	−9.8302	123.32$^{(iii)}$	119.60	−52.30	135.81 at 310 K
	443	−8.7702				
	453	−8.1101				
	463	−7.5902				

Notes: (i) Experimental data in units of T in K and of k in: s^{-1} (cases a, b, c, d, e, f, g, h, i, j, k, l, m, n, o, p) (ii) Calculated values; (iii) This work. **Important Note:** In the cases where our calculated values differ considerably from the values reported in the literature, we noticed that our difference was in the units of the rate constants. The unit of inverse time in k should be in s−1 since the units of the Planck's constant are in Js, i.e., time is in s (seconds). In some of the cases where our results are different, the unit of inverse time of the k was in min−1 or in h−1 (which is not correct).

In Figure 2, the barriers $\Delta G^{\neq}$ are equal to 92 $kJmol^{-1}$ plus the E_{act} of the reactants' diffusion. In the case of the biomolecules' reactions the E_{act} of the diffusion is bigger than the E_{act} of the diffusion of the antioxidants' reactions due to the nature of the corresponding medium (cell vs. water).

It must be pointed out that our calculated thermodynamic parameters of activation provide only information about the rate determining step (rds), and actually about the value of the free energy of activation. This free energy of activation is equal to 92 $kJmol^{-1}$ + the E_{act} for diffusion. So, we have evidence that singlet oxygen is produced during the rds. We have no evidence of what is next happening. Either a direct reaction of $^1O_2$ or a reaction by a secondary ROS (Reactive Oxygen Species) is taking place. The observations that are referred to Section 1.2, in paragraph "Singlet oxygen quenching" apply for our findings as well.

Also, our above derived conclusions are in perfect agreement with previous reports on the scavenging activity of certain antioxidants for singlet oxygen [8–10,12].

4.3. *Questions That Need to Be Answered*

If the above-suggested mechanism of the role of singlet oxygen, O_2 ($^1\Delta_g$) in the reactions of antioxidants is actually valid, then some questions arise that need to be answered: (1) which are the sources of singlet molecular oxygen in the biological systems? [1]; (2) where does the human body find the energy of 92 $kJmol^{-1}$ for ground state oxygen's excitation to the first excited state, i.e., to generate singlet oxygen state, $^1\Delta_g$ in a cell? [1]. It is known that the energy of the ATP (phosphoric) bond is 30.66 $kJmol^{-1}$. Can the excitation energy of O_2 be taken from the use of 3–4 ATP molecules? [1]; (3) is the generation of singlet oxygen increased selectively in neurons, and if so, how does this happen? [1]. The antioxidants must meet neurons if they are going to react with singlet oxygen generated in their environment. Can antioxidants meet neurons? Can they pass the Blood-Brain Barrier (BBB)?

Which are the sources of singlet molecular oxygen in the biological systems? Potential sources of singlet molecular oxygen in the biological systems have been in detail presented in [1]. Besides other sources, lipid, phospholipid and cholesterol hydroperoxides are sources of singlet molecular oxygen [1].

Where does the human body find the energy of 92 $kJmol^{-1}$ for ground state oxygen's excitation to the first excited state, i.e., to generate singlet oxygen state, $^1\Delta_g$ in a cell? This energy can be found in a cell according to Peter Mitchell's "the chemiosmotic hypothesis" [1].

Is the generation of singlet oxygen increased selectively in neurons and if so, how does this happen? This question has also been answered in [1]. The antioxidants must meet neurons if they are going to react with singlet oxygen generated in their environment. Can antioxidants meet neurons? Can they pass the BBB?

Blood–Brain Barrier (BBB), The BBB is an important filter that protects the brain [141,142] and the cells of the barrier allow, by passive diffusion, the passage of water, lipid-soluble molecules, and some gases, as well as the selective actively transport of molecules (metabolic products), such as glucose (across the barrier with specific proteins) [143] and amino acids that are necessary for neural function. It also prevents the entry of potential lipophilic neurotoxins by way of an active transport mechanism that is mediated by P-glycoprotein. Endothelial cells restrict the diffusion of microscopic objects (e.g., bacteria) and large or hydrophilic molecules into the cerebrospinal fluid (CSF), while they allow for the diffusion of hydrophobic molecules (O_2, CO_2, hormones) [144]. It is claimed that astrocytes are necessary to create the blood–brain barrier. A protective layer is played by a thick membrane and astrocytic end feet [145,146]. In addition to the above protection, cerebral endothelial cells have a defense system against oxidative stress, which includes GSH, glutathione peroxidase, glutathione reductase, and catalase when compared to the rest of the brain [147]. In particular, GSH is supported to play a role in maintenance of the BBB integrity [148]. All parts of the healthy brain contain antioxidants like superoxide dismutase (SOD) in order to balance against the produced high concentration of ROS and RNS [149]. Few regions in the brain do not have a BBB, including the circumventricular organs. The neuronal membrane contains polyunsaturated fatty acids especially docosahexaenoic acid. Polyunsaturated fatty acids undergo lipid peroxidation. Cerebral endothelial cells have a high concentration of mitochondria, leading to the generation of oxidative stress [150]. The high concentration of mitochondria is supported to play a role in maintenance of BBB. It has been reported [151] that with aging a decrease in mitochondrial number at cerebral endothelial cells and a subsequent loss of BBB integrity take place. The properties that can cause increase of oxidative stress lead not only to neurodegeneration and breakdown of the BBB via disruption of tight junction proteins, but can also affect blood flow [152]. The brain, particularly the cerebrovascular system, features many sources of producing oxidative stress as well as targets vulnerable to this stress allowing for a cycle of damage.

Does Disruption of the Blood–Brain Barrier Take Place in Alzheimer's Disease? There is evidence indicating that disruption of the blood–brain barrier in Alzheimer's disease patients allows blood plasma containing Aβ amyloid to enter the brain where the Aβ adheres preferentially to the surface of astrocytes [153]. These findings have led to some hypotheses about mechanisms in some cases of Alzheimer's disease. Thus, in some patients, Alzheimer's disease may be caused (or more likely, aggravated) by a breakdown in the blood–brain barrier [154].

4.4. Future Strategies

Having presented the above (possible) role of singlet oxygen (major component of oxidative stress) in the reactions of antioxidants, we conclude that antioxidant administration or donation of reagents bearing regions of high electron density (bases) may be useful in the prevention and treatment of neurodegenerative diseases and the other disorders that are mentioned above and in [1]. To obtain efficacy in delaying diseases progression, the candidate antioxidant or base must be given as early as possible, before irreversible neuronal loss. The antioxidant or base should also be tailored to the place of generation of $^1O_2$ ($^1\Delta_g$), i.e., to neurons that are rich in lipids and/or metal ions. The chosen antioxidant or the basic properties bearing reagent should also be able to penetrate the blood-brain barrier after systemic administration in order to attain a critical therapeutic level within the CNS [1].

The antioxidants should be ones that could prevent lipid, protein, DNA peroxidation, and thus prevent the production of the $^1O_2$ ($^1\Delta_g$). Suitable bases should be ones that could donate pair of electrons in the empty π^* orbital of the produced O_2 ($^1\Delta_g$) in order to prevent the reaction of it (π^* orbital) with protein, lipid, DNA, biomolecule in general.

The bases (reagents bearing regions of high electron density) and the antioxidants should react with the $^1O_2$ ($^1\Delta_g$) faster than lipids, proteins, DNA, etc. Thus,

$$V_{(\text{biomolecules+singlet oxygen's empty } \pi^* \text{ orbital})} < V_{(\text{antioxidants+singlet oxygen's empty } \pi^* \text{ orbital})}$$

The bases and the antioxidants must also meet neurons hence they must be able to pass the BBB. In order to achieve what we have found from our calculations, the solution is to increase the concentration of the antioxidants in order to create a higher rate of their reaction with the empty π^* orbital of the produced O_2 ($^1\Delta_g$).

Then, the antioxidants will win the competition with proteins, DNA, etc., in capturing singlet oxygen's empty π^* orbital. Thus we must find a way to increase the concentration of the antioxidants in the brain.

We are trying at the moment to find which antioxidants can have the best overlapping of their orbitals with the singlet oxygen's empty π^* orbital.

Computational studies have been reported in the literature [155] for the oxidation of guanine by singlet oxygen ($^1\Delta_g$) and formation of guanine: lysine cross-links. We have already referred to the molecule of guanine as being high electron density regions of DNA [1].

We are also studying aspirin as a candidate antioxidant since our preliminary calculations showed that the structure of its molecule having regions of high electron densities must have strong antioxidant properties. The valuable role of aspirin in tumor cells has been reported [156].

5. Conclusions

The values of $\Delta G^{\neq}$ suggest that singlet oxygen production ($^1O_2$, $^1\Delta_g$) from ground state oxygen (O_2, $^3\Sigma_g{}^-$) demanding 92 kJmol^{-1}, may be the crucial/decisive step in the common mechanism of reactions of the various antioxidants that were studied. About 10–30 kJmol^{-1} is the activation energy that is needed for the diffusion of reactants, where this is necessary, depending on the reaction and the medium. In aqueous solutions or in experiments in vitro, the E_{act} of diffusion of the reactants is smaller than in reactions in vivo. We attribute the common mechanism to the same role of oxidative stress and specifically of singlet oxygen to the above mentioned (studied) processes of antioxidants.

The ability of accepting a pair of electrons in the empty π^* orbital gives to the singlet oxygen species, $^1\Delta_g$, strong acidic properties meaning that it can react with antioxidants bearing regions of high electron density, that is, regions of high basicity.

Regions of high electron density in the various antioxidants that were studied are the double bonds, the lone pairs of electrons in O, N, S atoms, the aromatic rings etc., accommodating their free pair of electrons in the empty π^* orbital of singlet oxygen. The general reactions taking place could be represented as follows:

$$^1O_2\ (^1\Delta_g) = O_2\ [\pi^*\ \underline{\uparrow\downarrow}\ \ \underline{\ \ }\ \pi^*]\ \text{rate determining step—formation of singlet oxygen}$$

$$^1O_2(^1\Delta_g)\ +\ \text{antioxidant} \rightleftarrows \left[\text{adduct}\ (^1O_2/\text{antioxidant})\right]^{\neq} \rightleftarrows \text{oxidation products of antioxidants}$$

A similar mechanism has been proposed [1] for the reaction of singlet oxygen with biomolecules:

$$^1O_2\ (^1\Delta_g) = O_2\ [\pi^*\ \underline{\uparrow\downarrow}\ \ \underline{\ \ }\ \pi^*]\ \text{rate determining step—formation of singlet oxygen}$$

$$^1O_2(^1\Delta_g)\ +\ \text{biomolecule(s) bearing regions of high electron density} \rightleftarrows$$
$$\left[\text{adduct}(^1O_2/\text{biomolecule(s)})\right]^{\neq} \rightleftarrows \text{oxidation products of biomolecule(s)}$$

We have presented the regions of high electron density in the chemical structures of various antioxidants. There are not experimental data available for reactions of all of them with oxygen in order to use them for our calculations. Based on their structures, we can suggest that astaxanthin, carotenoids, vitamin K_2 are very suitable for the reactions with singlet oxygen.

We expect different behaviour of antioxidants in solution experiments (as are the experiments that provided us with the data that we have used for our calculations) and in the cells. We can expect different activation energies for the diffusion of the antioxidants in aqueous solutions and in the cells. E_{act} diffusion in aqueous media < E_{act} diffusion in cells. This explains the smaller $\Delta G^{\neq}$ that we found in our antioxidants' calculations.

There are common features in the structures of the antioxidants i.e., conjugated double bonds, C=O bonds, lone pairs of electrons in O, N, S atoms, etc.

Vitamin C, vitamin E, as well as vitamin K_1, are not the best antioxidants for the role that we expect them to play since they have very few sites that can overlap with singlet oxygen's empty π^* orbital, whereas astaxanthin, lycopene, beta-carotene etc., have a lot more sites available multiplying by this way their "concentration".

The competition between proteins, DNA, biomolecules in general and antioxidants for capturing singlet oxygen's empty π^* orbital could be successful for antioxidants by increasing their "useful concentration".

Acknowledgments: We thank the National and Kapodistrian University of Athens for financial support of this work. We thank all the authors that are included in the list of references, who, with their valuable data, the high-level scientific work both in experiments and in explanations have given us significant aid (a) in suggesting a possible role for singlet oxygen in the degradation of various antioxidants and (b) in pointing out that the Free Energy of Activation is the critical factor for all processes and not the E_{act}. We also thank the reviewers for constructive comments and suggestions that improved the manuscript. Thanks are also due to Esther Sakki for her valuable technical assistance in the preparation of this manuscript.

Author Contributions: Theodoros Ntanos and Antonis Liapis conducted the plots for the Arrhenius and the Eyring equations for data (k, T) that were found in the literature and were suggested by Athinoula L. Petrou. From the plots Theodoros Ntanos and Antonis Liapis performed the calculations of the thermodynamic parameters. Petros L. Petrou suggested the work with garlic and vitamin K2 providing also literature about garlic's effects in cardiovascular diseases. Athinoula L. Petrou conceived and designed the calculations analysed the data explaining the resulting thermodynamic activation parameters, proposed the mechanism and wrote the paper.

Conflicts of Interest: The authors declare no conflict of interest. The funding sponsor had no role in the design of the study; in the collection, analyses, or interpretation of data; in the writing of the manuscript, and in the decision to publish the results.

References

1. Petrou, A.L.; Terzidaki, A. A meta-analysis and review examining a possible role for oxidative stress and singlet oxygen in diverse diseases. *Biochem. J.* **2017**, *474*, 2713–2731. [CrossRef] [PubMed]
2. Freeman, L.R.; Keller, J.N. Oxidative stress and cerebral endothelial cells: Regulation of the blood-brain-barrier and antioxidant based interventions. *Biochim. Biophys. Acta* **2012**, *1822*, 822–829. [CrossRef] [PubMed]

3. Halliwell, B. Role of free radicals in the neurodegenerative diseases: Therapeutic implications for antioxidant treatment. *Drugs Aging* **2001**, *18*, 685–716. [CrossRef] [PubMed]
4. Halliwell, B. Antioxidants and human disease: A general introduction. *Nutr. Rev.* **1997**, *55*, S44–S49. [CrossRef] [PubMed]
5. Halliwell, B. Antioxidant defense mechanisms: From the beginning to the end (of the beginning). *Free Radic. Res.* **1999**, *31*, 261–272. [CrossRef] [PubMed]
6. Gorman, A.A.; Rodgers, M.A.J. Singlet Molecular Oxygen. *Chem. Soc. Rev.* **1981**, *10*, 205–231. [CrossRef]
7. Johnson, E.J. The role of carotenoids in human health. *Nutr. Clin. Care* **2002**, *5*, 56–65. [CrossRef] [PubMed]
8. Choe, E.; Min, D.B. Mechanisms of antioxidants in the oxidation of foods. *Compr Rev. Food Sci. Food Saf.* **2009**, *8*, 345–358. [CrossRef]
9. Tournaire, C.; Croux, S.; Maurette, M.-T.; Beck, I.; Hocquaux, M.; Braun, A.M.; Oliveros, E. Antioxidant activity of flavonoids: Efficiency of singlet oxygen ($^1\Delta_g$) quenching. *J. Photochem. Photobiol. B Biol.* **1993**, *19*, 205–215. [CrossRef]
10. Morales, J.; Gunther, G.; Zanacco, A.L.; Iemp, E. Singlet Oxygen reactions with flavonoids. A theoretical–experimental study. *PLoS ONE* **2012**. [CrossRef] [PubMed]
11. Ranal, F.; Birtic, S.; Cuine, S.; Triantaphylides, C.; Ravanat, J.-L.; Havaux, M. Chemical quenching of singlet oxygen by carotenoids in plants. *Plant Physiol.* **2012**, *158*, 1267–1278. [CrossRef]
12. Nishida, Y.; Yamashita, E.; Miki, W. Quenching activities of common hydrophilic and lipophilic antioxidants against singlet oxygen using chemiluminescence detection system. *Carotenoid Sci.* **2007**, *11*, 16–20.
13. Niedre, M.J.; Yu, C.S.; Patterson, M.S.; Wilson, B.C. Singlet oxygen luminescence as an in vivo photodynamic therapy dose metric: Validation in normal mouse skin with topical amino-levulinic acid. *Br. J. Cancer* **2005**, *92*, 298–304. [CrossRef] [PubMed]
14. Bellnier, D.A.; Wood, L.M.; Potter, W.R.; Weishaupt, K.R.; Oseroff, A.R. Design and construction of a light-delivery system for photodynamic therapy. *Med. Phys.* **1999**, *26*, 1552–1558. [CrossRef] [PubMed]
15. Dougherty, T.J.; Boyle, D.G.; Weishaupt, K.R.; Henderson, B.A.; Wityk, K.E. Photoradiation Therapy—Clinical and Drug Advances. *Adv. Exp. Med. Biol.* **1983**, *160*, 3–13. [CrossRef] [PubMed]
16. Tyrell, R.M.; Keyse, S.M. The interaction of UVA radiation with cultured cells. *J. Photochem. Photobiol.* **1990**, *4*, 349–361. [CrossRef]
17. Wyld, L.; Tomlinson, M.; Reed, M.W.R.; Brown, N.J. Aminolaevulinic acid-induced photodynamic therapy: Cellular responses to glucose starvation. *Br. J. Cancer* **2002**, *86*, 1343–1347. [CrossRef] [PubMed]
18. Petrou, A.L. The Free Energy of Activation as the critical factor in geochemical processes. *Chem. Geol.* **2012**, *308*, 50–59. [CrossRef]
19. Petrou, A.L.; Terzidaki, A. Calcium carbonate and calcium sulfate precipitation, crystallization and dissolution: Evidence for the activated steps and the mechanisms from the enthalpy and entropy of activation values. *Chem. Geol.* **2014**, *381*, 144–153. [CrossRef]
20. Katakis, D.; Gordon, G. *Mechanisms of Inorganic Reactions*; Wiley-Interscience: New York, NY, USA, 1987.
21. Petrou, A.L.; Economou-Eliopoulos, M. Platinum-group mineral formation: Evidence of an interchange process from the entropy of activation values. *Geochim. Cosmochim. Acta* **2009**, *73*, 5635–5645. [CrossRef]
22. Espenson, J.H. *Chemical Kinetics and Reaction Mechanisms*; Mc Graw-Hill: New York, NY, USA, 1981.
23. Johnson, H.A.; Pavelec, M. Thermal injury due to normal body temperature. *Am. J Pathol.* **1972**, *66*, 557–564. [PubMed]
24. Davies, K.M. *Plant Pigments and Their Manipulation*; Wiley-Blackwell: Boca Raton, FL, USA, 2004; p. 6. ISBN 1-4051-1737-0.
25. Archetti, M.; Döring, T.F.; Hagen, S.B.; Hughes, N.M.; Leather, S.R.; Lee, D.W.; Lev-Yadun, S.; Manetas, Y.; Ougham, H.J.; Schaberg, P.G.; et al. Unravelling the evolution of autumn colours: An interdisciplinary approach. *Trends Ecol. Evol.* **2011**, *24*, 166–173. [CrossRef] [PubMed]
26. Qiu, Z.; Wang, X.; Gao, J.; Guo, Y.; Huang, Z.; Du, Y. The Tomato Hoffman's Anthocyaninless Gene Encodes a bHLH Transcription Factor Involved in Anthocyanin Biosynthesis That Is Developmentally Regulated and Induced by Low Temperatures. *PLoS ONE* **2016**, *11*. [CrossRef] [PubMed]
27. Van Breusegem, F.; Dat, J.F. Reactive Oxygen Species in Plant Cell Death. *Plant Physiol.* **2006**, *141*, 384–390. [CrossRef] [PubMed]

28. Bernstein, P.S.; Li, B.; Vachali, P.P.; Gorusupudi, A.; Shyam, R.; Henriksen, B.S.; Nolan, J.M. Lutein, Zeaxanthin, and meso-Zeaxanthin: The Basic and Clinical Science Underlying Carotenoid-based Nutritional Interventions against Ocular Disease. *Prog. Retin. Eye Res.* **2015**, *50*, 34–66. [CrossRef] [PubMed]
29. Wang, W.D.; Xu, S.Y. Degradation kinetics of anthocyanins in blackberry juice and concentrate. *J. Food Eng.* **2007**, *82*, 271–275. [CrossRef]
30. Francis, F.J. Food colorants: Anthocyanins. *Crit. Rev. Food Sci. Nutr.* **1989**, *28*, 273–314. [CrossRef] [PubMed]
31. Cisse, M.; Vaillant, F.; Acosta, O.; Dhuique-Mayer, C.; Dornier, M. Thermal degradation kinetics of anthocyanins from blood orange, blackberry, and roselle using the Arrhenius, Eyring, and Ball Models. *J. Agric. Food Chem.* **2009**, *57*, 6285–6291. [CrossRef] [PubMed]
32. Beattie, J.; Crozier, A.; Duthie, G.G. Potential health benefits of berries. *Curr. Nutr. Food Sci.* **2005**, *1*, 71–86. [CrossRef]
33. Stintsing, F.C.; Reinhold, C. Functional properties of anthocyanins and betalains in plants, food, and in human nutrition. *Trends Food Sci. Technol.* **2004**, *15*, 19–38. [CrossRef]
34. Wrolstad, R.E. Anthocyanin pigments-Bioactivity and coloring properties. *J. Food Sci.* **2004**, *69*, 419–425. [CrossRef]
35. Susan, D.; Arnum, V. *Vitamin A in Kirk-Othmer Encyclopedia of Chemical Technology*; John Wiley: New York, NY, USA, 1998; pp. 99–107. [CrossRef]
36. Foods Highest in Lycopene, Nutrition Data, USDA Nutrient Database, Version SR-21. Available online: nutritiondata.com (accessed on 19 August 2014).
37. α-Carotene, β-carotene, β-Cryptoxanthin, Lycopene, Lutein, and Zeaxanthin. Available online: http://lpi.oregonstate.edu/mic/dietary-factors/phytochemicals/carotenoids (accessed on 29 May 2017).
38. Urrea, D.; Eim, V.S.; Gonzalez-Centeno, M.R.; Minjares-Fuentes, R.; Castell-Palou, A.; Juarez, M.D.; Rossello, C. Effects of air drying temperature on antioxidant activity and carotenoids content of carrots (Daucus carota). In Proceedings of the European Drying Conference-EuroDrying, Palma, Balearic Island, Spain, 26–28 October 2011.
39. Abdul-Hammed, M.; Bolarinwa, I.F.; Adebayo, L.O.; Akindele, S.L. Kinetics of the degradation of carotenoid antioxidants in tomato paste. *Adv. J. Food Sci. Technol.* **2016**, *11*, 734–741. [CrossRef]
40. Stefanovich, A.F.; Karel, M. Kinetics of beta-carotene degradation at temperatures typical of air drying of foods. *J. Food Process. Preserv.* **1982**, *6*, 227–242. [CrossRef]
41. Zaibunnisa, A.H.; Norashikin, S.; Mamot, S.; Osman, H. Stability of curcumin in turmeric oleoresin-β-cyclodextrin inclusion complex during storage. *Malays. J. Anal. Sci.* **2009**, *13*, 165–169.
42. Papadopoulou, A.; Frazier, R.A. Characterization of protein-polyphenol interactions. *Trends Food Sci. Technol.* **2004**, *15*, 186–190. [CrossRef]
43. Flavonoids. Available online: http://lpi.oregonstate.edu/mic/dietary-factors/phytochemicals/flavonoids (accessed on 26 February 2016).
44. Csepregi, K.; Neugart, S.; Schreiner, M.; Hideg, É. Comparative Evaluation of Total Antioxidant Capacities of Plant Polyphenols. *Molecules* **2016**, *21*, 208. [CrossRef] [PubMed]
45. Williams, R.J.; Spencer, J.P.; Rice-Evans, C. Flavonoids: Antioxidants or signalling molecules? *Free Radic. Biol. Med.* **2004**, *36*, 838–849. [CrossRef] [PubMed]
46. Arts, I.C.; Hollman, P.C. Polyphenols and disease risk in epidemiologic studies. *Am. J. Clin. Nutr.* **2005**, *81*, 317S–325S. [CrossRef] [PubMed]
47. Kumar, S.; Pandey, A.K. Chemistry and Biological Activities of Flavonoids: An overview. *Sci. World J.* **2013**. [CrossRef] [PubMed]
48. Lotito, S.B.; Frei, B. Consumption of flavonoid-rich foods and increased plasma antioxidant capacity in humans: Cause, consequence, or epiphenomenon? *Free Radic. Biol. Med.* **2006**, *41*, 1727–1746. [CrossRef] [PubMed]
49. D'Archivio, M.; Filesi, C.; Varì, R.; Scazzocchio, B.; Masella, R. Bioavailability of the Polyphenols: Status and Controversies. *Int. J. Mol. Sci.* **2010**, *11*, 1321–1342. [CrossRef] [PubMed]
50. Mennen, L.I.; Walker, R.; Bennetau-Pelissero, C.; Scalbert, A. Risks and Safety of Polyphenol Consumption. *Am. J. Clin. Nutr.* **2005**, *81*, 3265–3295. [CrossRef]
51. Solyom, K.; Sola, R.; Cocero, M.J.; Mato, R.B. Thermal degradation of grape marc polyphenols. *Food Chem.* **2014**. [CrossRef] [PubMed]

52. Zhang, Y.; Kensler, T.W.; Cho, C.G.; Posner, G.H.; Talalay, P. Anticarcinogenic activities of sulforafane and structurally related synthetic norbornyl isothiocyanates. *Proc. Natl. Acad. Sci. USA* **1994**, *91*, 3147–3150. [CrossRef] [PubMed]
53. Dashwood, R.H.; Ho, E. Dietary histone deacetylase inhibitors: From cells to mice to man. *Semin. Cancer Biol.* **2007**, *17*, 363–369. [CrossRef] [PubMed]
54. Ho, E.; Clarke, J.D.; Dashwood, R.H. Dietary sulforafane, a histone deacetylase inhibitor for cancer prevention. *J. Nutr.* **2009**, *139*, 2393–2396. [CrossRef] [PubMed]
55. Wu, Y.; Mao, J.; You, Y.; Liu, S. Study on degradation kinetics of sulforaphane in broccoli extract. *Food Chem.* **2014**, *155*, 235–239. [CrossRef] [PubMed]
56. Block, E. *Garlic and Other Alliums: The Lore and the Science*; The Royal Society of Chemistry: Cambridge, UK, 2010; ISBN 0-85404-190-7.
57. Germain, E.; Chevalier, J.; Siess, M.H.; Teyssier, C. Hepatic metabolism of diallyl disulphide in rat and man. *Xenobiotica* **2003**, *33*, 1185–1199. [CrossRef] [PubMed]
58. Tsai, C.W.; Yang, J.J.; Chen, H.W.; Sheen, L.Y.; Lii, C.K. Garlic organosulfur compounds upregulate the expression of the pi class of glutathione S-transferase in rat primary hepatocytes. *J. Nutr.* **2005**, *135*, 2560–2565. [CrossRef] [PubMed]
59. Wu, C.C.; Sheen, L.Y.; Chen, H.W.; Kuo, W.W.; Tsai, S.J.; Lii, C.K. Differential effects of garlic oil and its three major organosulfur components on the hepatic detoxification system in rats. *J. Agric. Food Chem.* **2002**, *50*, 378–383. [CrossRef] [PubMed]
60. Fukao, T.; Hosono, T.; Misawa, S.; Seki, T.; Ariga, T. The effects of allyl sulfides on the induction of phase II detoxification enzymes and liver injury by carbon tetrachloride. *Food Chem. Toxicol.* **2004**, *42*, 743–749. [CrossRef] [PubMed]
61. Lemar, K.M.; Aon, M.A.; Cortassa, S.; O'Rourke, B.; Müller, C.T.; Lloyd, D. Diallyl disulphide depletes glutathione in Candida albicans: Oxidative stress-mediated cell death studied by two-photon microscopy. *Yeast* **2007**, *24*, 695–706. [CrossRef] [PubMed]
62. Hu, Y.; Urig, S.; Koncarevic, S.; Wu, X.; Fischer, M.; Rahlfs, S.; Mersch-Sundermann, V.; Becker, K. Glutathione- and thioredoxin-related enzymes are modulated by sulfur-containing chemopreventive agents. *Biol. Chem.* **2007**, *388*, 1069–1081. [CrossRef] [PubMed]
63. Koh, S.H.; Kwon, H.; Park, K.H.; Ko, J.K.; Kim, J.H.; Hwang, M.S.; Yum, Y.N.; Kim, O.H.; Kim, J.; Kim, H.T.; et al. Protective effect of diallyl disulfide on oxidative stress-injured neuronally differentiated PC12 cells. *Brain Res. Mol. Brain Res.* **2005**, *133*, 17686. [CrossRef] [PubMed]
64. Kim, J.G.; Koh, S.H.; Lee, Y.J.; Lee, K.Y.; Kim, Y.; Kim, S.; Lee, M.K.; Kim, S.H. Differential effects of diallyl disulfide on neuronal cells depend on its concentration. *Toxicology* **2005**, *211*, 86–95. [CrossRef] [PubMed]
65. Iciek, M.; Marcinek, J.; Mleczko, U.; Włodek, L. Selective effects of diallyl disulfide, a sulfane sulfur precursor, in the liver and Ehrlich ascites tumor cells. *Eur. J. Pharmacol.* **2007**, *569*, 1–7. [CrossRef] [PubMed]
66. Iciek, M.; Bilska, A.; Ksiazek, L.; Srebro, Z.; Włodek, L. Allyl disulfide as donor and cyanide as acceptor of sulfane sulfur in the mouse tissues. *Pharmacol. Rep.* **2005**, *57*, 212–218. [PubMed]
67. Amonkar, S.V.; Banerji, A. Isolation and characterization of larvicidal principle of garlic. *Science* **1971**, *174*, 1343–1344. [CrossRef] [PubMed]
68. Avato, P.; Tursil, E.; Vitali, C.; Miccolis, V.; Candido, V. Allylsulfide constituents of garlic volatile oil as antimicrobial agents. *Phytomedicine* **2000**, *7*, 239–243. [CrossRef]
69. O'Gara, E.A.; Hill, D.J.; Maslin, D.J. Activities of garlic oil, garlic powder, and their diallyl constituents against Helicobacter pylori. *Appl. Environ. Microbiol.* **2000**, *66*, 2269–2273. [CrossRef] [PubMed]
70. Yu, J.; Xiao, Y.B.; Wang, X.Y. Effects of preoperatively selected gut decontamination on cardiopulmonary bypass-induced endotoxemia. *Chin. J. Traumatol.* **2007**, *10*, 131–137. [PubMed]
71. Glade, M.J. Food, nutrition, and the prevention of cancer: A global perspective. American Institute for Cancer Research/World Cancer Research Fund, American Institute for Cancer Research, 1997. *Nutrition* **1999**, *15*, 523–526. [PubMed]
72. Huang, Z.; Lei, X.; Zhong, M.; Zhu, B.; Tang, S.; Liao, D. Bcl-2 small interfering RNA sensitizes cisplatin-resistant human lung adenocarcinoma A549/DDP cell to cisplatin and diallyl disulfide. *Acta Biochim. Biophys. Sin.* **2007**, *39*, 835–843. [CrossRef] [PubMed]
73. Omar, S.H. Historical, chemical and cardiovascular perspectives on garlic: A review. *Pharmacogn. Rev.* **2007**, *1*, 80.

74. Bautista, D.M.; Movahed, P.; Hinman, A.; Axelsson, H.E.; Sterner, O.; Högestätt, E.D.; Julius, D.; Jordt, S.E.; Zygmunt, P.M. Pungent products from garlic activate the sensory ion channel TRPA1. *Proc. Natl Acad. Sci. USA* **2005**, *102*, 12248–12252. [CrossRef] [PubMed]

75. Mashour, N.H.; Lin, G.I.; Frishman, W.H. Herbal medicine for the treatment of cardiovascular disease (clinical consideration). *Arch. Intern. Med.* **1998**, *158*, 2225–2234. [CrossRef] [PubMed]

76. Berthold, H.K.; Sudhop, T.; von Bergmann, K. Effect of a garlic oil preparation on serum lipoproteins and cholesteol metabolism. *JAMA* **1998**, *279*, 1900–1902. [CrossRef] [PubMed]

77. Ackermann, R.T.; Mulrow, C.D.; Ramirez, G.; Gardner, C.D.; Morbidoni, L.; Lawrence, V.A. Promise for improving some cardiovascular risk factors garlic's properties. *Arch. Intern. Med.* **2001**, *161*, 813–824. [CrossRef] [PubMed]

78. Vastag, B. Garlic prevents plaque. *JAMA* **2002**, *288*, 11.

79. Nutrition Facts for Raw Garlic USDA National Nutrient Database, Version SR-21. Available online: nutritiondata.com (accessed on 2 November 2014).

80. Kinalski, T.; Norena, C.P.Z. Effect of blanching treatments on antioxidant activity and thiosulfinate degradation of garlic (*Allium sativum* L.). *Food Bioproc. Tech.* **2014**, *7*, 2152–2157. [CrossRef]

81. Banerjee, S.K.; Mukherjee, P.K.; Maulik, S.K. Garlic as an antioxidant: The good, the bad and the ugly. *Phytother. Res.* **2003**, *17*, 97–106. [CrossRef] [PubMed]

82. Staba, E.J.; Lash, L.; Staba, J.E. A commentary on the effects of garlic extraction and formulation on product composition. *J. Nutr.* **2001**, *131*, 1118–1119. [CrossRef]

83. Willett, C.W. Diet and health: What should we eat? *Science* **1994**, *264*, 532–537. [CrossRef] [PubMed]

84. Lin, C.H.; Chang, C.Y. Textural change and antioxidant properties of broccoli under different cooking treatments. *Food Chem.* **2005**, *46*, 1018–1021. [CrossRef]

85. Yin, M.C.; Cheng, W.S. Antioxidant and antimicrobial effects of four garlic-derived organosulfur compounds in ground beef. *Meat Sci.* **1991**, *63*, 23–28. [CrossRef]

86. Miron, T.; Rabinkov, A.; Mirelman, D.; Weiner, L.; Wilchek, M. A spectrophotometric assay for allicin and alliinase (alliin lyase) activity reaction of 2-nitro-5-thiobenzoate with thiosulfinates. *Anal. Biochem.* **1998**, *265*, 317–325. [CrossRef] [PubMed]

87. Smirnoff, N. L-ascorbic acid biosynthesis. *Vitam. Horm.* **2001**, *61*, 241–266. [CrossRef] [PubMed]

88. Linster, C.L.; Van Schaftingen, E. Vitamin C. Biosynthesis, recycling and degradation in mammals. *FEBS J.* **2007**, *274*, 1–22. [CrossRef] [PubMed]

89. Grudpan, K.; Kamfoo, K.; Jakmunee, J. Flow injection spectrophotometric or conductometric determination of ascorbic acid in a vitamin C tablet using permanganate or ammonia. *Talanta* **1999**, *49*, 1023–1026. [CrossRef]

90. Padayatty, S.J.; Katz, A.; Wang, Y.; Eck, P.; Kwon, O.; Lee, J.H.; Chen, S.; Corpe, C.; Dutta, A.; Dutta, S.K.; et al. Vitamin C as an antioxidant: Evaluation of its role in disease prevention. *J. Am. Coll. Nutr.* **2003**, *22*, 18–35. [CrossRef] [PubMed]

91. Matei, N.; Birghila, S.; Popescu, V.; Dobrinas, S.; Soceanu, A.; Oprea, C.; Magearu, V. Kinetic study of vitamin C degradation from pharmaceutical products. *Rom. J. Phys.* **2008**, *53*, 343–351.

92. Tola, Y.B.; Ramaswamy, H.S. Temperature and high pressure stability of lycopene and vitamin C of watermelon juice. *Afr. J. Food Sci.* **2015**, *9*, 351–358. [CrossRef]

93. Rahmawati, S.; Bundjali, B. Kinetics of the oxidation of vitamin C. *Indones. J. Chem.* **2012**, *12*, 291–296. [CrossRef]

94. Gold, R.; Kappos, L.; Arnold, D.L.; Bar-Or, A.; Giovannoni, G.; Selmaj, K.; Tornatore, C.; Sweetser, M.T.; Yang, M.; Sheikh, S.I.; et al. Placebo-Controlled Phase 3 Study of Oral BG-12 for Relapsing Multiple Sclerosis. *N. Engl. J. Med.* **2012**, *367*, 1098–1107. [CrossRef] [PubMed]

95. Dolinska, B.; Ryszka, F.; Ostrozka-Cieslik, A. The effect of selected antioxidants on the kinetics of changes in the stability of an HTK solution: A technical note. *AAPS PharmSciTech* **2006**, *7*, E144–E147. [CrossRef] [PubMed]

96. Nutrition Facts: Nuts, Walnuts, English Dried per 100 g. Condé Nast. Available online: http://nutritiondata.self.com/facts/nut-and-seed-products/3138/2 (accessed on 4 July 2014).

97. Gonabad, M.A.; Noghabi, M.S.; Niazmand, R. Estimation of kinetic parameters of walnut oil using rancimat test. *J. Appl. Environ. Biol. Sci.* **2015**, *4*, 28–32.

98. Gonzaga, F.B.; Pasquini, C.; Rodrigues, C.E.; Meirelles, A.J. Comparison of near-infrared emission spectroscopy and the Rancimat method for the determination of oxidative stability. *Eur. J. Lipid Sci. Technol.* **2007**, *109*, 61–65. [CrossRef]
99. Hasenhuettl, G.L.; Wan, P.J. Temperature effects on the determination of oxidative stability with the Metrohm Rancimat. *J. Am. Oil Chem. Soc.* **1992**, *69*, 525–527. [CrossRef]
100. Campo, P.; Zhao, Y.; Suidan, M.T.; Venosa, A.D.; Sorial, G.A. Biodegradation kinetics and toxicity of vegetable oil triacylglycerols under aerobic conditions. *Chemosphere* **2007**, *68*, 2054–2062. [CrossRef] [PubMed]
101. Lutterodt, H.; Slavin, M.; Whent, E.; Turner, E.; Yu, L. Fatty acid composition, oxidative stability, antioxidant and antiproliferative properties of selected cold-pressed grape seed oils and flours. *Food Chem.* **2011**, *128*, 391–399. [CrossRef] [PubMed]
102. Gholami, M.R.; Izadyar, M. Gas-phase kinetics and mechanism of diallyl sulphide thermal decomposition. *J. Phys. Org. Chem.* **2003**, *16*, 153–157. [CrossRef]
103. El-Bayoumy, K.; Sinha, R.; Pinto, J.T.; Rivlin, R.S. Cancer chemoprevention by garlic and garlic-containing sulfur and selenium compounds. *J. Nutr.* **2006**, *136*, 864S–869S. [CrossRef]
104. Brady, J.F.; Li, D.; Ishizaki, H.; Yang, C.S. Effect of Diallyl sulfide on rat liver microsomal nitrosamine metabolism and other monooxygenase activities. *Cancer Res.* **1988**, *48*, 5937–5940. [PubMed]
105. Mocek, M.; Richardson, P.J. Kinetics and mechanism of quercetin oxidation. *J. Inst. Brewing* **1972**, *78*, 459–465. [CrossRef]
106. Oberoi, D.P.S.; Sogi, D.S. Prediction of lycopene degradation during dehydration of watermelon pomace (*cv Sugar Baby*). *J. Saudi Soc. Agric. Sci.* **2017**, *16*, 97–103. [CrossRef]
107. Ax, K.; Mayer-Miebach, E.; Link, B.; Schuchmann, H.; Schubert, H. Stability of Lycopene in Oil-in-Water Emulsions. *Eng. Life Sci.* **2003**, *3*, 199–201. [CrossRef]
108. Naguib, Y.M. Antioxidant activities of astaxanthin and related carotenoids. *J. Agric. Food Chem.* **2000**, *48*, 1150–1154. [CrossRef] [PubMed]
109. Miki, W. Biological functions and activities of animal carotenoids. *Pure Appl. Chem.* **1991**, *63*, 141–146. [CrossRef]
110. Liu, X.; Osawa, T. *Cis* astaxanthin and especially 9-*cis* astaxanthin exhibits a higher antioxidant activity in vitro compared to the all-*trans* isomer. *Biochem. Biophys. Res. Commun.* **2007**, *357*, 187–193. [CrossRef] [PubMed]
111. Ambati, R.R.; Phang, S.M.; Ravi, S.; Aswathanarayana, R.G. Astaxanthin: Sources, Extraction, Stability, Biological Activities and Its Commercial Applications—A Review. *Mar. Drugs.* **2014**, *12*, 128–152. [CrossRef] [PubMed]
112. Pompella, A.; Visvikis, A.; Paolicchi, A.; De Tata, V.; Casini, A.F. The changing faces of glutathione, a cellular protagonist. *Biochem. Pharmacol.* **2003**, *66*, 1499–1503. [CrossRef]
113. Couto, N.; Malys, N.; Gaskell, S.J.; Barber, J. Partition and turnover of glutathione reductase from Saccharomyces cerevisiae: S proteomic approach. *J. Proteome Res.* **2013**, *12*, 2885–2894. [CrossRef] [PubMed]
114. Pastore, A.; Piemonte, F.; Locatelli, M.; Lo Russo, A.; Gaeta, L.M.; Tozzi, G.; Federici, G. Determination of blood total, reduced, and oxidized glutathione in pediatric subjects. *Clin. Chem.* **2001**, *47*, 1467–1469. [PubMed]
115. Lu, S.C. Glutathione synthesis. *Biochim. Biophys. Acta* **2013**, *1830*, 3143–3153. [CrossRef] [PubMed]
116. Meister, A.; Anderson, M.E. Glutathione. *Annual Review of Biochemistry.* **1983**, *52*, 711–760. [CrossRef] [PubMed]
117. McIlduff, C.E.; Rutkove, S.B. Critical appraisal of the use of alpha lipoic acid (thioctic acid) in the treatment of symptomatic diabetic polyneuropathy. *Ther. Clin. Risk Manag.* **2011**, *7*, 377–385. [CrossRef] [PubMed]
118. Ziegle, D.; Reljanovic, M.; Mehnert, H.; Gries, F.A. α-Lipoic acid in the treatment of diabetic polyneuropathy in Germany: Current evidence from clinical trials. *Exp. Clin. Endocrinol. Diabetes* **1999**, *107*, 421–430. [CrossRef] [PubMed]
119. Hardeland, R.; Pandi-Perumal, S.R.; Cardinali, D.P. Molecules in focus Melatonin. *Int. J. Biochem. Cell Biol.* **2006**, *38*, 313–316. [CrossRef] [PubMed]
120. Altun, A.; Ugur-Altun, B. Melatonin: Therapeutic and clinical utilization. *Int. J. Clin. Pract.* **2007**, *61*, 835–845. [CrossRef] [PubMed]
121. Hardeland, R. Antioxidative protection by melatonin: Multiplicity of mechanisms from radical detoxification to radical avoidance. *Endocrine* **2005**, *27*, 119–130. [CrossRef]

122. Reiter, R.J.; Acuña-Castroviejo, D.; Tan, D.X.; Burkhardt, S. Free radical-mediated molecular damage, Mechanisms for the protective actions of melatonin in the central nervous system. *Ann. N. Y. Acad. Sci.* **2001**, *939*, 200–215. [CrossRef] [PubMed]
123. Tan, D.X.; Manchester, L.C.; Terron, M.P.; Flores, L.J.; Reiter, R.J. One molecule, many derivatives: A never-ending interaction of melatonin with reactive oxygen and nitrogen species? *J. Pineal Res.* **2007**, *42*, 28–42. [CrossRef] [PubMed]
124. Tan, D.X.; Chen, L.D.; Poeggeler, B.; Manchester, L.C.; Reiter, R.J. Melatonin: A potent, endogenous hydroxyl radical scavenger. *Endocr. J.* **1993**, *1*, 57–60.
125. Reiter, R.J.; Paredes, S.D.; Manchester, L.C.; Tan, D.X. Reducing oxidative/nitrosative stress: A newly-discovered gene for melatonin. *Crit. Rev. Biochem. Mol. Biol.* **2009**, *44*, 175–200. [CrossRef] [PubMed]
126. Reiter, R.J.; Manchester, L.C.; Tan, D.X. Neurotoxins: Free radical mechanisms and melatonin protection. *Curr. Neuropharmacol.* **2010**, *8*, 194–210. [CrossRef] [PubMed]
127. Poeggeler, B.; Saarela, S.; Reiter, R.J.; Tan, D.X.; Chen, L.D.; Manchester, L.C.; Barlow-Walden, L.R. Melatonin—A highly potent endogenous radical scavenger and electron donor: New aspects of the oxidation chemistry of this indole accessed in vitro. *Ann. N. Y. Acad. Sci.* **1994**, *738*, 419–420. [CrossRef] [PubMed]
128. Arnao, M.B.; Hernández-Ruiz, J. The physiological function of melatonin in plants. *Plant Signal. Behav.* **2006**, *1*, 89–95. [CrossRef] [PubMed]
129. Tan, D.X.; Manchester, L.C.; Reiter, R.J.; Qi, W.B.; Karbownik, M.; Calvo, J.R. Significance of melatonin in antioxidative defense system: Reactions and products. *Biol. Signals Recept.* **2000**, *9*, 137–159. [CrossRef] [PubMed]
130. Pieri, C.; Marra, M.; Moroni, F.; Recchioni, R.; Marcheselli, F. Melatonin: A peroxyl radical scavenger more effective than vitamin E. *Life Sci.* **1994**, *55*, PL271–PL276. [CrossRef]
131. Lowes, D.A.; Webster, N.R.; Murphy, M.P.; Galley, H.F. Antioxidants that protect mitochondria reduce interleukin-6 and oxidative stress improve mitochondrial function, and reduce biochemical markers of organ dysfunction in a rat model of acute sepsis. *Br. J. Anaesth.* **2013**, *110*, 472–480. [CrossRef] [PubMed]
132. Herrera, E.; Barbas, C. Vitamin E: Action, metabolism and perspectives. *J. Physiol. Biochem.* **2001**, *57*, 43–56. [CrossRef] [PubMed]
133. Packer, L.; Weber, S.U.; Rimbach, G. Molecular aspects of alpha-tocotrienol antioxidant action and cell signaling. *J. Nutr.* **2001**, *131*, 369S–373S. [CrossRef] [PubMed]
134. Brigelius-Flohé, R.; Traber, M.G. Vitamin E: Function and metabolism. *FASEB J.* **1999**, *13*, 1145–1155. [CrossRef] [PubMed]
135. Traber, M.G.; Atkinson, J. Vitamin E, antioxidant and nothing more. *Free Radic. Biol. Med.* **2007**, *43*, 4–15. [CrossRef] [PubMed]
136. Wang, X.; Quinn, P.J. Vitamin E and its function in membranes. *Prog. Lipid Res.* **1999**, *38*, 309–336. [CrossRef]
137. Azzi, A. Molecular mechanism of alpha-tocopherol action. *Free Radic. Biol. Med.* **2007**, *43*, 16–21. [CrossRef] [PubMed]
138. Zingg, J.M.; Azzi, A. Non-antioxidant activities of vitamin E. *Curr. Med. Chem.* **2004**, *11*, 1113–1133. [CrossRef] [PubMed]
139. Sen, C.K.; Khanna, S.; Roy, S. Tocotrienols: Vitamin E beyond tocopherols. *Life Sci.* **2006**, *78*, 2088–2098. [CrossRef] [PubMed]
140. El Asmar, M.S.; Naoum, J.J.; Arbid, E.J. Vitamin K Dependent Proteins and the Role of Vitamin K2 in the Modulation of Vascular Calcification: A Review. *Oman Med. J.* **2014**, *29*, 172–177. [CrossRef] [PubMed]
141. Zlokovic, B.V. The blood-brain barrier in health and chronic neurodegenerative disorders. *Neuron* **2008**, *57*, 178–201. [CrossRef] [PubMed]
142. Liebner, S.; Czupalla, C.J. Wolburg, Current concepts of blood-brain barrier development. *Int. J. Dev. Biol.* **2011**, *55*, 467–476. [CrossRef] [PubMed]
143. Stamatovic, S.M.; Keep, R.F.; Andjelkovic, A.V. Brain Endothelial Cell-Cell Junctions: How to "Open" the Blood Brain Barrier. *Curr. Neuropharmacol.* **2008**, *6*, 179–192. [CrossRef] [PubMed]
144. Blood Brain Barrier Johns Hopkins University. Available online: https://www.bme.jhu.edu/about/awards-and-achievements/page/10/ (accessed on 7 May 2013).
145. Abbott, N.J.; Patabendige, A.A.; Dolman, D.E.; Yusof, S.R.; Begley, D.J. Structure and function of the blood-brain barrier. *Neurobiol. Dis.* **2010**, *37*, 13–25. [CrossRef] [PubMed]

146. Ballabh, P.; Braun, A.; Nedergaard, M. The blood-brain barrier: An overview Structure, regulation, and clinical implications. *Neurobiol. Dis.* **2004**, *16*, 1–13. [CrossRef] [PubMed]
147. Tayarani, I.; Chaudiere, J.; Lefauconnier, J.M.; Bourre, J.M. Enzymatic protection against peroxidative damage in isolated brain capillaries. *J. Neurochem.* **1987**, *48*, 1399–1402. [CrossRef] [PubMed]
148. Agarwal, R.; Shukla, G.S. Potential role of cerebral glutathione in the maintenance of blood-brain barrier integrity in rat. *Neurochem. Res.* **1999**, *24*, 1507–1514. [CrossRef] [PubMed]
149. Vatassery, G.T. Vitamin E and other endogenous antioxidants in the central nervous system. *Geriatrics* **1998**, *53*, S25–S27. [PubMed]
150. Grammas, P.; Martinez, J.; Miller, B. Cerebral microvascular endothelium and the pathogenesis of neurodegenerative diseases. *Expert Rev. Mol. Med.* **2011**, *13*. [CrossRef] [PubMed]
151. Mooradian, A.D. Effect of aging on the blood-brain barrier. *Neurobiol. Aging* **1988**, *9*, 31–39. [CrossRef]
152. Allen, C.L.; Bayraktutan, U. Oxidative stress and its role in the pathogenesis of ischaemic stroke. *Int. J. Stroke* **2009**, *4*, 461–470. [CrossRef] [PubMed]
153. Zipser, B.D.; Johanson, C.E.; Gonzalez, L.; Berzin, T.M.; Tavares, R.; Hulette, C.M.; Vitek, M.P.; Hovanesian, V.; Stopa, E.G. Microvascular injury and blood-brain barrier leakage in Alzheimer's disease. *Neurobiol. Aging* **2007**, *28*, 977–986. [CrossRef] [PubMed]
154. Clifford, P.M.; Zarrabi, S.; Siu, G.; Kinsler, K.J.; Koscink, M.C.; Venkataraman, V.; D'Andrea, M.R.; Dinsmore, S.; Nagele, R.G. Aβ peptides can enter the brain through a defective blood-brain barrier and bind selectively to neurons. *Brain Res.* **2007**, *1142*, 223–236. [CrossRef] [PubMed]
155. Thapa, B.; Munk, B.H.; Burrows, C.J.; Schlegel, H.B. Computational Study of Oxidation of Guanine by Singlet Oxygen ($^1\Delta_g$) and Formation of Guanine: Lysine Cross-Links. *Chem. Eur. J.* **2017**, *23*, 5804–5813. [CrossRef] [PubMed]
156. Scheit, K.; Bauer, G. Direct and indirect inactivation of tumor cell protective catalase by salicylic acid and anthocyanidins reactivates intercellular ROS signaling and allows for synergistic effects. *Carcinogenesis* **2015**, *36*, 400–411. [CrossRef] [PubMed]

4

Polyphenolic Composition and Antioxidant Activity of Aqueous and Ethanolic Extracts from *Uncaria tomentosa* Bark and Leaves

Mirtha Navarro-Hoyos [1,*], Diego Alvarado-Corella [2], Ileana Moreira-Gonzalez [3], Elizabeth Arnaez-Serrano [3] and Maria Monagas-Juan [4]

1 Department of Chemistry, University of Costa Rica (UCR), Sede Rodrigo Facio, San Pedro de Montes de Oca, San José 2060, Costa Rica
2 Department of Biology, University of Costa Rica (UCR), Sede Rodrigo Facio, San Pedro de Montes de Oca, San Jose 2060, Costa Rica; luis.alvaradocorella@ucr.ac.cr
3 Department of Biology, Technological University of Costa Rica (TEC), Cartago 7050, Costa Rica; imoreira@itcr.ac.cr (I.M.-G.), earnaez@itcr.ac.cr (E.A.-S.)
4 Institute of Food Science Research (CIAL), Spanish National Research Council (CSIC), C/Nicolás Cabrera 9, 28049 Madrid, Spain; mjm@usp.org
* Correspondence: mnavarro@codeti.org

Abstract: *Uncaria tomentosa* constitutes an important source of secondary metabolites with diverse biological activities mainly attributed until recently to alkaloids and triterpenes. We have previously reported for the first-time the polyphenolic profile of extracts from *U. tomentosa*, using a multi-step process involving organic solvents, as well as their antioxidant capacity, antimicrobial activity on aerial bacteria, and cytotoxicity on cancer cell lines. These promising results prompted the present study using food grade solvents suitable for the elaboration of commercial extracts. We report a detailed study on the polyphenolic composition of aqueous and ethanolic extracts of *U. tomentosa* bark and leaves (n = 16), using High Performance Liquid Chromatography coupled with Mass Spectrometry (HPLC-DAD/TQ-ESI-MS). A total of 32 compounds were identified, including hydroxybenzoic and hydroxycinnamic acids, flavan-3-ols monomers, procyanidin dimers and trimers, flavalignans–cinchonains and propelargonidin dimers. Our findings showed that the leaves were the richest source of total phenolics and proanthocyanidins, in particular propelargonidin dimers. Two-way Analysis of Variance (ANOVA) indicated that the contents of procyanidin and propelargonidin dimers were significantly different ($p < 0.05$) in function of the plant part, and leaves extracts showed higher contents. Oxygen Radical Absorbance Capacity (ORAC) and 2,2-diphenyl-1-picrylhidrazyl (DPPH) values indicated higher antioxidant capacity for the leaves ($p < 0.05$). Further, correlation between both methods and procyanidin dimers was found, particularly between ORAC and propelargonidin dimers. Finally, Principal Component Analysis (PCA) analysis results clearly indicated that the leaves are the richest plant part in proanthocyanidins and a very homogenous material, regardless of their origin. Therefore, our findings revealed that both ethanol and water extraction processes are adequate for the elaboration of potential commercial extracts from *U. tomentosa* leaves rich in proanthocyanidins and exhibiting high antioxidant activity.

Keywords: *U. tomentosa*; UPLC-DAD; TQ-ESI/MS; polyphenols; proanthocyanidins; propelargonidins; procyanidins; mass spectrometry; antioxidant

1. Introduction

Uncaria tomentosa L., commonly known as cat's claw, is a creeper vine typical of the rainy tropical forest that belongs to the Rubiaceae family. It is naturally distributed in South America, mainly in Peru and Brazil as well as in Central America, and it is traditionally used as a medicinal plant. Around 50 compounds have been isolated from *U. tomentosa*, from which approximately 35 chemical markers can be considered exclusive to this species, including triterpenes [1], alkaloids [2] and polyphenols [3]. The special interest on this plant is due to the fact that numerous scientific studies report a wide variety of biological activities [4], such as immunomodulatory properties [3], as well as their antioxidant, anti-inflammatory and cardiovascular effects and protective properties against cancer, among others [5].

Although originally attributed to alkaloids, recent studies suggest that the health effects derived from *U. tomentosa* could be attributed to a synergistic interaction among different chemical compounds present in this plant [6]. Of particular interest are polyphenols, for which there is strong evidence of having multiple molecular targets, modulating pro-inflammatory gene expression, interacting with phospholipid membranes [7] and modulating pathways related to chronic inflammation and energy metabolism [8].

Regarding polyphenols, *U. tomentosa* studies are scarce and mainly focused on a particular subclass, for instance on hydroxycinnamic acids [9,10], flavonols [11], flavan-3-ols [12,13] and cinchonains [14]. Recently, a detailed characterization of *U. tomentosa* leaves, bark, stem and wood has been reported indicating a high flavan-3-ol content, particularly in procyanidin dimers and trimers, propelargonidin dimers and cinchonain-type flavalignans [15] in leaves and bark. Also, assessment of biological activities of *U. tomentosa* proanthocyanidins showed evidence on the relationship between proanthocyanidin contents and antioxidant capacity, antimicrobial effect against *Staphylococcus aureus*, *Enterococcus faecalis* and *Pseudomonas aeruginosa* respiratory pathogens [16], and in vitro cytotoxicity, with high selectivity for AGS gastric and SW620 colon adenocarcinoma cell lines, mainly attributed to the content of propelargonidin dimers [17].

These promising results about the bioactivity of *U. tomentosa* proanthocyanidin extracts and their potential health effects were subject of an industrial patent [18] and prompted the need to further explore the viability of elaborating polyphenolic extracts form *U. tomentosa* using food-grade solvents (i.e., aqueous or ethanolic extracts) with potential use as Dietary Supplements.

Previous studies carried out with *U. tomentosa* aqueous and ethanolic extracts indicated antioxidant activity in vitro [2,19,20] and other biological activities such as important effects on mono- nuclear blood cells [21] with 95% ethanol extracts; however, detailed characterization of the extracts was not performed. Our present study focuses on the detailed phenolic characterization by HPLC-DAD/TQ-ESI-MS of aqueous and ethanolic extracts from both bark and leaves (n = 16) of *U. tomentosa* cultivated in Costa Rica, as well as to determine their antioxidant activity by Oxygen Radical Absorbance Capacity (ORAC) and 2,2-diphenyl-1-picrylhidrazyl (DPPH) methods. Finally, statistical analyses to determine the influence of factors, such as plant part and solvents, on the polyphenolic composition of *U. tomentosa* extracts were explored.

2. Results and Discussion

2.1. Phenolic Yield and Total Phenolic Content in U. tomentosa Extracts

The aqueous and ethanolic extraction methods described in Section 3, allowed to obtain extracts with yields as shown in Table 1. Considering the plant part, leaves exhibited the highest yields independently of the plant location with an overall average of 5.26%, whereas barks showed much lower yields with 2.28% average. For both parts, barks and leaves, ethanolic extraction yields were slightly higher (average: 2.54% and 5.88%, respectively) than those of aqueous extracts (average: 2.01% and 4.64%, respectively). In regards to total polyphenols (TP), leaves showed higher contents than barks and considering the geographical location, *U. tomentosa* leaves from Los Chiles showed the highest TP values in both aqueous and ethanolic solvents (385.6 and 387.6 mg gallic acid equivalents (GAE)/g extract respectively), followed by Asomat (335.0 and 362.4 mg GAE/g extract), whereas Sarapiqui showed the lowest values (218.2 and 321.0 mg GAE/g extract). In the case of barks, Asomat and Sarapiqui ethanolic extracts showed the highest TP values (295.2 and 321.0 mg GAE/g extract, respectively). Similar trends were observed for the flavan-3-ols (PRO) content.

Table 1. Extraction yield, total phenolic (TP) and flavan-3-ols (PRO) for aqueous and ethanolic extracts from *U. tomentosa*.

Samples	Extraction Yield (%) [1]	TP (mg/g) [2]	PRO (mg/g) [3]
Aqueous Extracts			
Leaves			
Asomat (AS)	4.95	335.2 ± 6.6	255.6 ± 6.5
Los Chiles (LC)	4.22	385.6 ± 1.1	304.9 ± 4.0
Palacios (PA)	3.95	311.0 ± 0.4	201.9 ± 2.6
Sarapiqui (SR)	5.45	218.2 ± 5.3	152.2 ± 2.9
Bark			
Asomat (AS)	1.93	236.0 ± 5.8	166.4 ± 2.3
Los Chiles (LC)	1.74	177.5 ± 1.6	108.4 ± 3.4
Palacios (PA)	1.71	138.2 ± 4.5	69.8 ± 1.9
Sarapiqui (SR)	2.65	201.5 ± 3.5	114.6 ± 2.2
Ethanolic extracts			
Leaves			
Asomat (AS)	5.99	362.4 ± 5.5	300.5 ± 6.0
Los Chiles (LC)	5.39	387.6 ± 3.0	298.6 ± 8.4
Palacios (PA)	6.12	340.4 ± 3.7	260.3 ± 3.7
Sarapiqui (SR)	6.03	342.1 ± 2.8	281.5 ±4.8
Bark			
Asomat (AS)	2.88	295.2 ± 3.1	198.3 ± 4.5
Los Chiles (LC)	1.26	196.2 ± 4.5	88.2 ± 3.3
Palacios (PA)	3.17	279.8 ± 6.2	194.8 ± 5.5
Sarapiqui (SR)	2.86	321.0 ± 3.6	216.7 ± 5.3

[1] g of extract/g of dry material expressed as %; [2] mg of gallic acid equivalent/g extract; [3] mg cyanidin chloride equivalents/g extract.

In order to assess the influence of plant part and extraction solvent on TP and PRO content, a two-way Analysis of Variance (ANOVA) was carried out. Results showed significant differences ($p < 0.05$) for both factors, plant part and solvent used, with ethanolic procedure yielding better TP and PRO values for both plant parts. In addition, importantly, findings indicated leaves extracts are richer in both contents than their bark counterparts, which is in agreement with a recent study on *U. tomentosa* phenolic extracts obtained through an extraction and purification method using different organic solvents [15].

2.2. UPLC-DAD/TQ-ESI-MS Analysis of U. tomentosa Polyphenolic Extracts

The UPLC-DAD/TQ-ESI-MS analysis was performed in the 16 aqueous and ethanolic extracts from *U. tomentosa*, as described in Section 3. Determination of 32 phenolic compounds was achieved, comprising non-flavonoid polyphenols, including seven hydroxybenzoic acids, namely benzoic, 4-hydroxybenzoic, salicylic, gallic, protocatechuic, syringic and vanillic acids; and four hydroxycinnamic acids, namely caffeic, *p*-coumaric, ferulic and isoferulic acids. Among flavonoid polyphenols, both flavan-3-ols monomers [(+)-catechin and (−)-epicatechin] were found, as well as eight procyanidin dimers, three procyanidin trimers, and four propelargonidin dimers. Also, four flavalignans-cinchonains were identified (Tables 2 and 3).

Multiple reaction monitoring (MRM) transitions under set tandem mass spectrometry (MS/MS) parameters were recorded for compounds found in extracts from *U. tomentosa* bark and leaves. For instance, at m/z 289/245 for flavan-3-ols monomers [(+)-catechin and (−)-epicatechin], at m/z 577/289 for procyanidin dimers, at m/z 561/289 for propelargonidin dimers, at m/z 865/577 for procyanidin trimers and at m/z 451/341 for flavalignans-cinchonains. As shown in Figure S1 (Supplementary Materials), MS/MS allowed to identify the different procyanidin dimers and propelargonidin dimers. These results constitute the first report, to our knowledge, of propelargonidins presence in *U. tomentosa* ethanolic and aqueous extracts.

In agreement with the TP and PRO determinations, the UPLC analysis revealed that the leaves have higher phenolic content (17,482.3–32,323.3 μg/g of extract) than the barks (5122.0–17,770.2 μg/g of extract). Differences in the distribution of phenolic compounds also occur. For example, in the case of flavan-3-ols (Figure 1) propelargonidin dimer (Rt = 4.43 min) (3067.8–4978.9 μg/g extract), propelargonidin dimer (Rt = 5.65 min) (2177.2–5209.1 μg/g extract) and procyanidin B4 (1771.8–3931.9 μg/g extract) are the most abundant flavan-3-ols in leaves, whereas in barks, procyanidin B2 (378.5–4011.4 μg/g extract) and (−)-epicatechin (712.6–3827.0 μg/g extract) appear to be more abundant. This latter flavan-3-ol monomer is found in larger concentration than (+)-catechin (66.4–1592.5 μg/g extract) in all leaves and bark samples.

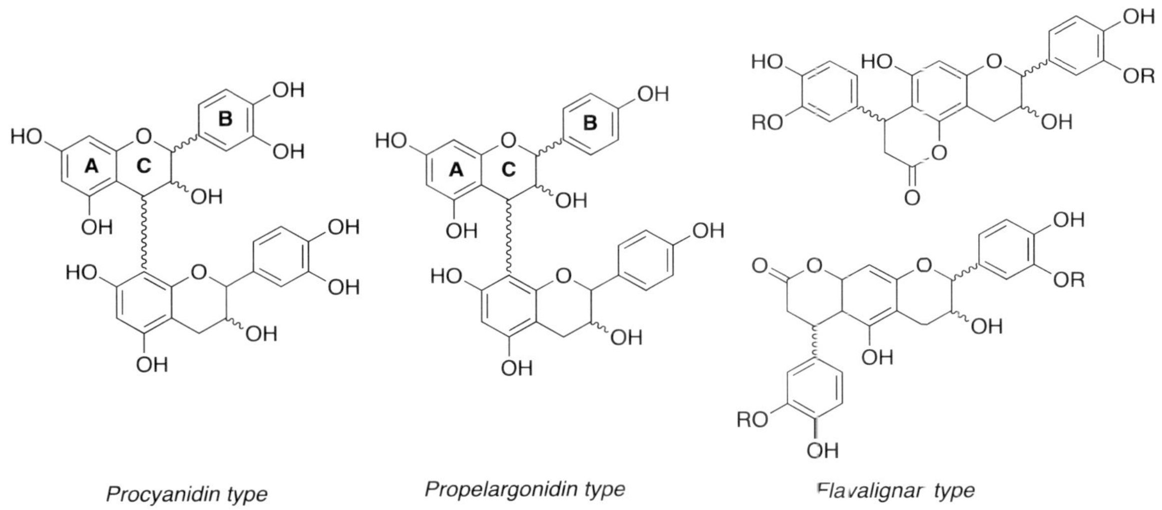

Figure 1. Procyanidin (PC), propelargonidin (PP) and flavalignans (FL) general chemical structures.

When considering subclasses of polyphenols (Figure 2), barks show variable contents, with procyanidin dimers as the most abundant group in Los Chiles (7971.4 μg/g of extract) aqueous extract, followed by Sarapiqui (6085.3–6464.1 μg/g of extract) in ethanolic and aqueous extracts, respectively. Los Chiles and Sarapiqui aqueous extracts exhibited the highest content of flavan-3-ols monomers (3994.4 and 4382.8 μg/g of extract, respectively), while hydroxybenzoic acids (HBA) is the third more abundant group, with the highest HBA contents in Los Chiles (6206.28 μg/g of extract) followed by Palacios (2772.6 μg/g of extract), both in ethanolic samples.

In contrast, extracts from leaves showed a more uniform subclass distribution, for instance, all extracts are particularly rich in propelargonidin dimers (7904.3–14,390.8 μg/g of extract), followed by procyanidin dimers (3593.1–9988.8 μg/g of extract) and flavalignans-cinchonains (1074.6–7058.0 μg/g of extract).

Table 2. Phenolic composition of aqueous extracts from bark and leaves of *U. tomentosa*.

	Leaves Extracts				Bark Extracts			
Compound	**AS**	**LC**	**PA**	**SR**	**AS**	**LC**	**PA**	**SR**
	Concentration (μg/g Extract)							
Hydroxybenzoic acids								
Benzoic acid	71.2 ± 6.9	50.3 ± 0.8	225.8 ± 7.6	120.0 ± 9.8	343.0 ± 23.2	60.3 ± 5.8	1181.6 ± 89.0	13.0 ± 0.5
Salicylic acid	27.7 ± 2.3	22.9 ± 0.4	24.7 ± 1.1	29.0 ± 1.9	20.1 ± 1.8	56.4 ± 0.9	105 ± 6.9	197.6 ± 1.4
4-hydroxybenzoic acid	35.2 ± 1.1	143.6 ± 3.2	200.0 ± 4.7	41.1 ± 1.1	113.7 ± 7.7	22.7 ± 1.1	164.7 ± 6.6	37.6 ± 1.9
Protocatechuic acid	60.5 ± 1.4	323.0 ± 5.5	495.5 ± 13.2	120.5 ± 6.9	983.8 ± 61.6	292.2 ± 9.6	696.5 ± 52.3	808.0 ± 18.7
Gallic acid	47.4 ± 1.2	188.5 ± 5.7	19.5 ± 1.4	10.7 ± 0.9	42.6 ± 3.3	25.3 ± 1.3	27.9 ± 2.9	28.3 ± 0.4
Vainillinic acid	5.8 ± 0.1	9.5 ± 0.9	10.7 ± 0.3	4.8 ± 0.1	94.8 ± 6.6	84.8 ± 8.3	136.7 ± 7.5	45.2 ± 2.3
Syringic acid	3.4 ± 0.0	6.9 ± 0.1	6.8 ± 0.1	4.4 ± 0.2	20.5 ± 1.0	26.8 ± 1.5	21.9 ± 0.5	12.7 ± 0.1
∑ *Hydroxybenzoic acids*	251.3	744.8	983.0	330.3	1618.5	568.5	2334.3	1142.5
Hydroxycinnamic acids								
p-cumaric acid	11.2 ± 1.1	42.9 ± 3.2	18.1 ± 4.7	37.5 ± 1.1	5.5 ± 7.7	5.2 ± 1.1	8.6 ± 6.6	2.2 ± 1.9
Caffeic acid	13.9 ± 0.7	91.4 ± 1.4	38.4 ± 0.9	15.3 ± 0.5	12.7 ± 0.6	15.9 ± 1.4	14.4 ± 1.3	7.3 ± 0.6
Ferulic acid	22.2 ± 0.7	46.1 ± 3.3	59.4 ± 2.0	31.2 ± 1.6	22.7 ± 1.1	12.2 ± 0.6	11.0 ± 0.5	14.3 ± 1.0
Isoferulic acid	15.4 ± 0.2	7.8 ± 0.7	12.0 ± 0.3	10.9 ± 1.0	nd	nd	nd	nd
∑ *Hydroxycinnamic acids*	62.7	188.3	128.0	94.9	40.9	33.2	34.1	23.8
Flavan-3-ols: monomers								
(+)-Catechin	1170.3 ± 30.5	947.2 ± 39.7	1181.0 ± 11.7	1592.5 ± 32.2	112.4 ± 2.8	691.5 ± 24.8	185.3 ± 18.4	555.8 ± 26.2
(−)-Epicatechin	3346.5 ± 46.6	1901.7 ± 39.6	2179.4 ± 68.8	2954.5 ± 73.0	835.1 ± 27.8	3302.9 ± 194.2	1032.9 ± 19.3	3827.0 ± 76.6
∑ *Monomers*	4516.8	2848.8	3360.4	4547.0	947.4	3994.4	1218.3	4382.8
Flavan-3-ols: procyanidin dimers								
Procyanidin B1	1233.6 ± 39.0	1536.6 ± 16.0	829.4 ± 16.3	887.1 ± 19.6	68.2 ± 1.8	587.2 ± 25.5	105.4 ± 10.8	327.4 ± 10.1
Procyanidin B2	2415.6 ± 35.6	1651.0 ± 26.9	1085.5 ± 24.9	1291.9 ± 29.8	1085.3 ± 20.8	4011.4 ± 297.6	1061.2 ± 78.3	3777.0 ± 68.0
Procyanidin B3	1119.1 ± 32.0	2417.8 ± 34.3	893.1 ± 36.3	1383.2 ± 32.7	53.2 ± 1.7	350.3 ± 17.5	70.2 ± 2.3	158.8 ± 9.5
Procyanidin B4	3642.9 ± 96.5	3888.7 ± 79.0	1886.0 ± 57.9	2979.5 ± 68.7	479.8 ± 5.5	2720.8 ± 159.0	681.5 ± 48.6	1715.3 ± 5.2
Procyanidin B5	317.1 ± 4.0	159.5 ± 7.4	137.6 ± 8.2	191.0 ± 7.3	72.6 ± 2.7	301.8 ± 18.9	50.4 ± 3.6	448.3 ± 12.2
Procyanidin B7	158.8 ± 12.2	164.2 ± 10.1	47.3 ± 2.7	118.4 ± 2.1	nd	nd	nd	nd
Procyanidin B (5.47 min)	154.8 ± 11.0	171.0 ± 12.9	63.2 ± 1.1	116.5 ± 6.7	nd	nd	nd	nd
Procyanidin B (9.27 min)	68.1 ± 2.4	nd	20.2 ± 1.4	79.0 ± 6.4	nd	nd	nd	37.3 ± 1.2
∑ *Procyanidin dimers*	9110.0	9988.8	4962.2	7046.6	1759.0	7971.4	1968.7	6464.1

Table 2. *Cont.*

Compound	Leaves Extracts				Bark Extracts			
	AS	LC	PA	SR	AS	LC	PA	SR
	Concentration (μg/g Extract)							
Flavan-3-ols: propelargonidin dimers								
Propelargonidin dimer (4.43 min)	4978.9 ± 161.5	4125.9 ± 84.3	4689.4 ± 185.5	4477.4 ± 235.3	22.3 ± 1.6	126.2 ± 6.6	46.8 ± 2.7	115.3 ± 2.1
Propelargonidin dimer (5.01 min)	3369.6 ± 102.6	2661.0 ± 39.5	3179.5 ± 23.3	2981.4 ± 52.4	118.3 ± 4.1	346.7 ± 15.7	94.2 ± 9.0	257.0 ± 4.7
Propelargonidin dimer (5.65 min)	5209.1 ± 59.9	2602.3 ± 23.3	2935.9 ± 60.4	2748.8 ± 69.6	238.5 ± 5.8	1135.2 ± 71.3	213.2 ± 19.7	1153.2 ± 13.6
Propelargonidin dimer (9.27 min)	833.2 ± 5.1	352.8 ± 2.8	298.9 ± 24.8	339.6 ± 3.1	17.6 ± 1.0	56.8 ± 2.7	9.2 ± 0.9	83.2 ± 4.5
∑ *Propelargonidin dimers*	14,390.8	9742.1	11,103.7	10,547.3	396.6	1664.9	363.3	1608.7
Flavan-3-ols: procyanidin trimers								
Trimer T2	nd	104.6 ± 11.3	nd	nd	nd	235.1 ± 25.2	nd	nd
Procyanidin C1	303.7 ± 9.0	190.7 ± 6.3	64.3 ± 0.6	106.3 ± 3.9	480.8 ± 45.4	2006.3 ± 169.3	323.2 ± 2.1	2148.3 ± 70.4
Trimer B (5.78 min)	176.6 ± 13.9	395.7 ± 15.4	101.3 ± 6.7	145.1 ± 8.5	86.6 ± 3.8	473.6 ± 16.9	54.5 ± 3.8	585.0 ± 13.9
∑ *Procyanidin trimers*	480.3	691.0	165.6	251.4	567.4	2715.1	377.7	2733.4
Flavalignans								
Cinchonain (7.37 min)	937.8 ± 21.5	325.4 ± 18.0	258.3 ± 11.3	354.8 ± 25.8	183.4 ± 6.9	391.8 ± 8.6	107.2 ± 4.2	213.1 ± 10.4
Cinchonain (9.05 min)	786.9 ± 9.8	420.4 ± 5.3	249.6 ± 20.9	522.8 ± 19.8	18.9 ± 1.1	49.5 ± 2.8	22.5 ± 1.2	15.3 ± 0.3
Cinchonain (9.30 min)	977.6 ± 20.8	565.4 ± 17.4	335.5 ± 16.7	570.8 ± 20.2	24.7 ± 0.6	55.7 ± 2.6	24.0 ± 1.2	21.4 ± 1.1
Cinchonain (12.27 min)	809.3 ± 11.3	301.3 ± 7.4	231.2 ± 11.9	337.9 ± 19.1	189.3 ± 2.6	325.7 ± 11.9	115.6 ± 9.3	207.9 ± 7.3
∑ *Flavalignans*	3511.6	1612.4	1074.6	1786.3	416.3	822.7	269.4	457.7

AS—Asomat; LC—Los Chiles; PA—Palacios; SR—Sarapiquí; nd—not detected.

Table 3. Phenolic composition of ethanolic extracts from bark and leaves of *U. tomentosa*.

Compound	Leaves Extracts				Bark Extracts			
	AS	LC	PA	SR	AS	LC	PA	SR
	Concentration (μg/g Extract)							
Hydroxybenzoic acids								
Benzoic acid	46.3 ± 0.2	88.9 ± 9.8	165.9 ± 8.8	64.8 ± 4.3	1053.4 ± 41.9	5102.6 ± 69.5	1567.6 ± 22.0	20.1 ± 1.4

Table 3. *Cont.*

Compound	Leaves Extracts AS	Leaves Extracts LC	Leaves Extracts PA	Leaves Extracts SR	Bark Extracts AS	Bark Extracts LC	Bark Extracts PA	Bark Extracts SR
	Concentration (μg/g Extract)							
Salicylic acid	12.0 ± 1.1	10.0 ± 0.5	12.4 ± 0.6	12.0 ± 0.6	27.6 ± 0.5	175.4 ± 2.3	100.8 ± 7.1	110.0 ± 3.3
4-hydroxybenzoic acid	19.9 ± 0.7	23.2 ± 1.3	124.3 ± 4.4	26.2 ± 1.4	203.0 ± 6.2	117.2 ± 4.6	176.2 ± 15.3	42.2 ± 2.2
Protocatechuic acid	25.7 ± 1.8	61.4 ± 1.0	118.4 ± 3.3	48.5 ± 2.8	932.9 ± 21.5	283.8 ± 4.3	742.1 ± 61.7	326.5 ± 9.2
Gallic acid	5.8 ± 0.3	10.5 ± 0.1	11.5 ± 0.6	2.8 ± 0.1	28.1 ± 1.7	32.5 ± 1.1	15.8 ± 1.1	15.4 ± 0.2
Vainillinic acid	3.5 ± 0.0	5.8 ± 0.2	12.6 ± 0.6	4.4 ± 0.1	150.3 ± 6.6	412.1 ± 16.7	147.7 ± 10.5	47.0 ± 1.8
Syringic acid	nd	3.4 ± 0.3	5.3 ± 0.2	nd	40.9 ± 2.1	82.7 ± 3.0	22.4 ± 1.3	12.5 ± 0.1
∑ *Hydroxybenzoic acids*	113.2	203.2	450.4	158.6	2436.1	6206.3	2772.6	573.8
Hydroxycinnamic acids								
p-cumaric acid	4.6 ± 0.7	8.1 ± 1.3	22.5 ± 4.4	22.1 ± 1.4	9.9 ± 6.2	7.6 ± 4.6	4.8 ± 15.3	2.6 ± 2.2
Caffeic acid	5.3 ± 0.5	7.5 ± 0.3	7.4 ± 0.4	5.4 ± 0.3	9.0 ± 0.6	7.5 ± 0.7	10.8 ± 1.0	4.5 ± 0.2
Ferulic acid	10.2 ± 1.0	17.9 ± 0.9	30.1 ± 1.9	16.7 ± 1.5	31.5 ± 1.1	32.4 ± 3.2	11.8 ± 0.9	21.7 ± 0.8
Isoferulic acid	14.4 ± 0.1	nd	7.7 ± 0.2	nd	21.0 ± 1.5	38.9 ± 4.0	nd	nd
∑ *Hydroxycinnamic acids*	34.5	33.6	67.7	44.3	71.3	86.4	27.4	28.8
Flavan-3-ols: monomers								
(+)-Catechin	615.1 ± 6.7	674.2 ± 16.0	412.0 ± 14.1	1173.2 ± 33.4	66.4 ± 5.5	67.7 ± 4.7	100.7 ± 8.4	181.1 ± 11.3
(−)-Epicatechin	2163.7 ± 62.3	1554.3 ± 52.9	1097.2 ± 31.8	2159.0 ± 45.3	712.6 ± 44.0	978.3 ± 38.9	1444.3 ± 142.2	3148.6 ± 64.9
∑ *Monomers*	2778.8	2228.5	1509.2	3332.2	779.0	1046.0	1545.0	3329.6
Flavan-3-ols: procyanidin dimers								
Procyanidin B1	621.5 ± 13.4	1114.6 ± 40.6	313.6 ± 8.4	769.6 ± 27.9	23.2 ± 0.9	21.8 ± 1.5	99.0 ± 8.2	170.5 ± 5.8
Procyanidin B2	1363.7 ± 35.7	1399.3 ± 24.3	539.1 ± 18.2	992.1 ± 36.8	527.4 ± 19.8	378.5 ± 20.2	1592.3 ± 55.9	2792.9 ± 83.7
Procyanidin B3	830.0 ± 26.6	2353.2 ± 16.1	687.6 ± 11.4	1708.5 ± 93.7	19.2 ± 1.0	14.2 ± 0.2	69.3 ± 1.6	68.3 ± 3.4
Procyanidin B4	2476.6 ± 41.9	3931.9 ± 108.9	1711.8 ± 13.6	3172.6 ± 73.6	370.9 ± 15.7	319.1 ± 17.0	1866.0 ± 86.1	2015.7 ± 10.4
Procyanidin B5	291.0 ± 6.4	268.7 ± 8.3	122.6 ± 9.9	217.2 ± 3.4	72.9 ± 2.8	53.9 ± 0.1	292.0 ± 5.6	744.6 ± 13.6
Procyanidin B7	161.4 ± 9.3	267.6 ± 6.1	85.5 ± 4.8	170.5 ± 14.5	nd	nd	nd	112.2 ± 5.5
Procyanidin B (5.47 min)	137.8 ± 9.6	263.3 ± 7.5	96.0 ± 10.6	184.3 ± 13.2	nd	nd	65.1 ± 4.3	123.1 ± 9.4
Procyanidin B (9.27 min)	53.4 ± 2.2	nd	36.8 ± 2.8	76.0 ± 9.4	nd	nd	nd	58.0 ± 3.3
∑ *Procyanidin dimers*	5935.4	9598.5	3593.1	7290.8	1013.6	787.4	3983.8	6085.3
Flavan-3-ols: propelargonidin dimers								
Propelargonidin dimer (4.43 min)	3239.3 ± 63.1	3067.8 ± 72.3	3644.5 ± 59.8	4660.6 ± 105.0	9.9 ± 1.0	22.0 ± 0.8	16.4 ± 2.4	68.7 ± 5.7
Propelargonidin dimer (5.01 min)	2503.6 ± 26.9	2179.3 ± 22.1	2926.1 ± 37.8	3343.7 ± 57.1	85.7 ± 6.0	58.0 ± 5.1	153.6 ± 6.4	231.7 ± 18.0

Table 3. *Cont.*

	Leaves Extracts				Bark Extracts			
Compound	**AS**	**LC**	**PA**	**SR**	**AS**	**LC**	**PA**	**SR**
	Concentration (μg/g Extract)							
Propelargonidin dimer (5.65 min)	3253.4 ± 12.5	2177.2 ± 33.1	2178.4 ± 82.6	2480.8 ± 38.0	112.8 ± 4.3	77.6 ± 2.4	308.0 ± 13.8	895.5 ± 24.3
Propelargonidin dimer (9.27 min)	795.7 ± 30.3	480.0 ± 15.5	471.1 ± 20.5	576.8 ± 21.0	12.2 ± 1.2	12.4 ± 0.8	42.3 ± 1.3	143.8 ± 5.7
∑ *Propelargonidin dimers*	9792.0	7904.3	9220.2	11,061.9	220.6	169.9	520.2	1339.7
Flavan-3-ols: procyanidin trimers								
Trimer T2	nd	nd	nd	nd	nd	nd	nd	nd
Procyanidin C1	243.4 ± 25.4	260.6 ± 13.2	69.7 ± 0.4	181.2 ± 9.1	37.8 ± 0.4	nd	744.6 ± 10.8	1636.2 ± 76.2
Trimer B (5.78 min)	nd	nd	nd	nd	nd	nd	nd	nd
∑ *Procyanidin trimers*	243.4	260.6	69.7	181.2	37.8	0.0	744.6	1636.2
Flavalignans								
Cinchonain (7.37 min)	1723.6 ± 23.5	1011.9 ± 17.8	567.2 ± 14.4	773.0 ± 33.1	236.0 ± 15.1	170.7 ± 9.8	745.7 ± 20.4	447.7 ± 2.5
Cinchonain (9.05 min)	2010.3 ± 17.0	1816.3 ± 48.4	744.3 ± 23.4	1544.1 ± 77.1	19.7 ± 1.2	20.7 ± 2.6	63.8 ± 5.1	28.4 ± 1.4
Cinchonain (9.30 min)	1795.3 ± 31.1	1901.5 ± 32.5	773.9 ± 23.1	1358.0 ± 65.7	22.7 ± 2.0	25.8 ± 0.9	56.0 ± 2.5	34.6 ± 1.9
Cinchonain (12.27 min)	1528.8 ± 20.7	900.5 ± 14.5	486.7 ± 16.2	727.2 ± 23.3	285.3 ± 10.1	217.3 ± 12.9	710.2 ± 25.7	471.9 ± 17.3
∑ *Flavalignans*	7058.0	5630.1	2572.0	4402.1	563.7	434.4	1575.7	982.6

AS—Asomat; LC—Los Chiles; PA—Palacios; SR—Sarapiquí; nd—not detected

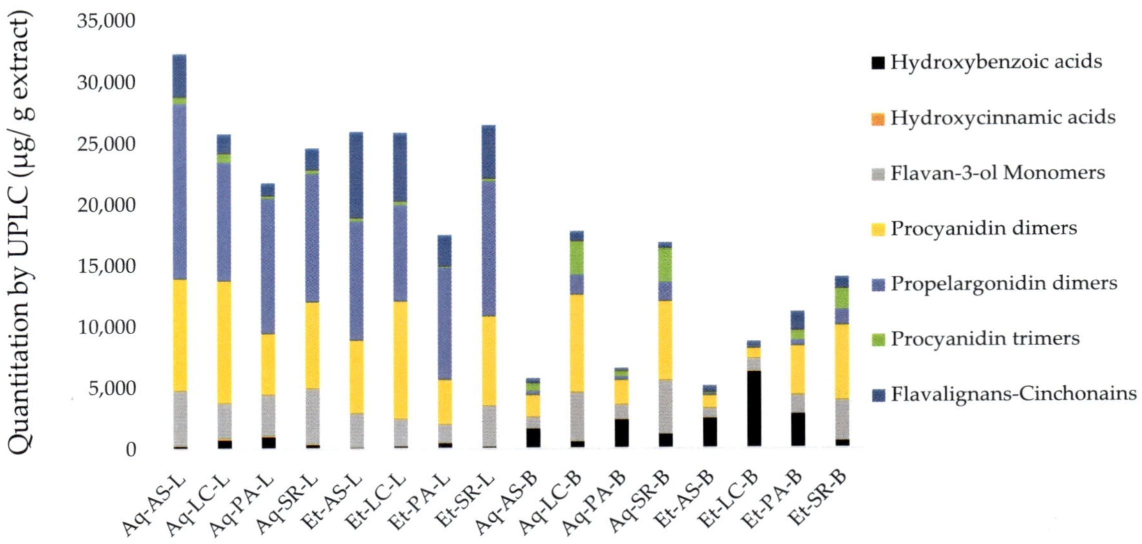

Figure 2. Quantification of polyphenols subclasses by Ultra Performance Liquid Chromatography coupled with Mass Spectrometry (UPLC-DAD/TQ-ESI-MS) for aqueous and ethanolic extracts of *U. tomentosa* leaves (L) and barks (B). Solvent: Aq—aqueous, Et—ethanolic; Origin: AS—Asomat; LC—Los Chiles; PA—Palacios; SR—Sarapiqui.

In order to identify the influence of plant part and extraction procedure on phenolic content and distribution, a two-way ANOVA was performed in the 16 extracts. This analysis showed significant differences ($p < 0.05$) in the content of flavalignans-cinchonains in function of both factors, plant part and solvent, with leaves and ethanol rendering the highest results. On the other hand, flavan-3-ols monomers, procyanidin trimers and hydroxycinnamic acids contents were not influenced by neither factor, plant parts or solvent. In contrast, hydroxybenzoic acids, procyanidin dimers and propelargonidin dimers showed significant differences ($p < 0.05$) only when considering *U. tomentosa* part material, with hydroxybenzoic acids being more abundant in barks, while procyanidin and propelargonidin dimers being predominant in leaves. A similar trend was observed when comparing these results with previous findings reported in a detailed study on *U. tomentosa* phenolic extracts obtained through extraction and purification with organic solvents [15], which reported a higher presence of hydroxybenzoic acids in barks and a higher propelargonidin dimers content in leaves.

In sum, our study shows that independently of the plant origin, leaves extracts exhibit high contents of phenolic compounds and more importantly high contents of proanthocyanidins derivatives, mainly propelargonidin dimers and procyanidin dimers. These compounds are linked to diverse bioactivities, for instance due to their antioxidant capacity, as shown in reports for commercial dietary products from grape [22] and cocoa [23], which suggest these *U. tomentosa* extracts' potential for further studies.

2.3. *Evaluation of Antioxidant Capacity of U. tomentosa Polyphenolic Extracts*

Evaluation of the antioxidant capacity of the 16 samples was performed through Oxygen Radical Absorbance Capacity (ORAC) and DPPH methods (Table 4).

Table 4. Oxygen Radical Absorbance Capacity (ORAC) and 2,2-diphenyl-1-picrylhidrazyl (DPPH) antioxidant activity of aqueous and ethanolic extracts from bark and leaves of *U. tomentosa*.

	ORAC (μmol TE/mg) [1]		**DPPH IC_{50} (μg/mL)**	
Extraction	**Leaves**	**Bark**	**Leaves**	**Bark**
		Aqueous		
AS	12.06 ± 0.36	5.22 ± 0.10	5.23 ± 0.02	8.83 ± 0.21
LC	10.53 ± 0.43	5.27 ± 0.15	5.81 ± 0.01	6.66 ± 0.15
PA	9.65 ± 0.44	4.07 ± 0.15	7.84 ± 0.03	8.98 ± 0.06
SR	6.66 ± 0.13	6.22 ± 0.28	10.13 ± 0.15	7.31 ± 0.16
		Ethanolic		
AS	9.48 ± 0.40	4.47 ± 0.15	5.95 ± 0.05	7.88 ± 0.18
LC	11.57 ± 0.33	3.48 ±0.13	5.56 ± 0.10	11.52 ± 0.05
PA	8.01 ± 0.28	6.65 ± 0.26	9.05 ± 0.23	7.47 ± 0.17
SR	11.27 ± 0.51	7.23 ± 0.19	5.98 ± 0.03	6.34 ± 0.07

[1] μmol Trolox equivalents/mg extract. Origin: AS—Asomat, LC—Los Chiles, PA—Palacios, SR—Sarapiqui.

Among leaves, Asomat (12.06 μmol Trolox equivalents (TE)/mg extract) aqueous extract showed the highest antioxidant activity in ORAC methodology, followed by Los Chiles (11.57 μmol TE/mg extract) ethanolic extract, while the lowest value was obtained for Sarapiqui (6.66 μmol TE/mg extract) aqueous extract. In the case of bark samples, Sarapiqui (7.23 μmol TE/mg extract) ethanolic extract showed the highest values followed by Palacios (6.65 μmol TE/mg extract) in the same conditions, while the lowest value was found for Los Chiles (3.48 μmol TE/mg extract) aqueous extract. DPPH values for leaves followed the same trend as ORAC results, showing that Asomat aqueous extract yielded the highest value (IC_{50} = 5.23 μg/mL) followed by Los Chiles ethanolic extract (IC_{50} = 5.56 μg/mL), while Sarapiqui aqueous extract showed the lowest value (IC_{50} = 10.13 μg/mL). Referring to bark samples, DPPH values also followed a similar trend as ORAC results, with Sarapiquí ethanolic extract yielding the highest antioxidant value (IC_{50} = 6.34 μg/mL) and Los Chiles ethanolic extract showing the lowest antioxidant result (IC_{50} = 11.52 μg/mL). These values are slightly better than previous DPPH reported results [2,24] for *U. tomentosa* extracts.

To evaluate the influence of both factors, plant part and extraction solvent on ORAC and DPPH, a two-way ANOVA analysis was performed for both methods. Results indicated no significant differences for DPPH. However, ORAC antioxidant capacity was influenced by *U. tomentosa* plant part ($p < 0.05$), with leaves materials rendering better results when compared to bark samples. Considering the extraction solvent, ethanolic extracts provided slightly better results than aqueous extracts but these results were not significantly different. Literature reports on *U. tomentosa* bark and leaves extracts using aqueous and organic solvents show variable results, depending upon radical scavenging methods used, for instance some indicating better results for leaves [21] and ethanolic extraction [19] in agreement with our results. Our findings indicate both solvents yield interesting polyphenolic composition and antioxidant values, thus studies could be carried out using hydro-alcoholic mixtures to explore if results and processes could be further optimized for industrial application.

A correlation analysis was performed between both antioxidant methods and extracts phenolic contents. Results show a positive correlation between ORAC values and total phenolics determined by UPLC ($r = 0.809$, $p < 0.05$) and by the Folin–Ciocalteau method ($r = 0.883$, $p < 0.05$). Similarly, a positive correlation was found with the PRO method ($r = 0.822$, $p < 0.05$). These results are in agreement with other reports that indicate correlation between total polyphenolic content and ORAC values for several plants [25,26].

Further, Figure 3 shows the correlation analysis performed for proanthocyanidin subclasses, including total flavan-3-ols, procyanidin monomers, procyanidin dimers, propelargonidin dimers, and flavalignans-cinchonains. It should be noted the significant positive correlation with total flavan-3-ols ($r = 0.846$, $p < 0.05$) (Figure 3A), procyanidin dimers ($r = 0.766$, $p < 0.05$) (Figure 3B), flavalignans ($r = 0.729$, $p < 0.05$) (Figure 3C) and propelargonidin dimers ($r = 0.854$, $p < 0.05$) (Figure 3D), while no correlation was found for flavan-3-ol monomers. Our findings are in agreement with other studies, reporting that the antioxidant activity was lower for flavan-3-ol monomers in comparison with flavan-3-ols of higher degree of polymerization [27,28]. Also, previous studies have revealed that properlagonidin dimers from *U. tomentosa* may play a major role in conferring antioxidant capacity [17]. Furthermore, ORAC values obtained are similar to those of proanthocyanidin extracts from grape seeds [22], indicating the potential commercial value of these *U. tomentosa* extracts.

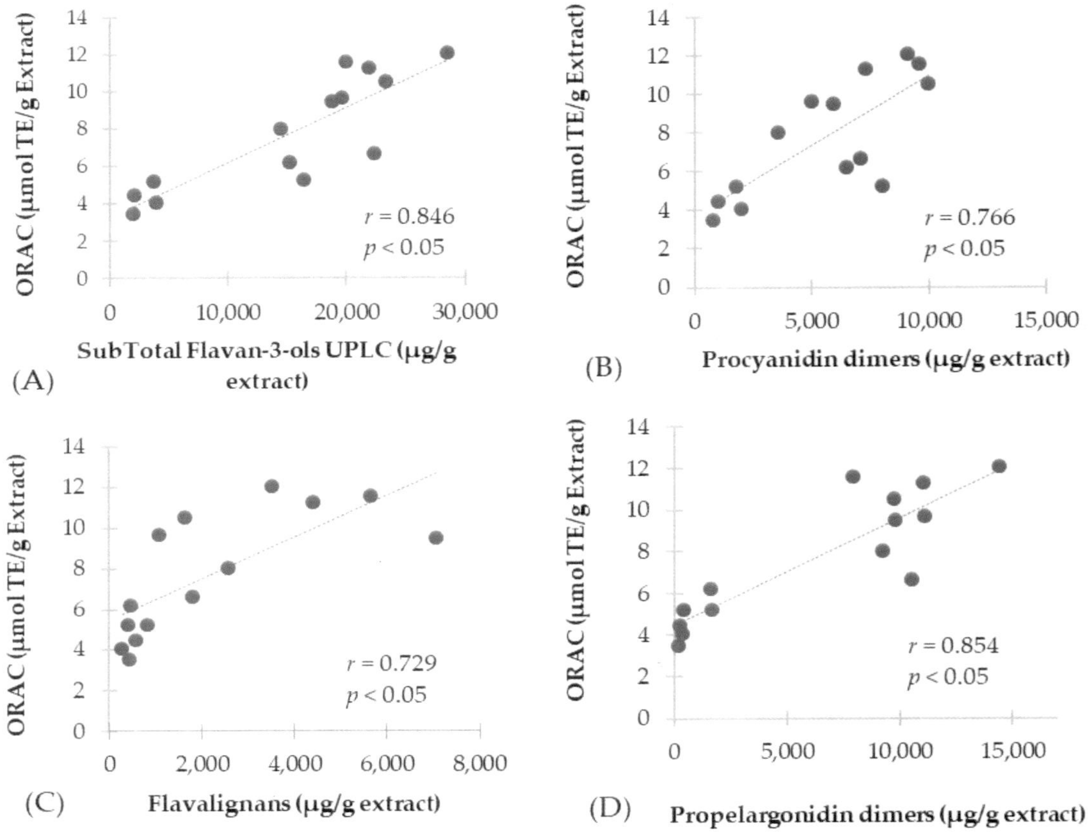

Figure 3. Correlation of antioxidant scavenging activity assessed by ORAC method with UPLC quantification: (**A**) Total flavan-3-ols; (**B**) Procyanidin dimers; (**C**) Flavalignans-cinchonains and (**D**) Propelargonidin dimers.

In respect to DPPH, results show correlation between total phenolics determined by UPLC ($r = -0.596$, $p < 0.05$) and antioxidant activity measured through DPPH, as well as between Folin–Ciocalteau values ($r = -0.635$, $p < 0.05$) and DPPH antioxidant values. Similarly, a correlation was found between these antioxidant results and the PRO values ($r = -0.670$, $p < 0.05$). These results are in agreement with a report on *U. tomentosa,* showing correlation between antioxidant potency of cat's claw preparations and their protective ability against DPPH [24].

Further, Figure 4 shows the correlation analysis performed for proanthocyanidin subclasses. Results show a negative correlation with total flavan-3-ols ($r = -0.601$, $p < 0.05$) (Figure 4A), procyanidin dimers ($r = -0.734$, $p < 0.05$) (Figure 4B), flavalignans ($r = -0.551$, $p < 0.05$) (Figure 4C), while no correlation was found for flavan-3-ol monomers and propelargonidin dimers. Finally, Figure 4D shows negative correlation results between the antioxidant capacity evaluated through ORAC method and DPPH results ($r = -0.735$, $p < 0.05$).

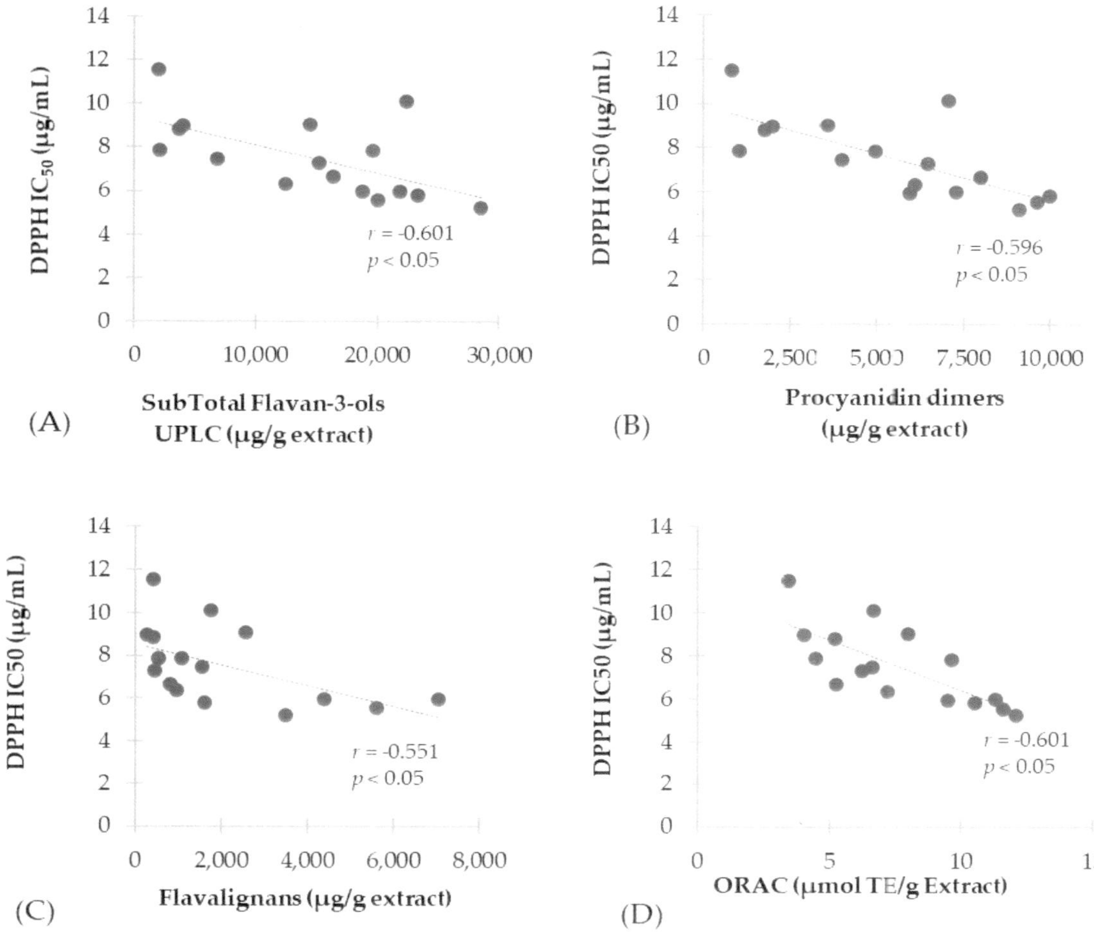

Figure 4. Correlation of antioxidant scavenging activity assessed by DPPH with: (**A**) Total flavan-3-ols; (**B**) Procyanidin dimers; (**C**) Flavalignans-cinchonains and (**D**) ORAC antioxidant capacity.

2.4. Principal Component Analysis for Polyphenolic Extracts of U. tomentosa

To summarize the findings, a statistical Principal Component Analysis (PCA) was performed (n = 16) considering 32 individual phenolic compounds as well as TP, PRO, DPPH and ORAC values. Two components (PC1 and PC2) were obtained (loadings > 0.18). The first component (PC1) represented 44.9% of total variance and showed positive correlation to various proanthocyanidin compounds, including procyanidin B1, B3, B4, B7 dimers, all four propelargonidin dimers and two flavalignans-cinchonains (at *Rt* 8.99 and 9.25 min) as well as TP, PRO and ORAC values. The second component (PC2) accounted for 16.5% of the total variance and was positively correlated to four acids, namely benzoic acid, 4-hydroxybenzoic acid, ferulic acid and isoferulic acid.

As illustrated in the plane represented by the two components (Figure 5), bark samples showed low scores in PC1, representing their lower values for these variables, and they are distributed along the second component (PC2) indicating high variability in the contents of the hydroxybenzoic and hydroxycinnamic acids previously cited. In contrast, leaves samples are grouped in the higher score in PC1 with larger content of polyphenols (TP), proanthocyanidin (PRO) and ORAC capacity, as well as all four propelargonidin dimers, procyanidin B1, B3, B4, B7 dimers and the two flavalignans-cinchonains derivatives mentioned above, independently of the extraction procedure.

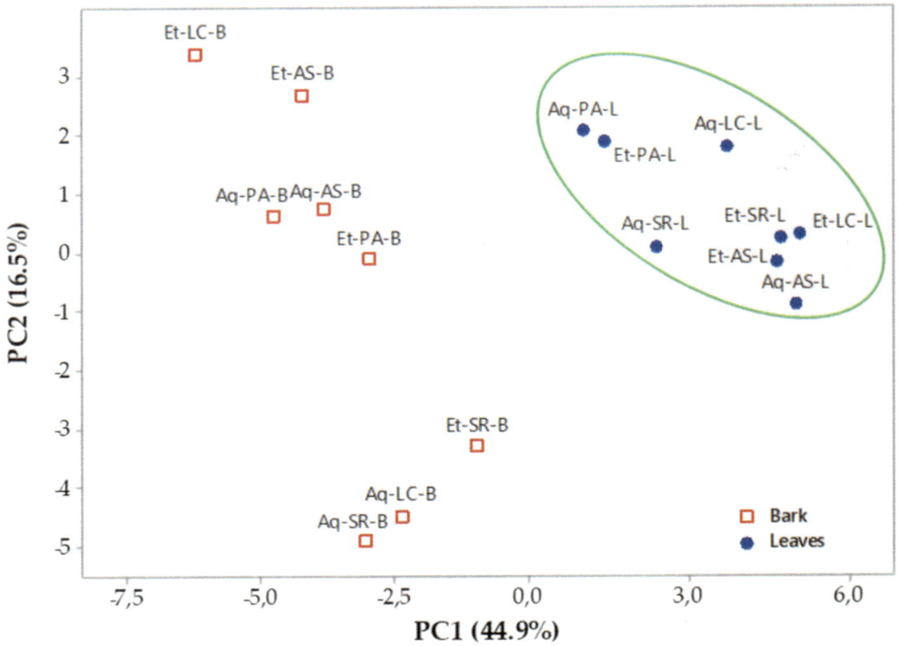

Figure 5. Plane defined by two first principal components (PC1 and PC2) resulting from the Principal component analysis (PCA) of individualized phenolic composition of *U. tomentosa* phenolic extracts (n = 16). Extraction: Aq—Aqueous, Et—Ethanolic. Origin: AS—Asomat, LC—Los Chiles, PA—Palacios, SR—Sarapiqui. Plant part: B—Bark, L—Leaves.

In sum, our results, using solvents and process adequate for the development of commercial products for human consumption, clearly indicate that leaves are the most valuable sources of functional polyphenols. Even though most of the commercial preparations are derived from bark material, our findings suggest that leaves represent a more valuable source of proanthocyanidins linked to important antioxidant activity and other potential bioactivities [16,17,22].

3. Materials and Methods

3.1. Plant Material, Chemicals and Reagents

Uncaria tomentosa samples were collected from different places in Costa Rica: Asomat (El Amparo) and Los Chiles (northern part), as well as Palacios (Aprolece) and Sarapiqui (Caribbean part). Vouchers for all plants are deposited in the Costa Rican National Herbarium, under series no. AQ2953, AQ3331, AQ3332 and AQ3510, respectively. The plant material studied consisted of bark (B) and leaves (L) for each location. The material was separated and dried in a stove at 40 °C, being turned over every 24 h for a week until totally dry. The dried material was then ground and preserved in plastic recipients. Solvents such as ethanol, methanol, and acetonitrile were purchased from Baker (Center Valley, PA, USA). Reagents such as AAPH (2,2-azobis(2-amidinopropane) dihydrochloride), sodium molibdate, gallic acid, Trolox (6-hydroxy-2,5,7,8-tetramethylchroman-2-carboxylic acid), fluorescein, and sodium tungstate were provided by Sigma-Aldrich (St. Louis, MO, USA).

3.2. Extraction of Phenolic Compounds from Bark and Leaves of U. tomentosa

The ground dried material from *U. tomentosa* bark and leaves (n = 8) was extracted (0.05 g/mL) separately in ethanol at 25 °C during 24 h. Afterwards the solvent was removed by filtration and the extraction process was repeated three times under the same conditions. The filtrates were concentrated to dryness using a Buchi™ 215 (Flawil, Switzerland) rotavapor, and the ethanolic extracts were preserved at −20 °C until extraction. In turn, to obtain the aqueous extracts, each ground dried material from bark and leaves ($n = 8$) was extracted (0.05 g/mL) in distilled water, under stirring and heating until reaching 80 °C. After cooling at 25 °C, the solvent was removed by filtration and the extraction procedure was repeated once. The filtrates were freeze-dried in a Free Zone −105 °C, 4.5 L, Cascade Benchtop Freeze Dry System (Labconco, Kansas, MO, USA), and the freeze-dried extracts were preserved at −20 °C until extraction.

3.3. Determination of Total Phenolic Content

Total polyphenolic contents were evaluated through a variation of the Singleton and Rossi method, as previously described [15], using the Folin–Ciocalteu (FC) reagent, which consists of a mixture of phosphomolybdic and phosphotungstic acids. Briefly, 0.5 mL of a dissolution from each *U. tomentosa* extract in MeOH (0.1% HCl) was mixed with FC reagent (0.5 mL) and 10 mL of Na_2CO_3 (7.5%). Water was added to complete 25 mL. A similar process was followed to prepare the blank, using 0.5 mL of MeOH (0.1% HCl) instead of extract. Both, extract and blank mixtures were left standing in the dark for 1 h, and afterwards absorbance was measured at 750 nm. Values of total polyphenolic content were obtained by extrapolating absorbances in a gallic acid calibration curve. Analyses were performed in triplicate. Values are expressed as mg gallic acid equivalents (GAE)/g of *U. tomentosa* extract.

3.4. Total Proanthocyanidin Determination

Evaluation of total proanthocyanidin contents was performed through a variation of the Bate–Smith method, consisting of C–C interflavanic bond oxidative cleavage, as described early [16]. Briefly, 0.2 mL of a dissolution from each *U. tomentosa* extract was mixed with 20 mL of butanol/HCl (50:50) and 0.54 mM $FeSO_4$. The mixture was incubated at 90 °C for 1 h, and then left cooling to 25 °C. Afterwards, butanol-HCl mixture was added to complete 25 mL. A similar process was followed to prepare the blank, but without heating. The absorbance of each *U. tomentosa* extract mixture was measured at 550 nm against the blank. Values of total proanthocyanidin content were obtained by extrapolating absorbances in a cyanidin chloride calibration curve. Values are expresses as mg of cyanidin chloride equivalents/g of *U. tomentosa* extract.

3.5. Analysis of Phenolic Compounds by UPLC-DAD-ESI-TQ MS

To analyze the phenolic composition of *U. tomentosa* bark and leaves extracts, an UPLC-DAD-ESI-TQ MS system was used, consisting of an UPLC coupled to an Acquity PDA eλ photodiode array detector (DAD), as well as an Acquity tandem quadrupole (TQD) mass spectrometer equipped with Z-spray electrospray interface (Waters, Milford, MA, USA) *U. tomentosa* extracts were dissolved in acetonitrile:H_2O (1:4), for separation on a Waters® BEH C18 column (2.1 × 100 mm; 1.7 μm) at 40 °C. The flow rate was 0.5 mL/min and the eluent system consisted of a gradient of solvent A—water:acetic acid (98:2, v/v)—and B—acetonitrile:acetic acid (98:2, v/v)—in the following order [15]: 0–1.5 min: 0.1% B, 1.5–11.17 min: 0.1–16.3% B, 11.17–11.5 min: 16.3–18.4% B, 11.5–14 min: 18.4% B, 14–14.1 min: 18.4–99.9% B, 14.1–15.5 min: 99.9% B, 15.5–15.6 min: 0.1% B, 15.6–18 min: 0.1% B. DAD was functioning at 250–420 nm, 1.2 nm resolution and at a 20 point/s rate. ESI was operated in negative mode and ESI parameters comprised: source temperature of 130 °C; capillary voltage of 3 kV; desolvation temperature of 400 °C; cone and desolvation gas (N_2) with flow rates of 60 L/h and 750 L/h respectively.

Data were collected in the MRM mode, with specific transitions of parent and product ions for each compound, whereas external calibration curves were used. Main transitions corresponded to flavan-3-ol monomers (+)-catechin and (−)-epicatechin) at m/z 289/245, to dimers of procyanidins at m/z 577/289 and of propelargonidins at m/z 561/289. Also, transitions for procyanidin trimers at m/z 865/577), and finally for flavanolignans-cinchonains at m/z 451/341. For optimizations, mass detector parameters and calibration curves, commercial standards were used for both flavan-3-ol monomers [(−) epicatechin and (+)-catechin] and two procyanidin dimers, namely B1 [(−)-epicatechin-(4β → 8)-(+)-catechin] and B2 [(−)-epicatechin-(4β → 8)-(−)-epicatechin], as well as for procyanidin trimer C1

[(−)-epicatechin-(4β → 8)-(−)-epicatechin-(4β → 8)-(−)-epicatechin]. For other procyanidin structures such as dimer B3 [(+)-catechin-(4α → 8)-(+)-catechin], B5 [(−)-epicatechin-(4β → 6)-(−)-epicatechin], and B7 [(−)-epicatechin-(4β → 6)-(+)-catechin] work was carried out with standards isolated from other plants and with confirmation by MS/MS spectrum. This method was also applied for procyanidin trimer T2 [(−)-epicatechin-(4β → 8)-(−)-epicatechin-(4β → 8)-(+)-catechin]. To confirm the structure of flavanolignans and propelargonidins, because of the absence of commercial standards, MS/MS spectrum was achieved for molecular ions at m/z 451 and m/z 561 respectively. In respect to quantification for these two types of molecules, this was carried out on the calibration curve of (−)-epicatechin and that of procyanidin dimer B1 respectively. Finally, calibration curve of procyanidin B1 was used for quantification of procyanidin dimers B2 and B3. The limit of quantification (LOQ) and the limit of detection (LOD) of the different standards are published elsewhere [29,30]. The analyses were carried out in triplicate.

3.6. Oxygen Radical Absorbance Capacity (ORAC)

The radical scavenging activity of the *U. tomentosa* phenolic extracts was evaluated through the ORAC method [31]. Briefly, 0.05 g of each *U. tomentosa* leaves and bark extracts were dissolved in 10 mL of methanol/HCl (1000:1, v/v), then centrifuged (3024 g, 5 min, 5 °C) and filtered (0.45 μm). The reaction was performed at 37 °C in 75 mM phosphate buffer (pH 7.4), whereas the final reaction mixture (200 μL) comprised fluorescein (70 nM, used as a fluorescence probe), antioxidant (Trolox (1–8 μM) or *U. tomentosa* extract (at different concentrations)) and AAPH (12 mM). AAPH and Trolox solutions were freshly prepared while a fluorescein stock solution (1.17 mM) served to prepare dilutions using 75 mM phosphate buffer (pH 7.4). Black 96-well untreated microplates (Nunc, Denmark) were used for fluorescence determinations in a Polarstar Galaxy plate reader with 520-P emission and 485-P excitation filters, as well as a Fluorstar Galaxy version v.4.11-0 software (BMG Labtechnologies GmbH, Offenburg, Germany). The 96-well microplate was automatically shaken before the first fluorescence reading and afterwards readings were recorded every minute for 98 min. The curve of the blank (no antioxidant) served to normalize the fluorescence measurements. The area under the decay curve (AUC) was calculated from the fluorescence normalized curve, and each sample net AUC was calculated using the formula: Net AUC = $AUC_{antioxidant} - AUC_{blank}$. Afterwards, the regression equation between the antioxidant concentration and the net AUC was estimated. The actual ORAC value for each sample was calculated by dividing the slope of the later equation by the slope of the Trolox equation attained for the same assay. ORAC values were expressed as mmol of Trolox equivalents (TE)/g of *U. tonentosa* extract. Besides each reaction mixture being performed in duplicate, three independent runs were carried out for each sample.

3.7. DPPH Radical-Scavenging Activity

To assess the radical scavenging activity through DPPH method, a 0.25 mM solution of 2,2-diphenyl-1-picrylhidrazyl (DPPH) was prepared in methanol. Then, 0.5 mL of this solution were mixed with 1 mL of polyphenolic samples at different concentrations and the mixture was incubated at 25 °C in the dark for 30 min. Blanks were prepared using 1 mL of samples but using 0.5 mL of methanol instead of DPPH. Finally, DPPH absorbance was measured at 517 nm. Each sample was analyzed in three independent assays. Curves of absorbance vs. concentration were plotted to obtain IC_{50}, which is the concentration sample needed to get 50% of radical-scavenging activity.

3.8. Statistical Analysis

Two-way analyses of variance (ANOVA) were applied to subtotals of phenolic subclasses in order to determine differences in quantitative values in respect to both factors, part of plant and extraction solvents used. On the other hand, in order to evaluate if the total phenolic contents (TP, PRO) and the phenolic subclasses measured by UPLC-DAD/TQ-ESI-MS contribute to the antioxidant activity, a Pearson correlation analysis was carried out between such variables and ORAC values. Finally, a Principal component analysis (PCA) was applied to summarize the data from the leaves and bark extracts ($n = 16$) from *U. tomentosa* taking in consideration 32 individual phenolic contents, TP, PRO, DPPH and ORAC, using the above mentioned Statistical program.

4. Conclusions

This paper describes successful methods to obtain enriched polyphenolic extracts of *U. tomentosa* bark and leaves with solvents adequate for human consumption. Using advanced analytical techniques such as UPLC-DAD/TQ-ESI-MS, results showed selective distribution of 32 non-flavonoid and flavonoid phenolics among the different samples, proanthocyanidins being predominant in leaves, independently of their origin or solvent used. Among proanthocyanidins, propelargonidin dimers are characteristic marker compounds in leaves, showing significant correlation with ORAC and DPPH antioxidant activity. PCA analysis also revealed that the phenolic composition of the leaves tends to be less variable than that of barks, also suggesting that leaves constitute a more homogenous material for extraction procedures like the ones used in this study. While most of products already commercialized are pulverized bark material, our results suggest that leaves constitute the part of *U. tomentosa* more suitable for use in the elaboration of standardize phenolic extracts with potential applications in the nutraceutical industry.

Author Contributions: M.N.-H. and M.M.-J. participated in the conception and design of the study. M.N.-H., M.M.-J., and D.A.-C. were involved in samples preparation, technical work and interpretation of data. I.M.-G. and E.A.-S. were involved in samples acquisition and preparation as well as initial analysis. M.N.-H. drafted the manuscript that was revised and approved by all the authors.

Funding: This project was partially funded by grant from the Spanish International Development Cooperation Agency (AECID) (Ref. A/023397/09 and A/030037/10) and a joint grant from the Costa Rica-USA Foundation (CRUSA) and the Spanish Scientific Research Council (CSIC) (Ref. CR0024).

Acknowledgments: Authors also thank financial support from the University of Costa Rica and Technological University of Costa Rica. Special thanks are due to Juan Manuel Cordero and Alonso Quesada from Costa Rican National Herbarium for his support with the plant vouchers.

Conflicts of Interest: The authors declare no conflicts of interest.

References

1. Rizzi, R.; Re, F.; Bianchi, A.; De Feo, V.; De Simone, F.; Bianchi, L.; Stivala, L.A. Mutagenic and antimutagenic activities of *Uncaria tomentosa* and its extracts. *J. Ethnopharmacol.* **1993**, *38*, 63–77. [CrossRef]
2. Sandoval, M.; Okuhama, N.N.; Zhang, X.J.; Condezo, L.A.; Lao, J.; Angeles, F.M.; Musah, R.A.; Bobrowski, P.; Miller, J.S. Anti-inflammatory and antioxidant activities of cat's claw (*Uncaria tomentosa* and *Uncaria guianensis*) are independent of their alkaloid content. *Phytomedicine* **2002**, *9*, 325–337. [CrossRef] [PubMed]
3. Steinberg, P.N. Cat's Claw: An herb from the Peruvian Amazon. *Sidahora* **1995**, *4–5*, 35–36.
4. Heitzman, M.E.; Neto, C.C.; Winiarz, E.; Vaisberg, A.J.; Hammond, G.B. Ethnobotany, Phytochemistry and Pharmacology of Uncaria (*Rubiaceae*). *Phytochemistry* **2005**, *66*, 5–29. [CrossRef] [PubMed]
5. Zhang, Q.; Zhao, J.J.; Xu, J.; Feng, F.; Qu, W. Medicinal uses, phytochemistry and pharmacology of the genus Uncaria. Review. *J. Ethnopharmol.* **2015**, *173*, 48–80. [CrossRef] [PubMed]
6. Falkiewicz, B.; Lukasiak, J. Vilcacora [Uncaria tomentosa (Willd.) DC and *Uncaria guianensis* (Aublet) Gmell.]—A review of published scientific literature. *Case Rep. Clin. Pract. Rev.* **2001**, *2*, 305–316.
7. Funes, L.; Laporta, O.; Cerdán-Calero, M.; Micol, V. Effects of verbascoside, a phenylpropanoid glycoside from lemon verbena, on phospholipid model membranes. *Chem. Phys. Lipids* **2010**, *163*, 190–199. [CrossRef] [PubMed]

8. Hernandez-Aguilera, A.; Rull, A.; Rodriguez-Gallego, E.; Riera-Borrull, M.; Luciano-Mateo, F.; Camps, J.; Menéndez, J.; Joven, J. Mitochondrial dysfunction: A basic mechanism in inflammation-related non-communicable diseases and therapeutic opportunities. *Mediat. Inflamm.* **2013**, 135698. [CrossRef] [PubMed]
9. Wu, T.S.; Chan, Y.Y. Constituents of leaves of *Uncaria hirsute* Haviland. *J. Chin. Chem. Soc.* **1994**, *41*, 209–212. [CrossRef]
10. Pavei, C.; Kaiser, S.; Borre, G.L.; Ortega, G.G. Validation of a LC Method for Polyphenols Assay in Cat's Claw (*Uncaria tomentosa*). *J. Liquid Chromatogr. Relat. Technol.* **2010**, *33*, 1551–1561. [CrossRef]
11. Desmarchelier, C.; Mongelli, E.; Coussio, J.; Ciccia, G. Evaluation of the in vitro antioxidant activity in extracts of *Uncaria tomentosa* (willd.) DC. *Phytother. Res.* **1997**, *11*, 254–256. [CrossRef]
12. De Matta, M.; Delle Monache, F.; Ferrari, F.; Marini-Bettolo, G.B. Alkaloids and procyanidins in *Uncaria* sp. from Peru. *Farm. Sci.* **1976**, *31*, 527–535.
13. Gonçalves, C.; Dinis, T.; Batista, M.T. Antioxidant properties of proanthocyanidins of *Uncaria tomentosa* bark decoction: A mechanism for anti-inflammatory activity. *Phytochemistry* **2005**, *66*, 89–98. [CrossRef] [PubMed]
14. Wirth, C.; Wagner, H. Pharmacologically active procyanidines from the bark of *Uncaria tomentosa*. *Phytomedicine* **1997**, *4*, 265–266. [CrossRef]
15. Navarro-Hoyos, M.; Sanchez, F.; Murillo, R.; Martín, P.; Zamora, W.; Monagas, M.; Bartolomé, B. Phenolic assesment of *Uncaria tomentosa* L. (Cat's Claw): Leaves, Stem, Bark and Wood Extracts. *Molecules* **2015**, *20*, 22703–22717. [CrossRef] [PubMed]
16. Navarro-Hoyos, M.; Lebrón-Aguilar, R.; Quintanilla-López, J.E.; Cueva, C.; Hevia, D.; Quesada, S.; Azofeifa, G.; Moreno-Arribas, M.V.; Monagas, M.; Bartolomé, B. Proanthocyanidin Characterization and Bioactivity of Extracts from Different Parts of *Uncaria tomentosa* L. (Cat's Claw). *Antioxidants* **2017**, *6*, 12. [CrossRef] [PubMed]
17. Navarro, M.; Zamora, W.; Quesada, S.; Azofeifa, G.; Alvarado, D.; Monagas, M. Fractioning of proanthocyanidins of *Uncaria tomentosa*. Composition and structure-bioactivity relationship. *Antioxidants* **2017**, *6*, 60. [CrossRef] [PubMed]
18. Monagas, M.; Sánchez-Patán, F.; Quintanilla, J.E.; Lebrón-Aguilar, R.; Bartolomé, B.; Navarro, M. Phenolic extracts of *Uncaria tomentosa* L. (Cat's claw) Containing Procyanidins, Propelargonidins and Flavanolignans, Method for the Production Thereof, and Applications of Same. Patent WO2014/096488 A1, 24 June 2014.
19. Pilarski, R.; Zielinski, H.; Ciesiołka, D.; Gulewicz, K. Antioxidant activity of ethanolic and aqueous extracts of *Uncaria tomentosa* (Willd.) DC. *J. Ethnopharm.* **2006**, *104*, 18–23. [CrossRef] [PubMed]
20. Amaral, S.; Mira, L.; Nogueira, J.M.; da Silva, A.P.; Florêncio, H.M. Plant extracts with anti-inflammatory properties. A new approach for characterization of their bioactive compounds and establishment of structure-antioxidant activity relationships. *Bioorg. Med. Chem.* **2009**, *17*, 1876–1883. [CrossRef] [PubMed]
21. Bors, M.; Bukowska, B.; Pilarski, R.; Gulewicz, K.; Oszmianski, J.; Michałowicz, J.; Koter-Michalak, M. Protective activity of the *Uncaria tomentosa* extracts on human erythrocytes in oxidative stress induced by 2,4-dichlorophenol (2,4-DCP) and catechol. *Food Chem. Toxicol.* **2011**, *49*, 2202–2211. [CrossRef] [PubMed]
22. Monagas, M.; Hernandez, B.; Garrido, I.; Martin-Álvarez, P.J.; Gomez, C.; Bartolomé, B. Quality assessment of commercial dietary antioxidant products from *Vitis vinifera* L. grape seeds. *Nutr. Cancer* **2005**, *53*, 244–254. [CrossRef] [PubMed]
23. Cádiz-Gurrea, M.L.; Lozano-Sanchez, J.; Contreras-Gámez, M.; Legeai-Mallet, L.; Fernández-Arroyo, S.; Segura-Carretero, A. Isolation, comprehensive characterization and antioxidant activities of *Theobroma cacao* extract. *J. Funct. Foods* **2014**, *10*, 485–498. [CrossRef]
24. Sandoval, M.; Charbonnet, R.M.; Okuhama, N.N.; Roberts, J.; Krenova, Z.; Trentacosti, A.M.; Miller, J.S. Cat's claw inhibits TNF-α production and scavenges free radicals: Role in cytoprotection. *Free Radic. Biol. Med.* **2000**, *29*, 71–78. [CrossRef]
25. Lizcano, L.J.; Bakkali, F.; Ruiz-Larrea, B.; Ruiz-Sanz, J.I. Antioxidant activity and polyphenol content of aqueous extracts from Colombia Amazonian plants with medicinal use. *Food Chem.* **2010**, *119*, 1566–1570. [CrossRef]
26. Dudonné, S.; Vitrac, X.; Coutière, P.; Woillez, M.; Mérillon, J.M. Comparative Study of Antioxidant Properties and Total Phenolic Content of 30 Plant Extracts of Industrial Interest Using DPPH, ABTS, FRAP, SOD, and ORAC Assays. *J. Agric. Food Chem.* **2009**, *57*, 1768–1774. [CrossRef] [PubMed]

27. Spranger, I.; Sun, B.; Mateus, A.M.; Freitas, V.; Ricardo-da-Silva, J.M. Chemical characterization and antioxidant activities of oligomeric and polymeric procyanidin fractions from grape seeds. *Food Chem.* **2008**, *108*, 519–532. [CrossRef] [PubMed]
28. Es-Safi, N.E.; Guyot, S.; Ducrot, P.H. NMR, ESI/MS, and MALDI-TOF/MS analysis of pear juice polymeric proanthocyanidins with potent free radical scavenging activity. *J. Agric. Food Chem.* **2006**, *54*, 6969–6977. [CrossRef] [PubMed]
29. Sánchez-Patán, F.; Monagas, M.; Moreno-Arribas, M.V.; Bartolome, B. Determination of microbial phenolic acids in human faeces by UPLC-ESI-TQ MS. *J. Agric. Food Chem.* **2011**, *59*, 2241–2247. [CrossRef] [PubMed]
30. Sánchez-Patán, F.; Cueva, C.; Monagas, M.; Walton, G.E.; Gibson, G.R.; Martin-Alvarez, P.J.; Moreno-Arribas, M.V.; Bartolome, B. Gut microbial catabolism of grape seed flavan-3-ols by human faecal microbiota. Targetted analysis of precursor compounds, intermediate metabolites and end-products. *Food Chem.* **2012**, *131*, 337–347. [CrossRef]
31. Dávalos, A.; Gomez-Cordoves, C.; Bartolome, B. Extending applicability of the oxygen radical absorbance capacity (ORAC-Fluorescein) assay. *J. Agric. Food Chem.* **2004**, *52*, 48–54. [CrossRef] [PubMed]

5

Phytochemical Profile of Brown Rice and its Nutrigenomic Implications

Keneswary Ravichanthiran [1,†], Zheng Feei Ma [2,3,*,†], Hongxia Zhang [4,†], Yang Cao [5], Chee Woon Wang [6], Shahzad Muhammad [7], Elom K. Aglago [8], Yihe Zhang [9], Yifan Jin [2] and Binyu Pan [10]

1 Faculty of Food Science and Nutrition, Universiti Malaysia Sabah, Kota Kinabalu 2073, Sabah, Malaysia; rkeneswary@yahoo.com
2 Department of Public Health, Xi'an Jiaotong-Liverpool University, Suzhou 215123, China; Yifan.Jin14@student.xjtlu.edu.cn
3 School of Medical Sciences, Universiti Sains Malaysia, Kota Bharu 15200, Kelantan, Malaysia
4 Department of Food Science, University of Otago, Dunedin 9016, New Zealand; zhanghongxia326@hotmail.com
5 Department of Health Promotion, Pudong Maternal and Child Health Care Institution, Shanghai 201399, China; evacaoyang@163.com
6 Department of Biochemistry, Faculty of Medicine, MAHSA University, Bandar Saujana Putra 42610, Jenjarom, Selangor, Malaysia; wang.chee@mahsa.edu.my
7 Institute of Basic Medical Sciences, Khyber Medical University, Peshawar 25100, Pakistan; shahzad.ibms@kmu.edu.pk
8 Joint Unit of Research in Nutrition and Food Science, Ibn Tofail University, Kenitra 14000, Morocco; aglagoelom@gmail.com
9 Division of Medicine, School of Life and Medical Sciences, University College London, London WC1E6BT, UK; yihe.zhang.16@ucl.ac.uk
10 Department of Clinical Nutrition, The First People's Hospital of Wujiang District, Suzhou 215200, China; panbinyu19881102@126.com
* Correspondence: Zhengfeei.Ma@xjtlu.edu.cn
† These authors contributed equally to this work.

Abstract: Whole grain foods have been promoted to be included as one of the important components of a healthy diet because of the relationship between the regular consumption of whole-grain foods and reduced risk of chronic diseases. Rice is a staple food, which has been widely consumed for centuries by many Asian countries. Studies have suggested that brown rice is associated with a wide spectrum of nutrigenomic implications such as anti-diabetic, anti-cholesterol, cardioprotective and antioxidant. This is because of the presence of various phytochemicals that are mainly located in bran layers of brown rice. Therefore, this paper is a review of publications that focuses on the bioactive compounds and nutrigenomic implications of brown rice. Although current evidence supports the fact that the consumption of brown rice is beneficial for health, these studies are heterogeneous in terms of their brown rice samples used and population groups, which cause the evaluation to be difficult. Future clinical studies should focus on the screening of individual bioactive compounds in brown rice with reference to their nutrigenomic implications.

Keywords: brown rice; nutrigenomics; phenolics; rice

---

1. Introduction

For centuries, rice (*Oryza sativa* L.), one of the most well-known cereal foods, has been a primary food for many people around the world and is known to feed half of the population [1]. Therefore, the role of rice as a staple food in providing nutrition to populations has been acknowledged. In 2015, the global rice paddy production was 739.1 million tonnes, yielding 490.5 million tonnes of white rice after milling. The rice paddy production in Asia was 668.4 million tonnes, accounting for 90% of the global production, indicating that rice consumption occurs mostly in Asian countries. The environmental flexibility of culturing rice paddies at various temperatures, humidities and soil conditions allows rice to become a globally-viable crop [2]. However, the health benefits of rice were never considered because rice is considered as a staple food based on the palatability and availability. The major producers of rice are China, India and Indonesia [3].

There are more than 8000 varieties of rice, which have different types of quality and nutritional content. After the post-harvest process, all the varieties of rice can be categorised as either white or brown rice [4]. The aromatic rice varieties, known collectively as "Basmati rice", have been sourced by people from Asian and European countries, because aroma has been considered as the highest preferred characteristic of cereal grain. Basmati rice possesses unique cereal quality features, such as long, supreme grains, characteristic aroma, swelling on cooking and tenderness of cooked rice. Basmati rice with a high amylose to amylopectin ratio and a medium glycaemic index is suitable for staple diets of diabetics [5].

Rough rice can be separated into husk and brown rice through a threshing process. The components in brown rice that was hulled from rough rice are bran layers (6–7%), an embryo (2–3%) and an endosperm (about 90%) [6]. Brown rice can be further separated into polished rice, commonly called white rice, which is obtained by removing the bran. Minor differences may exist in the degree of milling. Brown rice has a nutty flavour, chewier than white rice, but more easily goes rancid, as well [7]. The difference between brown rice and white rice can be obtained through milling [7]. White rice contains mainly the starchy endosperm. The removal of rice bran leads to a loss of nutrients. During milling, about 85% of the fat, 15% of protein, 75% of phosphorus, 90% of calcium and 70% of B vitamins (including B_1, B_2 and B_3) are removed [7].

As the degree of milling increases, the loss of phytochemical compounds beneficial to health occurs, and cellular antioxidant activity decreases. Furthermore, the contents of phenolic compounds have also been shown to decrease by increasing the degree of milling. Thus, by carefully controlling the degree of milling during rice processing, both the sensory quality and nutritional composition could be optimized. Thus, brown rice with a low degree of milling (<2.7%) exhibits a more ideal balance between sensory quality and retention of beneficial phytochemicals [8]. Brown rice is a rich source of various bioactive compounds, such as γ-oryzanol, tocopherol, tocotrienol, amino acids, dietary fibres and minerals. It is less consumed than white rice because its cooking is more difficult than white rice due to its slow water absorption, and the palatability quality of brown rice is inferior to white rice [9].

There are two types of brown rice, which are germinated and non-germinated. Germinated brown rice is obtained by immersing the brown rice grain in water to initiate germination [10]. The benefits of germinated brown rice are that the nutrients found in brown rice are more easily digested and the texture of brown rice is better [10]. Germination has been employed to improve the texture of cooked brown rice. It also initiates numerous changes in the composition and chemical structure of the bioactive components. Germination could induce the formation of new bioactive compounds, such as gamma-aminobutyric acid (GABA). The consumption of germinated brown rice is increasing in many Asian countries because of its improved palatability quality and potential health-promoting functions [11].

Advances in the human genome era have shown that diet plays an important factor in the health and the causation chronic diseases such as type 2 diabetes. This is because the diet-genome interactions can result in changes especially in the proteome, transcriptome and metabolome. For example, current healthcare practitioners recommend brown rice to be consumed rather than white rice. This is due to the fact that brown rice is more nutritious. One common trait between white rice and brown rice is that they are both gluten free and contain no trans fat or cholesterol [7]. Encouraging people to eat brown rice more is a difficult challenge due to its taste, which is less likeable compared to the taste of white rice [7]. In the United States, more than 70% of rice consumed is white rice, and rice consumption has reached 9.3 kg per capita since the 1930s [1]. In addition, the consumption of brown rice is beneficial for postprandial blood glucose control because brown rice has a lower glycaemic index than white rice (55 vs. 64) [12].

Rice is the main staple food for more than half of the world's population. The cereal was also utilised as a popular remedy since ancient times for several therapeutic purposes. Rice or rice-based products were also well documented in the traditional medicines of different Asian countries. The well-known popular uses are anti-diabetic, anti-inflammatory for the airway, ailment of gastrointestinal disorders and diarrhoea, diuretic, source of vitamins and skin preparations [13,14]. One of the rice varieties, red rice Rakthashali, is a staple food in India and has been described by Ayurveda practitioners as a functional food for a number of medications [15]. The medicinal rice Kullakar has high thiamine content, while the Karikalaveya variety is high in riboflavin and niacin [16].

Therefore, the aim of our work is to review the phytochemical constituents and nutrigenomic implications of brown rice in relation to animal and human studies. In addition, our work has also contributed significantly to the current understandings of brown rice with reference to the nutrigenomic implications of brown rice shown in human intervention studies. Therefore, this mini-review will provide a valuable reference resource for future studies in such areas.

Search Strategy

An electronic literature search was conducted using PubMed, Medline (OvidSP) Cochrane CENTRAL and Web of Science until December 2017. Additional articles were identified from references in the retrieved articles. Search terms included combinations of the following: rice, brown rice, phytochemicals, nutrigenomics and bioactives. The search was restricted to articles in English that addressed the phytochemical constituents and nutrigenomic implications of brown rice.

2. Phytochemical Compounds in Brown Rice

The advantages for health with the consumption of brown rice mainly come from the phytochemicals found in its bran layers [17]. Figure 1 shows the various parts of the rice grain. The phytochemical composition of brown rice cannot be dissociated from the scientific work of the Dutch Nobel prize scientist Christiaan Eijkman who initially reported the potential of brown rice and the story behind beriberi in humans in the previous centuries. Table 1 show the major phytochemical composition of brown rice. In addition to B vitamins, phytochemicals found in brown rice include dietary fibre, functional lipids, essential amino-acids, phytosterols, phenolic acids, flavonoids, anthocyanins, proanthocyanins, tocopherols, tocotrienols, minerals, gamma aminobutyric acid (GABA) and γ-oryzanol [11,17]. Brown rice also contains high levels of phytic acid [18].

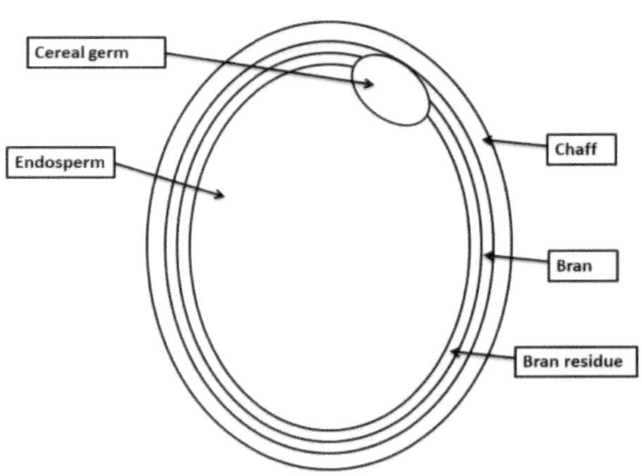

Figure 1. The various parts of the rice grain.

Table 1. Summary of the major phytochemical composition of brown rice.

Family	Compounds
Phenolics	Gallic acid, protocatechuic acid, *p*-hydroxybenzoic acid, vanillic acid, syringic acid, chlorogenic acid, caffeic acid, *p*-coumaric acid, sinapic acid, ferulic acid, cinnamic acid, ellagic acid
Flavonoids	Luteolin, apigenin, tricin, quercetin, kaempferol, isorhamnetin, myricetin
Anthocyanins and proanthocyanins	Peonidin-3-*O*-glucoside, cyanidin-3-*O*-glucoside, cyanidin-3-*O*-galactoside, cyanidin-3-*O*-rutinoside, catechin, epicatechin
Vitamins	Tocopherols, tocotrienols, B vitamins (B1, B3, B6)
Amino acids	Alanine, arginine, aspartic acid, cystine, glutamic acid, glycine, histidine, isoleucine, leucine, lysine, methionine, phenylalanine, proline, serine, threonine, tryptophan, tyrosine, valine
Phytosterols	Stigmasterol, stigmastanol, β-sitosterol, campesterol, δ5-avenasterol, δ7-avenasterol
γ-Oryzanol	Cycloartanyl ferulate, 24-methylene cycloartanyl ferulate, campesteryl ferulate, β-sitosteryl ferulate
Others	Dietary fibre, phytic acid, minerals

Amongst these nutritional factors, phenolic acids are the most common substances found in brown rice [19]. Phenolics are classified under phytochemicals having one or more aromatic rings with one or more hydroxyl groups [20]. Phenolic compounds are associated with diverse human health benefits including anti-inflammatory, hypoglycaemic, anticarcinogenic, antiallergenic and antiatherosclerotic properties [20]. Examples of phenolics are phenolic acids, flavonoids, tannins, coumarins and stilbenes [21]. In rice, phenolics are found in three distinct forms, which are free, soluble-conjugated and bound forms, and the bound form is the main form among the three [22]. High levels of phenolics exist in the germ and bran layers [23]. Since brown rice does not undergo any polishing or milling, these phenolics found in the germ and bran layers are easily preserved. Free phenolics are the most readily available for absorption in the small intestine, while bound phenolics tend to be preserved throughout the intestinal tract and released in the bowel, where they interact with the microbiome to favour the Firmicutes/Bacteroidetes ratio [24]. The two main groups of phenolic acids are p-hydroxybenzoic acid and p-hydroxycinnamic acid derivatives [21]. The primary phenolic compound found in brown rice is *trans*-ferulic acid (range: 161.42–374.81 μg/g), a hydroxycinnamic acid that exists in the bound form [19]. The second major phenolic acid found in brown rice is *trans-p*-coumaric acid (range: 35.49–81.52 μg/g), which is a hydroxycinnamic acid derivative with its bound form making up about 98% [19]. Another component that is widely found is *cis*-ferulic acid (range: 20.76–83.02 μg/g), an isomer of *trans*-ferulic acid, which is found abundantly in the bound form [19].

Soluble phenolic compounds consist of free phenolic acids and hydroxycinnamate sucrose esters [25]. The main soluble phenolic compounds in brown rice are feruloylsucrose, sinapoyl sucrose and ferulic acid [25]. The components that are notable in brown rice in bound forms are 8-*O*-4′ diferulic acid (DFA) (range: 13.88–22.61 μg/g), 8-5′ benzofuran DFA (range: 9.28–14.79 μg/g), 5-5′ DFA (range: 7.29–13.86 μg/g) and 8-5′ DFA (range: 3.26–8.79 μg/g) [19]. The three other hydroxycinnamic acid derivatives that were found in brown rice in small amounts are caffeic acid (range: 0.00–1.44 μg/g), sinapic acid (range: 1.19–1.25 μg/g) and chlorogenic acid (0.63 μg/g) [19]. Two examples of hydroxybenzoic acid derivatives that were found are vanillic acid (range: 2.65–4.74 μg/g) and syringic acid (range: 0.47–2.52 μg/g) [19]. In brown rice, catechin (range: 4.06–8.92 μg/g), quercetin (range: 3.27–6.53 μg/g) and kaempferol (range: 1.30–3.04 μg/g) are the three main flavonoids that are usually found in the free form [19].

In contrast to white rice, brown rice is still constituted by the germ and the bran layers, which contain diverse nutritional compounds, including anti-oxidants [26]. Therefore, despite its high nutritional value, brown rice is consumed less than white rice mainly due to its appearance, longer cooking time, cost, limited availability and bioavailability and poor appreciation of its nutritional value [27]. Apart from cooking, several approaches, including germination, have been emphasized to improve the palatability and the bioavailability of the nutrients present in brown rice. Germination improves the texture and the bioavailability of the nutrients and the phytochemicals [25,28].

In germinated (sprouted) brown rice, about a 70% drop is found in feruloylsucrose (from 1.09–0.27 mg/100 g of flour) and sinapoyl sucrose (from 0.41–0.13 mg/100 g of flour), whereas free ferulic acid content increased (0.48 mg/100 g of flour) when compared to brown rice [25]. However, in general germinated brown rice contains less soluble phenolic compounds when compared to brown rice (1.45 vs. 2.17 mg/100 g of flour) [25]. Apart from that, the sinapinic acid level also increases ten-fold in germinated brown rice (0.21 mg/100 g of flour) compared to brown rice (0.02 mg/100 g of flour) [25]. Germination also increases the levels of the GABA in brown rice [28]. Inositol hexaphosphate is a naturally-occurring molecule found in brown rice [18]. This compound has demonstrated anti-cancer properties [18]. Selenium is a trace mineral, which is found abundantly in brown rice [29]. The function of selenium is to induce DNA repair and combine in damaged cells to promote apoptosis, which is the self-destruction of the cells in the body to remove damaged and worn out cells [29]. Selenium also functions as a cofactor of glutathione peroxidase, which is an enzyme used in the liver to detoxify many possible harmful molecules [29]. Plant lignans are one type of phytonutrient that is found widely in brown rice, which are then converted to mammalian lignan, called enterolactone [30]. Brown rice also serves as a rich source of magnesium. Magnesium plays an important role in our body, as it works as a cofactor of more than 300 enzymes [31]. About 21% of the daily value of magnesium can be obtained by consuming a cup of brown rice [31].

Brown rice contains a high amount of dietary fibre, which has been shown to protect against colorectal cancer [32] and breast cancer [33]. In an animal study, rice bran from brown rice was shown to be beneficial against the development of polyps in the bowel [34]. Due to its high content in fibre, brown rice has a lower glycaemic index, compared to white rice [12]. Consumption of brown rice compared to white rice results in improved endothelial function, without changes in HbA1c levels, possibly through reducing glucose excursions [35]. Vitamin E is also found in brown rice, mainly in two types of structure, which are tocopherols (α, β, γ and δ forms) and tocotrienols (α, β, γ and δ forms) [17]. The function of vitamin E is antioxidant activity, maintenance of membrane integrity, DNA repair, immune support and metabolic processes [21].

Regarding insoluble phenolic compounds, germinated brown rice has at least twice the total content value of insoluble phenolic compounds than brown rice [25]. Ferulic acid and *p*-coumaric acid are found in the highest quantity in white rice, brown rice and germinated brown rice [25]. Generally, in germinated brown rice (24.78 mg/100 g of flour), insoluble phenolic compounds are 1–2-times more when compared to brown rice (18.47 mg/100 g of flour) [25]. The high levels of phenolic compounds in germinated brown rice are due to the increase in the free forms with alkaline hydrolysis, and this is because of the dismantling of the cell wall during germination [25]. The high levels of insoluble phenolic compounds can enhance the availability of hydrolyzable insoluble phenolic compounds during the germination of brown rice [25].

Amongst other antioxidants that constitute brown rice are the flavonoids. The chemical structure of flavonoids is constituted of a 15-carbon skeleton, which itself is constituted of two aromatic rings interlinked by a heterocyclic ring. The antioxidant activity of the flavonoids stems from the phenolic hydroxyls. Flavones are the most common flavonoids found in brown rice, and tricin is the major flavonoid, accounting for more than 75% of the flavonoids in brown rice [36]. Other flavonoids such as luteolin, apigenin, quercetin, isorhamnetin, kaempferol and myricetin are at relatively low concentrations, as well as isovitexin, naringenin, hesperidin, rutin, luteolin-7-*O*-glucoside, apigenin-7-*O*-glucoside and quercetin-3-*O*-glucoside, amongst others that have been reported [36].

Brown rice also contains sterols present in the bran. The most common sterol is γ-oryzanol, a ferulic acid ester of major phytosterols: campesterol, stigmasterol and β-sitosterol or triterpene alcohols [36]. The γ-oryzanol exhibits several physiological properties including effects on the anthropometry and muscles, cholesterol levels and potential anti-cancer properties [37]. Several analytical methods have been used for the determination of the phytochemical compounds in rice [38–47] (Table 2).

Table 2. Summary of analytical methods used to identify the phytochemical compounds in rice.

Phytochemical Compounds in Rice	Analytical Methods	References
Phenolic acids	Microwave-assisted extraction (MAE) Ultrasound-assisted extraction (UAE)	Sato et al. (2004) [38]
Antioxidants	Microwave-assisted extraction (MAE) Ultrasound-assisted extraction (UAE)	Sato et al. (2004) [38]
Anthocyanins and proanthocyanins	UV-visible spectroscopy	Sato et al. (2004) [38]
Dietary fibre	Enzymatic-gravimetric method	Tiansawang et al. (2016) [39]
Functional lipid	Gravimetric method	Zhou et al. (2003) [40]
Essential amino acid	HPLC method	Naomi et al. (2014) [41]
Phytosterols	Gas chromatography	Zubair et al. (2012). [42]
Flavonoids	Fluorescent DCF	Srisawat et al. (2011) [43]
Tocopherols and tocotrienols	Fluorescent DCF	Srisawat et al. (2011) [43]
Minerals	Ashing method	Horwitz (2000) [44]
Gamma aminobutyric acid (GABA)	Amino acid auto analyser	Cao et al. (2015) [45]
γ-oryzanol	Reversed-phase HPLC method	Xu and Godber (1999) [47]
Phytic acid	UV-Vis spectroscopy	Perera et al. (2018) [46]

Microbial Profiling in Brown Rice

Since the bran and embryo of brown rice are rich in vitamins and fibre, brown rice has the capacity to harbour more microbial association than white rice [48]. During germination, the quality of rice will be improved because the high molecular weight polymers undergo hydrolysis to produce GABA, amino acids, fibres and other bioactive compounds [9]. The germination usually takes place in a warm and humid condition, which favours the growth of microorganisms [49]. The germination of brown rice is initiated when soaking of brown rice occurs. This process involves fermentation because the microbial flora of the environment act upon it after the brown rice is soaked in the water for a certain period of time [50]. Some of these microorganisms can be either harmful or beneficial for consumers [51–55]. For example, some lactic acid bacteria including *Lactobacillus fermentum, Pediococcus pentosaceus* and *Weissella confuse* are detected in germinated brown rice [56]. Table 3 shows the types of microbial association in rice.

Table 3. Summary of major microbial association in rice.

Group	Microbes	Microbial Association	References
Gram positive bacteria	*Brevibacillus laterosporus, Brevibacillus brevis, Brevibacterium* spp.	Production of amino acids	Cottyn et al. [51]
	Cellulomonas flavigena	Degradation of cellulose	Cottyn et al. [51]
	Bacillus thuringiensis and *Bacillus cereus*	Production of enterotoxin	Kim et al. [52]
	Staphylococcus saprophyticus	Food-borne pathogen	Cottyn et al. [51]
Fungi	*Monascus purpureus*	Production of red pigment	Pengnoi et al. [53]
	Fusarium fujikuroi, Aspergillus flavus and *Candida*	Production of toxin	Tanaka et al. [54]
Yeast	*Torulopsis etchellsii, Hansenula anomala, Trichosporon pullulans, Geotrichum candidum, Saccharomyces* sp.	An increase in the essential amino acids; a decrease in phytic acid and enzyme inhibitors	Panneerselvam et al. [2]; Shortt [55]

3. Nutrigenomic Implications of Brown Rice

Similar to other plants [57–60], although the review of the literature has reported on the health benefits of brown rice, these studies often cannot provide the direct causal relationship between a bioactive compound of brown rice and the observed health benefits. Therefore, it is important to note that these studies should not be over-interpreted because this might be the simplification of the complicated mechanisms in the body that lead to such observed health benefits related to the consumption of brown rice. For example, the review of the literature has shown that brown rice is associated with a wide range of pharmacological properties such as anti-diabetic, anti-cholesterol, anti-hyperlipidemic, cardioprotective and antioxidant [61–67]. Table 4 shows the summary of some important nutrigenomic mechanisms involved in brown rice

Table 4. Summary of some important nutrigenomic mechanisms involved in brown rice.

Property	Potential Underlying Nutrigenomic Mechanism	References
Antioxidative	An increase in antioxidant status and a reduction in oxidative stress via v-akt murine thyromoma viral oncogene (AKT), nuclear factor beta (NF-Kβ), mitogen activated protein kinase (p38 MAPK), c-Jun N-terminal kinase (JNK), extracellular signal-regulated kinase (ERK1/2), p53 tumour suppressor genes, catalase, insulin-like growth factor 2 (IGF2) and superoxide dismutase (SOD)	Azmi et al. (2013) [61]; Imam et al. (2013) [62]; Imam et al. (2012a) [63]; Imam et al. (2012b) [64]
Anti-hyperglycemia	A decrease in the level of blood glucose via the suppression of fbp and pck genes, which are gluconeogenic	Imam and Ismail [62]
Anti-hypocholesterolaemia	A decrease in low density lipoprotein (LDL) and total cholesterol, as well as an increase in high density lipoprotein (HDL) via the transcriptional regulation of hepatic LDL receptor, lipoprotein lipase (LPL), adiponectin, peroxisome proliferator-activator receptor (PPAR) γ, ATP binding cassette (ABCA) 1, AKT and apolipoprotein genes	Imam et al. (2013) [66]; Imam et al. [67]

3.1. Anti-Diabetic Effect

Type 2 diabetes is a worldwide epidemic affecting millions of people across the world and associated with significant morbidity and mortality. Diet and life style factors play an important role in the pathogenicity of type 2 diabetes. Therapeutic management of the disease is only partially effective, costly and associated with adverse side effects. Therefore, scientists and healthcare professionals are looking for alternative management approaches that are safe, affordable and easily accessible to people, especially those residing in the low and middle income countries. In recent years, a considerable increase in scientific research has been observed regarding the use of brown rice for effective management of diabetes mellitus since it is the main staple food in many parts of the world, especially developing countries of Asia and Africa.

Several population-based studies have shown increased risk of type 2 diabetes associated with the intake of white rice, while higher dietary intake or substitution of white rice with brown rice in the diet may decrease the risk [1,27]. In the same context, results of clinical studies are also encouraging. Recently, a research group in Japan has reported a significant decrease in postprandial glucose level in diabetic patients following consumption of glutinous brown rice for one day [68]. The same group has also reported improved glycaemic control in diabetic patients even after eight weeks of ingestion of glutinous brown rice [69]. Using an open-labelled, randomized cross-over study design, they observed a significant decrease in postprandial plasma glucose, haemoglobin A1c (HbA1c) and glycoalbumin levels in patients who ate glutinous brown rice twice a day compared to those on white rice. Another study of similar duration and dietary intervention on Japanese diabetic patients has also reported decreased levels of postprandial plasma glucose levels and improved endothelial function. However, no significant changes were observed in the HbA1c level [35]. Similarly, a randomized controlled trial on Korean type 2 diabetic patients who followed a brown rice-based vegan diet for 12 weeks have also shown improved glycaemic control (larger reductions in HbA1c level) compared to those who followed the conventional diabetic diet [70].

Several other clinical studies have also reported a decreased glycaemic index and better glycaemic and insulin responses in healthy, diabetic and overweight subjects following consumption of brown rice [71–74]. All these beneficial effects are mainly attributed to several bioactive compounds present in brown rice. Brown rice has been shown to prevent type 2 diabetes in several studies [68,69,75]. Brown rice has a crucial role in lowering postprandial blood glucose levels in humans [75]. Apart from that, it also helped in weight management and ameliorated glucose and lipid dysmetabolism in individuals with metabolic syndrome. Brown rice contains high amounts of dietary fibre and other polysaccharides such as arabinoxylan and β-glucan. These fibres and polysaccharides help in regulating glucose absorption in the intestine, thus lowering the glycaemic index [76,77]. It also acts as growth substrates for these components to help in the growth of beneficial bacteria in the gut such as *Lactobacillus* and *Bifidobacterium* [78], thus modulating the gut microbial composition and helping in the prevention of diabetes and obesity [75,79]. It is found that in a recent study, there was a significant relationship between the composition of the intestinal microbiota, obesity and type 2 diabetes [75]. Brown rice is proven to have an important effect on the gut microbial composition in humans. This further supports that there is a relationship between the profile and activity of the intestinal microbiota with the anti-obesity and anti-diabetic effects of brown rice [75].

The rice bran in brown rice is rich in γ-oryzanol, which is responsible for many pharmacological properties, such as cholesterol lowering, anti-inflammatory, anti-cancer, anti-diabetic and antioxidant activities. Brown rice ameliorated glucose tolerance and insulin resistance. A lower glycaemic index was observed in healthy (12.1% lower) and diabetic subjects (35.6% lower) due to consumption of brown rice, and this could help to avoid type 2 diabetes and control glycemia, respectively [74]. These effects are due to the rich bioactive content found in brown rice [63]. A study by Sun et al. [1] has proven that consumption of white rice increased the chances of type 2 diabetes, while substituting one third of the daily serving with brown rice lowered the risk of type 2 diabetes in 200,000 subjects. Brown rice that undergoes germination also has differences in its properties, whereby it is less chewy and richer in bioactive compounds [63]. In germinated brown rice, the high content of dietary fibre helps to decrease the glycaemic index by regulating the absorption of glucose in the intestines [76]. Hypoadiponectinemia, which is implicated in reduced insulin sensitivity in diabetes, can be stopped by γ-oryzanol that is found in brown rice [80]. It also acts on pancreatic islets and increases glucose-stimulated insulin secretion [75]. In addition, GABA, another important bioactive present in brown rice, also has shown a similar effect against hypoadiponectinemia [81].

Similarly, acylated steryl glycoside (ASG), a component found in brown rice, regenerates sodium potassium adenosine triphosphatase and homocysteine thiolactonase enzymes with potential to reverse diabetic neuropathy and oxidative changes on biomolecules [82]. It also enhanced the overall metabolic condition in diabetes as a result of the induction of insulin-like growth factor-1 and reduced oxidative stress, which is a problem in type 2 diabetes [83]. The molecular targets of all these bioactive compounds discussed above are not known. However, it is believed that dysregulation of peroxisome proliferator-activated receptors gamma (PPARγ) is linked to the development of metabolic conditions including type 2 diabetes. Thus, PPARs can be a potential target for bioactive compounds, including those present in germinated brown rice. Indeed, a study by Imam et al. has already reported upregulation of PPARγ following treatment of HEP-G2 cells with germinated brown rice bioactive compounds. Upregulation of PPARγ has therapeutic potential in the management of diabetes.

3.2. *Anti-Dyslipoproteinemia*

Dyslipoproteinemia is a group of heterogeneous disorders characterized by elevated plasma cholesterol, triglycerides and lipoproteins level. Dyslipoproteinemia is an important risk factor for an array of clinical conditions including atherosclerosis, cardiovascular diseases and acute pancreatitis [84]. Diet plays an important role in inducing dyslipoproteinemia as evident by the rise in the incidence of the disease due to the intake of modern diets high in fats, sugars and refined grain products. Many studies have demonstrated that brown rice also has anti-dyslipoproteinemia and cholesterol lowering effects in animal models. A study by Shen et al. [85] reported an improved lipid profile (significantly decreased level of triglycerides, total cholesterol, high density lipoprotein and non-high density lipoprotein) in mice fed with pre-germinated brown rice-containing high fat diet for 16 weeks. The authors reported that feeding mice with a high fat diet induced dyslipidemia, which can be successfully averted when the mice were fed a high fat diet supplemented with pre-germinated brown rice [85]. The exact mechanisms are not known; however, this might be achieved by decreasing lipid absorption and synthesis and increasing lipid metabolism. The germinated brown rice extract administration in high fat diet-induced obese mice resulted in a significant reduction in serum triglycerides and total cholesterol levels by suppressing lipogenesis via downregulation of genes involved in lipid synthesis [86].

Another pre-clinical study by Miura et al. [87] reported that feeding hepatoma-bearing rats with white rice resulted in hypercholesteremia, which could be successfully suppressed when the rats were fed with a diet containing germinated brown rice. They probably do so by upregulating cholesterol catabolism. Other studies have also reported anti-dyslipoproteinemia and cholesterol lowering effects of germinated brown rice [88,89]. Human clinical studies evaluating the effects of germinated brown rice on dyslipoproteinemia are limited. In a clinical study involving sixty Vietnamese women (aged 45–65 years) with impaired glucose tolerance, the impact of germinated brown rice and white rice intake on blood glucose and lipid profile was evaluated. Following four months of intervention, Bui et al. [90] observed an improvement in blood glucose and lipid level in the pre-germinated brown rice diet group compared to the white rice group.

Similarly, a randomized control trial on 11 diabetic patients also reported a significant reduction in serum total cholesterol and triglyceride level following consumption of pre-germinated brown rice for 14 weeks compared to white rice group [91]. However, no such improvement in serum lipid profile and other metabolic parameters was observed in healthy volunteers who followed either a white rice diet or a white rice plus germinated brown rice diet (1:1, w/w) for 11–13 months [92]. However, this may be due to the presence of white rice in the diet, which diminishes the beneficial effects of germinated brown rice [72]. Hypercholesterolemia induced by hepatoma growth can be suppressed by means of upregulating cholesterol metabolism. Germinated brown rice also has a greater effect on the restorative effects on cholesterol levels compared to brown rice. This proves that germinated brown rice has a greater impact on high blood cholesterol [88]. All these beneficial activities of brown rice are mainly attributed to the presence of the high concentration of various biologically-active components such as GABA, dietary fibre, γ-oryzanol and other antioxidants in brown rice that help in preventing hyperlipidaemia. The risk of atherogenesis and coronary artery disease through its protection against LDL oxidation can be reduced by the antioxidant contents in brown rice and germinated brown rice [10,93].

3.3. Anti-Cancer Effect

Recent studies have reported the chemo-preventive and anticancer potential of some biologically-active molecules present in germinated brown rice. These molecules can prevent or suppress cancer development. Chemopreventive activities of germinated rough rice have been demonstrated in a recent study [94]. Using azoxymethane, colon cancer was induced in six-week-old male Sprague-Dawley rats followed by oral administration of either control diet or different doses of germinated rough rice crude extract (2000, 1000 and 5000 mg/kg body weight) once daily for eight weeks. The study showed a dose-dependent reduction in the size and number of aberrant crypt foci formation and β-catenin expression in rats fed with germinated rough rice crude extract.

Similarly, a study by Latifah et al. [95] also showed a significant decrease in aberrant crypt foci formation and β-catenin and cox-2 expression when azoxymethane-induced colon cancer rats were fed with different doses of germinated brown rice (2.5, 5 and 10 g/kg body weight). From germinated brown rice, GABA-enhanced parts were extracted, and they portrayed inhibitory action on the reproduction of some cancer cells and a stimulatory action on immune responses. GABA-enriched extracts from germinated brown rice had also been shown to inhibit effects on leukemic cells' proliferation and to stimulate cancer cells in terms of apoptosis [96]. GABA may also play a role in protecting smokers from pulmonary adenocarcinoma due to the reported tumour suppression activity in small airway epithelia [97]. Besides GABA, other bioactive compounds such as tocopherols and tocotrienols present in brown rice may also exhibit anticancer potential [98]. All these studies suggest the potential role of germinated brown rice in cancer prevention. However, further epidemiological and clinical studies are required in order to utilize germinated brown rice as a staple food in cancer prevention activity and for its inhibitory effect. The leukaemia cells that were treated with germinated brown rice extract showed greater DNA fragmentation compared to leukaemia cells treated with brown rice [11]. Apart from that, immunoregulatory activities found in germinated brown rice enhance the cell proliferation of mesenteric lymph node cells in vitro and also increase murine splenic B, T-helper cell subpopulations and nitric oxide c- interferon production [96].

3.4. Lowering Cholesterol

GABA found in brown rice also helps to nourish blood vessels, regulate insulin secretion, avoid increasing blood cholesterol, reduce emotional unrest, improvement from stroke better the kidney and liver function and prevent chronic alcohol disease [11]. The rice bran oil (RBO) found in brown rice can help to reduce the atherogenic level and increase HDL cholesterol. The cholesterol-reducing activity induced by RBO was due to the decreased absorption-reabsorption of cholesterol and the interference of the plant sterols in cholesterol metabolism. When the unsaponifiable matters of rice bran were fed to hamsters in a study, the faecal fat and neutral sterol excretion was greater. This shows that there is a decrease in fat digestibility [11].

3.5. Cardio-Protective Effect

Cardiovascular disease (CVD) includes diseases of the heart and circulatory system including angina, hypertension, heart attack, congenital heart disease and stroke. On a global scale, CVD is the most common cause of death with an estimated 17.7 million people dying because of CVD in 2015 [99]. To reduce the risk and increase protection against CVD, effective nutritional intervention has always been a focus of public health strategies. In this regard, brown rice and its bioactive compounds have been reported to possess anti-hyperlipidemic, anti-hypercholesteraemic and antihypertensive potential and thus have a role in preventing CVD.

Recently, a randomized cross-over clinical trial was conducted to evaluate the effect of brown rice consumption on inflammatory markers and cardiovascular risk factors [100]. Forty non-menopausal overweight or obese women (BMI > 25) were recruited and divided into two groups. Participants in both groups were asked to consume 150 g cooked brown rice or white rice for six weeks, followed by a two-week wash out period and switching over to an alternate diet for six weeks. Results of the study revealed that consumption of brown rice can significantly reduce inflammatory markers (CRP) and other risk factors (weight, BMI, waist, diastolic blood pressure) associated with CVD.

Another clinical study on healthy female university students revealed that ingestion of brown rice as a staple food for 10 weeks improved general health and prevented hyperlipidaemia, thus protecting against CVD [101]. Several pre-clinical studies have also reported anti-hypertensive effects of germinated brown rice in spontaneously hypertensive rats [102,103]. Mechanistic studies revealed that the antihypertensive effects may be due to the presence of several bioactive compounds in brown rice such as GABA, dietary fibres and ferulic acids [104,105]. On this basis, germinated brown rice can be a good choice as a staple diet or functional food to prevent CVD.

3.6. Antioxidant Effect

Brown rice contains many types of phenolic acids, which are well known for their antioxidant activities and one of the most common antioxidants in our diet. They can protect cells against oxidative damage, thereby reducing the risk of diseases associated with oxidative damage. Prevention of diseases such as cardiovascular disease, type 2 diabetes, obesity and cancer is possible due to the high antioxidant levels found in brown rice. The phenolic acids from brown rice also are assumed to contain chemopreventive properties for breast and colon cancer [106]. Based on the sensory attributes, the whole rice grain is harder to chew and has less taste qualities. Thus, pre-germinated rice is favoured. Brown rice is first soaked in water to initiate germination and contains a higher nutritional value. It is also shown that pre-germinated brown rice increases mental health and immunity. It also helps to prevent diabetic decline [107]. Hepatic fibrosis is one of the most prevalent health problems, and it can be prevented by consuming brown rice. Ferulic acid, *p*-coumaric acid, γ-oryzanol, γ-tocotrienol, GABA and other components in pre-germinated brown rice can decrease liver inflammation and fibrosis and hence reduce the risk of liver cirrhosis and cancer [108].

4. Conclusions and Future Research

Our review has highlighted that brown rice contains certain bioactive phytochemical compounds that might be associated with some important nutrigenomic implications. Therefore, brown rice has received increasing attention from consumers who are health-conscious. In addition, our review also suggests that there are several opportunities for the food industry to develop a wide range of food products using brown rice as the main ingredient. Similar to other plants [59,60,109], future research should be designed to screen for the individual bioactive components that might be associated with the nutrigenomic implications of brown rice.

Author Contributions: The project idea was developed by Z.F.M., K.R. and Z.F.M. wrote the first draft of the manuscript. K.R., Z.F.M., H.Z., Y.C., C.W.W., S.M., E.K.A., Y.Z., Y.J. and B.P. conducted the literature review and revised the manuscript.

Funding: This research received no external funding.

Acknowledgments: Zheng Feei Ma would like to thank Siew Poh Tan, Peng Keong Ma and Zheng Xiong Ma for their active encouragement and support of this work. The authors received no specific funding for this work.

Conflicts of Interest: The authors declare no conflict of interest.

References

1. Sun, Q.; Spiegelman, D.; van Dam, R.M.; Holmes, M.D.; Malik, V.S.; Willett, W.C.; Hu, F.B. White rice, brown rice, and risk of type 2 diabetes in US men and women. *Arch. Intern. Med.* **2010**, *170*, 961–969. [CrossRef] [PubMed]
2. Panneerselvam, P.; Binodh, A.K.; Kumar, U.; Sugitha, T.; Anandan, A. Microbial association in brown rice and their influence on human health. In *Brown Rice*; Manickavasagan, A., Santhakumar, C., Venkatachalapathy, N., Eds.; Springer International Publishing: Cham, Switzerland, 2017; pp. 159–181.
3. Fairhurst, T.; Dobermann, A. Rice in the global food supply. *Better Crops Int.* **2002**, *16*, 3–6.
4. Zareiforoush, H.; Minaei, S.; Alizadeh, M.R.; Banakar, A. Qualitative classification of milled rice grains using computer vision and metaheuristic techniques. *J. Food Sci. Technol.* **2016**, *53*, 118–131. [CrossRef] [PubMed]
5. Kale, S.J.; Jha, S.K.; Jha, G.K.; Sinha, J.P.; Lal, S.B. Soaking induced changes in chemical composition, glycemic index and starch characteristics of basmati rice. *Rice Sci.* **2015**, *22*, 227–236. [CrossRef]
6. Chen, H.; Siebenmorgen, T.J.; Griffin, K. Quality characteristics of long-grain rice milled in two commercial systems. *Cereal Chem. J.* **1998**, *75*, 560–565. [CrossRef]
7. Vetha Varshini, P.; Azhagu Sundharam, K.; Vijay Praveen, P. Brown rice—Hidden nutrients. *J. Biosci. Tech.* **2013**, *4*, 503–507.
8. Liu, L.; Guo, J.; Zhang, R.; Wei, Z.; Deng, Y.; Guo, J.; Zhang, M. Effect of degree of milling on phenolic profiles and cellular antioxidant activity of whole brown rice. *Food Chem.* **2015**, *185*, 318–325. [CrossRef] [PubMed]

9. Ohtsubo, K.I.; Suzuki, K.; Yasui, Y.; Kasumi, T. Bio-functional components in the processed pre-germinated brown rice by a twin-screw extruder. *J. Food Compos. Anal.* **2005**, *18*, 303–316. [CrossRef]
10. Wu, F.; Yang, N.; Touré, A.; Jin, Z.; Xu, X. Germinated brown rice and its role in human health. *Crit. Rev. Food Sci. Nutr.* **2013**, *53*, 451–463. [CrossRef] [PubMed]
11. Cho, D.H.; Lim, S.T. Germinated brown rice and its bio-functional compounds. *Food Chem.* **2016**, *196*, 259–271. [CrossRef] [PubMed]
12. Foster-Powell, K.; Holt, S.H.; Brand-Miller, J.C. International table of glycemic index and glycemic load values: 2002. *Am. J. Clin. Nutr.* **2002**, *76*, 5–56. [CrossRef] [PubMed]
13. Umadevi, M.; Pushpa, R.; Sampathkumar, K.; Bhowmik, D. Rice—Traditional medicinal plant in India. *J. Pharmacogn. Phytochem.* **2012**, *1*, 6–12.
14. Burlando, B.; Cornara, L. Therapeutic properties of rice constituents and derivatives (*Oryza sativa* L.): A review update. *Trends Food Sci. Technol.* **2014**, *40*, 82–98. [CrossRef]
15. Hegde, S.; Yenagi, N.; Kasturiba, B. Indigenous knowledge of the traditional and qualified ayurveda practitioners on the nutritional significance and use of red rice in medications. *Indian J. Tradit. Knowl.* **2013**, *12*, 506–511.
16. Isaac, R.S.R.; Nair, A.S.; Varghese, E.; Chavali, M. Phytochemical, antioxidant and nutrient analysis of medicinal rice (*Oryza sativa* L.) varieties found in south India. *Adv. Sci. Lett.* **2012**, *11*, 86–90. [CrossRef]
17. Okarter, N.; Liu, R.H. Health benefits of whole grain phytochemicals. *Crit. Rev. Food Sci. Nutr.* **2010**, *50*, 193–208. [CrossRef] [PubMed]
18. Babu, P.D.; Subhasree, R.; Bhakyaraj, R.; Vidhyalakshmi, R. Brown rice-beyond the color reviving a lost health food—A review. *Am.-Eurasian J. Agron.* **2009**, *2*, 67–72.
19. Gong, E.S.; Luo, S.J.; Li, T.; Liu, C.M.; Zhang, G.W.; Chen, J.; Zeng, Z.C.; Liu, R.H. Phytochemical profiles and antioxidant activity of brown rice varieties. *Food Chem.* **2017**, *227*, 432–443. [CrossRef] [PubMed]
20. Tan, B.L.; Norhaizan, M.E. Scientific evidence of rice by-products for cancer prevention: Chemopreventive properties of waste products from rice milling on carcinogenesis in vitro and in vivo. *BioMed Res. Int.* **2017**, *2017*, 9017902. [CrossRef] [PubMed]
21. Liu, R.H. Whole grain phytochemicals and health. *J. Cereal Sci.* **2007**, *46*, 207–219. [CrossRef]
22. Adom, K.K.; Liu, R.H. Antioxidant activity of grains. *J. Agric. Food Chem.* **2002**, *50*, 6182–6187. [CrossRef] [PubMed]
23. Adom, K.K.; Sorrells, M.E.; Liu, R.H. Phytochemicals and antioxidant activity of milled fractions of different wheat varieties. *J. Agric. Food Chem.* **2005**, *53*, 2297–2306. [CrossRef] [PubMed]
24. Martínez, I.; Lattimer, J.M.; Hubach, K.L.; Case, J.A.; Yang, J.; Weber, C.G.; Louk, J.A.; Rose, D.J.; Kyureghian, G.; Peterson, D.A.; et al. Gut microbiome composition is linked to whole grain-induced immunological improvements. *ISME J.* **2013**, *7*, 269–280. [CrossRef] [PubMed]
25. Tian, S.; Nakamura, K.; Kayahara, H. Analysis of phenolic compounds in white rice, brown rice, and germinated brown rice. *J. Agric. Food Chem.* **2004**, *52*, 4808–4813. [CrossRef] [PubMed]
26. Cáceres, P.J.; Peñas, E.; Martinez-Villaluenga, C.; Amigo, L.; Frias, J. Enhancement of biologically active compounds in germinated brown rice and the effect of sun-drying. *J. Cereal Sci.* **2017**, *73*, 1–9. [CrossRef]
27. Adebamowo, S.N.; Eseyin, O.; Yilme, S.; Adeyemi, D.; Willett, W.C.; Hu, F.B.; Spiegelman, D.; Adebamowo, C.A. A mixed-methods study on acceptability, tolerability, and substitution of brown rice for white rice to lower blood glucose levels among Nigerian adults. *Front. Nutr.* **2017**, *4*, 33. [CrossRef] [PubMed]
28. Patil, S.B.; Khan, M.K. Germinated brown rice as a value added rice product: A review. *J. Food Sci. Technol.* **2011**, *48*, 661–667. [CrossRef] [PubMed]
29. Vogt, T.M.; Ziegler, R.G.; Graubard, B.I.; Swanson, C.A.; Greenberg, R.S.; Schoenberg, J.B.; Swanson, G.M.; Hayes, R.B.; Mayne, S.T. Serum selenium and risk of prostate cancer in U.S. blacks and whites. *Int. J. Cancer* **2003**, *103*, 664–670. [CrossRef] [PubMed]
30. Anderson, J.W.; Hanna, T.J. Whole grains and protection against coronary heart disease: What are the active components and mechanisms? *Am. J. Clin. Nutr.* **1999**, *70*, 307–308. [CrossRef] [PubMed]
31. Jiamyangyuen, S.; Ooraikul, B. The physico-chemical, eating and sensorial properties of germinated brown rice. *J. Food Agric. Environ.* **2008**, *6*, 119–124.
32. Aune, D.; Chan, D.S.M.; Lau, R.; Vieira, R.; Greenwood, D.C.; Kampman, E.; Norat, T. Dietary fibre, whole grains, and risk of colorectal cancer: Systematic review and dose-response meta-analysis of prospective studies. *Br. Med. J.* **2011**, *343*, d6617. [CrossRef] [PubMed]

33. Aune, D.; Chan, D.S.; Greenwood, D.C.; Vieira, A.R.; Rosenblatt, D.A.; Vieira, R.; Norat, T. Dietary fiber and breast cancer risk: A systematic review and meta-analysis of prospective studies. *Ann. Oncol.* **2012**, *23*, 1394–1402. [PubMed]
34. Verschoyle, R.D.; Greaves, P.; Cai, H.; Edwards, R.E.; Steward, W.P.; Gescher, A.J. Evaluation of the cancer chemopreventive efficacy of rice bran in genetic mouse models of breast, prostate and intestinal carcinogenesis. *Br. J. Cancer* **2007**, *96*, 248–254. [CrossRef] [PubMed]
35. Kondo, K.; Morino, K.; Nishio, Y.; Ishikado, A.; Arima, H.; Nakao, K.; Nakagawa, F.; Nikami, F.; Sekine, O.; Nemoto, K.I.; et al. Fiber-rich diet with brown rice improves endothelial function in type 2 diabetes mellitus: A randomized controlled trial. *PLoS ONE* **2017**, *12*, e0179869. [CrossRef] [PubMed]
36. Goufo, P.; Trindade, H. Rice antioxidants: Phenolic acids, flavonoids, anthocyanins, proanthocyanidins, tocopherols, tocotrienols, gamma-oryzanol, and phytic acid. *Food Sci. Nutr.* **2014**, *2*, 75–104. [CrossRef] [PubMed]
37. Cicero, A.F.; Gaddi, A. Rice bran oil and gamma-oryzanol in the treatment of hyperlipoproteinaemias and other conditions. *Phytother. Res.* **2001**, *15*, 277–289. [PubMed]
38. Sato, S.; Soga, T.; Nishioka, T.; Tomita, M. Simultaneous determination of the main metabolites in rice leaves using capillary electrophoresis mass spectrometry and capillary electrophoresis diode array detection. *Plant J.* **2004**, *40*, 151–163. [CrossRef] [PubMed]
39. Tiansawang, K.; Luangpituksa, P.; Varanyanond, W.; Hansawasdi, C. GABA production, antioxidant activity in some germinated dietary seeds and the effect of cooking on their GABA content. *Food Sci. Technol.* **2016**, *36*, 313–321. [CrossRef]
40. Zhou, Z.; Blanchard, C.; Helliwell, S.; Robards, K. Fatty acid composition of three rice varieties following storage. *J. Cereal Sci.* **2003**, *37*, 327–335. [CrossRef]
41. Eshun Naomi, A.; Emmanuel, A.; Barimah, J.; VM, D.; Van Twisk, C. Amino acid profiles of some varieties of rice, soybean and groundnut grown. *J. Food Process. Technol.* **2015**, *6*, 420.
42. Zubair, M.; Anwar, F.; Ashraf, M.; Uddin, M.K. Characterization of high-value bioactives in some selected varieties of Pakistani Rice (*Oryza sativa* L.). *Int. J. Mol. Sci.* **2012**, *13*, 4608–4622. [CrossRef] [PubMed]
43. Srisawat, U.; Panunto, W.; Kaendee, N.; Tanuchit, S.; Itharat, A.; Lerdvuthisopon, N.; Hansakul, P. Determination of phenolic compounds, flavonoids, and antioxidant activities in water extracts of Thai red and white rice cultivars. *J. Med. Assoc. Thail.* **2010**, *93*, S83–S91.
44. Horwitz, W. *Official Methods of Analysis of AOAC International*; AOAC International: Gaithersburg, MD, USA, 2000.
45. Cao, Y.; Jia, F.; Han, Y.; Liu, Y.; Zhang, Q. Study on the optimal moisture adding rate of brown rice during germination by using segmented moisture conditioning method. *J. Food Sci. Technol.* **2015**, *52*, 6599–6606. [CrossRef] [PubMed]
46. Perera, I.; Seneweera, S.; Hirotsu, N. Manipulating the phytic acid content of rice grain toward improving micronutrient bioavailability. *Rice* **2018**, *11*, 4. [CrossRef] [PubMed]
47. Xu, Z.; Godber, J.S. Purification and identification of components of γ-oryzanol in rice bran oil. *J. Agric. Food Chem.* **1999**, *47*, 2724–2728. [CrossRef] [PubMed]
48. Cui, L.; Pan, Z.; Yue, T.; Atungulu, G.G.; Berrios, J. Effect of ultrasonic treatment of brown rice at different temperatures on cooking properties and quality. *Cereal Chem. J.* **2010**, *87*, 403–408. [CrossRef]
49. Lu, Z.H.; Zhang, Y.; Li, L.T.; Curtis, R.B.; Kong, X.L.; Fulcher, R.G.; Zhang, G.; Cao, W. Inhibition of microbial growth and enrichment of gamma-aminobutyric acid during germination of brown rice by electrolyzed oxidizing water. *J. Food Prot.* **2010**, *73*, 483–487. [CrossRef] [PubMed]
50. Puri, S.; Dhillon, B.; Sodhi, N.S. Effect of degree of milling (Dom) on overall quality of rice—A review. *Int. J. Adv. Biotechnol. Res.* **2014**, *5*, 474–489.
51. Cottyn, B.; Regalado, E.; Lanoot, B.; De Cleene, M.; Mew, T.W.; Swings, J. Bacterial populations associated with rice seed in the tropical environment. *Phytopathology* **2001**, *91*, 282–292. [CrossRef] [PubMed]
52. Kim, B.; Bang, J.; Kim, H.; Kim, Y.; Kim, B.S.; Beuchat, L.R.; Ryu, J.H. *Bacillus cereus* and *Bacillus thuringiensis* spores in Korean rice: Prevalence and toxin production as affected by production area and degree of milling. *Food Microbiol.* **2014**, *42*, 89–94. [CrossRef] [PubMed]
53. Pengnoi, P.; Mahawan, R.; Khanongnuch, C.; Lumyong, S. Antioxidant properties and production of monacolin k, citrinin, and red pigments during solid state fermentation of purple rice (*Oryzae sativa*) varieties by *Monascus purpureus*. *Czech J. Food Sci.* **2017**, *35*, 32–39.

54. Tanaka, K.; Sago, Y.; Zheng, Y.; Nakagawa, H.; Kushiro, M. Mycotoxins in rice. *Int. J. Food Microbiol.* **2007**, *119*, 59–66. [CrossRef] [PubMed]
55. Shortt, C. Living it up for dinner. *Chem. Ind.* **1998**, *8*, 300–303.
56. Kim, K.-S.; Kim, B.-H.; Kim, M.-J.; Han, J.-K.; Kum, J.-S.; Lee, H.-Y. Quantitative microbiological profiles of brown rice and germinated brown rice. *Food Sci. Biotechnol.* **2012**, *21*, 1785–1788. [CrossRef]
57. Ma, Z.F.; Zhang, H. Phytochemical constituents, health benefits, and industrial applications of grape seeds: A mini-review. *Antioxidants* **2017**, *6*, 71. [CrossRef] [PubMed]
58. Ma, Z.F.; Lee, Y.Y. Virgin coconut oil and its cardiovascular health benefits. *Nat. Prod. Commun.* **2016**, *11*, 1151–1152.
59. Zhang, H.; Ma, Z.F. Phytochemical and pharmacological poperties of *Capparis spinosa* as a medicinal plant. *Nutrients* **2018**, *10*, 116. [CrossRef] [PubMed]
60. Cao, Y.; Ma, Z.; Zhang, H.; Jin, Y.; Zhang, Y.; Hayford, F. Phytochemical properties and nutrigenomic implications of yacon as a potential source of prebiotic: Current evidence and future directions. *Foods* **2018**, *7*, 59. [CrossRef] [PubMed]
61. Azmi, N.H.; Ismail, N.; Imam, M.U.; Ismail, M. Ethyl acetate extract of germinated brown rice attenuates hydrogen peroxide-induced oxidative stress in human SH-SY5Y neuroblastoma cells: Role of anti-apoptotic, pro-survival and antioxidant genes. *BMC Complement. Altern. Med.* **2013**, *13*, 177. [CrossRef] [PubMed]
62. Imam, M.U.; Ismail, M. Nutrigenomic effects of germinated brown rice and its bioactives on hepatic gluconeogenic genes in type 2 diabetic rats and HEPG2 cells. *Mol. Nutr. Food Res.* **2013**, *57*, 401–411. [CrossRef] [PubMed]
63. Imam, M.U.; Musa, S.N.A.; Azmi, N.H.; Ismail, M. Effects of white rice, brown rice and germinated brown rice on antioxidant status of type 2 diabetic rats. *Int. J. Mol. Sci.* **2012**, *13*, 12952–12969. [CrossRef] [PubMed]
64. Imam, M.U.; Ismail, M.; Omar, A.R. Nutrigenomic effects of germinated brown rice bioactives on antioxidant genes. *Free Radic. Biol. Med.* **2012**, *53*, S105–S106. [CrossRef]
65. Imam, M.U.; Azmi, N.H.; Ismail, M. Upregulation of superoxide dismutase gene is involved in antioxidant effects of germinated rown rice. *Free Radic. Biol. Med.* **2012**, *53*, S84. [CrossRef]
66. Imam, M.U.; Ismail, M.; Omar, A.R.; Ithnin, H. The hypocholesterolemic effect of germinated brown rice involves the upregulation of the apolipoprotein A1 and low-density lipoprotein receptor genes. *J. Diabetes Res.* **2013**, *2013*, 134694. [CrossRef] [PubMed]
67. Imam, M.U.; Ishaka, A.; Ooi, D.-J.; Zamri, N.D.M.; Sarega, N.; Ismail, M.; Esa, N.M. Germinated brown rice regulates hepatic cholesterol metabolism and cardiovascular disease risk in hypercholesterolaemic rats. *J. Funct. Foods* **2014**, *8*, 193–203. [CrossRef]
68. Terashima, Y.; Nagai, Y.; Kato, H.; Ohta, A.; Tanaka, Y. Eating glutinous brown rice for one day improves glycemic control in Japanese patients with type 2 diabetes assessed by continuous glucose monitoring. *Asia Pac. J. Clin. Nutr.* **2017**, *26*, 421–426. [PubMed]
69. Nakayama, T.; Nagai, Y.; Uehara, Y.; Nakamura, Y.; Ishii, S.; Kato, H.; Tanaka, Y. Eating glutinous brown rice twice a day for 8 weeks improves glycemic control in Japanese patients with diabetes mellitus. *Nutr. Diabetes* **2017**, *7*, e273. [CrossRef] [PubMed]
70. Lee, Y.M.; Kim, S.A.; Lee, I.K.; Kim, J.G.; Park, K.G.; Jeong, J.Y.; Jeon, J.H.; Shin, J.Y.; Lee, D.H. Effect of a brown rice based vegan diet and conventional diabetic diet on glycemic control of patients with type 2 diabetes: A 12-week randomized clinical trial. *PLoS ONE* **2016**, *11*, e0155918. [CrossRef] [PubMed]
71. Shobana, S.; Lakshmipriya, N.; Bai, M.R.; Gayathri, R.; Ruchi, V.; Sudha, V.; Malleshi, N.G.; Krishnaswamy, K.; Henry, C.K.; Anjana, R.M.; et al. Even minimal polishing of an Indian parboiled brown rice variety leads to increased glycemic responses. *Asia Pac. J. Clin. Nutr.* **2017**, *26*, 829–836. [PubMed]
72. Ito, Y.; Mizukuchi, A.; Kise, M.; Aoto, H.; Yamamoto, S.; Yoshihara, R.; Yokoyama, J. Postprandial blood glucose and insulin responses to pre-germinated brown rice in healthy subjects. *J. Med. Investig.* **2005**, *52*, 159–164. [CrossRef]
73. Mohan, V.; Spiegelman, D.; Sudha, V.; Gayathri, R.; Hong, B.; Praseena, K.; Anjana, R.M.; Wedick, N.M.; Arumugam, K.; Malik, V.; et al. Effect of brown rice, white rice, and brown rice with legumes on blood glucose and insulin responses in overweight Asian Indians: A randomized controlled trial. *Diabetes Technol. Ther.* **2014**, *16*, 317–325. [CrossRef] [PubMed]
74. Panlasigui, L.N.; Thompson, L.U. Blood glucose lowering effects of brown rice in normal and diabetic subjects. *Int. J. Food Sci. Nutr.* **2006**, *57*, 151–158. [CrossRef] [PubMed]

75. Kozuka, C.; Yabiku, K.; Takayama, C.; Matsushita, M.; Shimabukuro, M. Natural food science based novel approach toward prevention and treatment of obesity and type 2 diabetes: Recent studies on brown rice and gamma-oryzanol. *Obes. Res. Clin. Pract.* **2013**, *7*, e165–e172. [CrossRef] [PubMed]
76. Ou, S.; Kwok, K.; Li, Y.; Fu, L. In vitro study of possible role of dietary fiber in lowering postprandial serum glucose. *J. Agric. Food Chem.* **2001**, *49*, 1026–1029. [CrossRef] [PubMed]
77. Seki, T.; Nagase, R.; Torimitsu, M.; Yanagi, M.; Ito, Y.; Kise, M.; Mizukuchi, A.; Fujimura, N.; Hayamizu, K.; Ariga, T. Insoluble fiber is a major constituent responsible for lowering the post-prandial blood glucose concentration in the pre-germinated brown rice. *Biol. Pharm. Bull.* **2005**, *28*, 1539–1541. [CrossRef] [PubMed]
78. Jaskari, J.; Kontula, P.; Siitonen, A.; Jousimies-Somer, H.; Mattila-Sandholm, T.; Poutanen, K. Oat beta-glucan and xylan hydrolysates as selective substrates for *Bifidobacterium* and *Lactobacillus* strains. *Appl. Microbiol. Biotechnol.* **1998**, *49*, 175–181. [CrossRef] [PubMed]
79. Benno, Y.; Endo, K.; Miyoshi, H.; Okuda, T.; Koishi, H.; Mitsuoka, T. Effect of rice fiber on human fecal microflora. *Microbiol. Immunol.* **1989**, *33*, 435–440. [CrossRef] [PubMed]
80. Nagasaka, R.; Yamsaki, T.; Uchida, A.; Ohara, K.; Ushio, H. Gamma-oryzanol recovers mouse hypoadiponectinemia induced by animal fat ingestion. *Phytomedicine* **2011**, *18*, 669–671. [CrossRef] [PubMed]
81. Ohara, K.; Kiyotani, Y.; Uchida, A.; Nagasaka, R.; Maehara, H.; Kanemoto, S.; Hori, M.; Ushio, H. Oral administration of gamma-aminobutyric acid and gamma-oryzanol prevents stress-induced hypoadiponectinemia. *Phytomedicine* **2011**, *18*, 655–660. [CrossRef] [PubMed]
82. Usuki, S.; Ito, Y.; Morikawa, K.; Kise, M.; Ariga, T.; Rivner, M.; Yu, R.K. Effect of pre-germinated brown rice intake on diabetic neuropathy in streptozotocin-induced diabetic rats. *Nutr. Metab.* **2007**, *4*, 25. [CrossRef] [PubMed]
83. Usuki, S.; Tsai, Y.Y.; Morikawa, K.; Nonaka, S.; Okuhara, Y.; Kise, M.; Yu, R.K. IGF-1 induction by acylated steryl beta-glucosides found in a pre-germinated brown rice diet reduces oxidative stress in streptozotocin-induced diabetes. *PLoS ONE* **2011**, *6*, e28693. [CrossRef] [PubMed]
84. Nordestgaard, B.G.; Varbo, A. Triglycerides and cardiovascular disease. *Lancet* **2014**, *384*, 626–635. [CrossRef]
85. Shen, K.-P.; Hao, C.-L.; Yen, H.-W.; Chen, C.-Y.; Chen, J.-H.; Chen, F.-C.; Lin, H.-L. Pre-germinated brown rice prevented high fat diet induced hyperlipidemia through ameliorating lipid synthesis and metabolism in C57BL/6J mice. *J. Clin. Biochem. Nutr.* **2016**, *59*, 39–44. [CrossRef] [PubMed]
86. Ho, J.N.; Son, M.E.; Lim, W.C.; Lim, S.T.; Cho, H.Y. Anti-obesity effects of germinated brown rice extract through down-regulation of lipogenic genes in high fat diet-induced obese mice. *Biosci. Biotechnol. Biochem.* **2012**, *76*, 1068–1074. [CrossRef] [PubMed]
87. Miura, D.; Ito, Y.; Mizukuchi, A.; Kise, M.; Aoto, H.; Yagasaki, K. Hypocholesterolemic action of pre-germinated brown rice in hepatoma-bearing rats. *Life Sci.* **2006**, *79*, 259–264. [CrossRef] [PubMed]
88. Roohinejad, S.; Omidizadeh, A.; Mirhosseini, H.; Saari, N.; Mustafa, S.; Yusof, R.M.; Hussin, A.S.; Hamid, A.; Abd Manap, M.Y. Effect of pre-germination time of brown rice on serum cholesterol levels of hypercholesterolaemic rats. *J. Sci. Food Agric.* **2010**, *90*, 245–251. [CrossRef] [PubMed]
89. Albarracin, M.; Weisstaub, A.R.; Zuleta, A.; Drago, S.R. Extruded whole grain diets based on brown, soaked and germinated rice. Effects on cecum health, calcium absorption and bone parameters of growing Wistar rats. Part I. *Food Funct.* **2016**, *7*, 2722–2728. [CrossRef] [PubMed]
90. Bui, T.N.; Le, T.H.; Nguyen, D.H.; Tran, Q.B.; Nguyen, T.L.; Le, D.T.; Do, V.A.; Vu, A.L.; Aoto, H.; Okuhara, Y.; et al. Pre-germinated brown rice reduced both blood glucose concentration and body weight in Vietnamese women with impaired glucose tolerance. *J. Nutr. Sci. Vitaminol.* **2014**, *60*, 183–187. [CrossRef] [PubMed]
91. Hsu, T.F.; Kise, M.; Wang, M.F.; Ito, Y.; Yang, M.D.; Aoto, H.; Yoshihara, R.; Yokoyama, J.; Kunii, D.; Yamamoto, S. Effects of pre-germinated brown rice on blood glucose and lipid levels in free-living patients with impaired fasting glucose or type 2 diabetes. *J. Nutr. Sci. Vitaminol.* **2008**, *54*, 163–168. [CrossRef] [PubMed]
92. Morita, H.; Uno, Y.; Umemoto, T.; Sugiyama, C.; Matsumoto, M.; Wada, Y.; Ishizuka, T. Effect of gamma-aminobutyric acid-rich germinated brown rice on indexes of life-style related diseases. *Nihon Ronen Igakkai Zasshi* **2004**, *41*, 211–216. [CrossRef] [PubMed]
93. Wu, C.; Ye, Z.; Li, H.; Wu, S.; Deng, D.; Zhu, Y.; Wong, M. Do radial oxygen loss and external aeration affect iron plaque formation and arsenic accumulation and speciation in rice? *J. Exp. Bot.* **2012**, *63*, 2961–2970. [CrossRef] [PubMed]

94. Saki, E.; Saiful Yazan, L.; Mohd Ali, R.; Ahmad, Z. Chemopreventive effects of germinated rough rice crude extract in inhibiting azoxymethane-induced aberrant crypt foci formation in sprague-dawley rats. *BioMed Res. Int.* **2017**, *2017*, 9517287. [CrossRef] [PubMed]
95. Latifah, S.Y.; Armania, N.; Tze, T.H.; Azhar, Y.; Nordiana, A.H.; Norazalina, S.; Hairuszah, I.; Saidi, M.; Maznah, I. Germinated brown rice (GBR) reduces the incidence of aberrant crypt foci with the involvement of beta-catenin and COX-2 in azoxymethane-induced colon cancer in rats. *Nutr. J.* **2010**, *9*, 16. [CrossRef] [PubMed]
96. Oh, C.H.; Oh, S.H. Effects of germinated brown rice extracts with enhanced levels of GABA on cancer cell proliferation and apoptosis. *J. Med. Food* **2004**, *7*, 19–23. [CrossRef] [PubMed]
97. Schuller, H.M.; Al-Wadei, H.A.; Majidi, M. Gamma-aminobutyric acid, a potential tumor suppressor for small airway-derived lung adenocarcinoma. *Carcinogenesis* **2008**, *29*, 1979–1985. [CrossRef] [PubMed]
98. Har, C.H.; Keong, C.K. Effects of tocotrienols on cell viability and apoptosis in normal murine liver cells (BNL CL.2) and liver cancer cells (BNL 1ME A.7R.1), in vitro. *Asia Pac. J. Clin. Nutr.* **2005**, *14*, 374–380. [PubMed]
99. Go, A.S.; Mozaffarian, D.; Roger, V.L.; Benjamin, E.J.; Berry, J.D.; Blaha, M.J.; Dai, S.; Ford, E.S.; Fox, C.S.; Franco, S.; et al. Heart Disease and Stroke Statistics—2014 Update: A Report From the American Heart Association. *Circulation* **2014**, *129*, e28–e292. [CrossRef] [PubMed]
100. Kazemzadeh, M.; Safavi, S.M.; Nematollahi, S.; Nourieh, Z. Effect of brown rice consumption on inflammatory marker and cardiovascular risk factors among overweight and obese non-menopausal female adults. *Int. J. Prev. Med.* **2014**, *5*, 478–488. [PubMed]
101. Ebizuka, H.; Sasaki, C.; Kise, M.; Arita, M. Effects of retort pouched rice containing pre-germinated brown rice on daily nutrition and physical status in healthy subjects. *J. Integr. Study Diet. Habits* **2007**, *18*, 216–222. [CrossRef]
102. Ebizuka, H.; Ihara, M.; Arita, M. Antihypertensive effect of pre-germinated brown rice in spontaneously hypertensive rats. *Food Sci. Technol. Res.* **2009**, *15*, 625–630. [CrossRef]
103. Choi, H.-D.; Kim, Y.-S.; Choi, I.-W.; Park, Y.-K.; Park, Y.-D. Hypotensive effect of germinated brown rice on spontaneously hypertensive rats. *Korean J. Food Sci. Technol.* **2006**, *38*, 448–451.
104. Suzuki, A.; Kagawa, D.; Fujii, A.; Ochiai, R.; Tokimitsu, I.; Saito, I. Short- and long-term effects of ferulic acid on blood pressure in spontaneously hypertensive rats. *Am. J. Hypertens.* **2002**, *15*, 351–357. [CrossRef]
105. Ohsaki, Y.; Shirakawa, H.; Koseki, T.; Komai, M. Novel effects of a single administration of ferulic acid on the regulation of blood pressure and the hepatic lipid metabolic profile in stroke-prone spontaneously hypertensive rats. *J. Agric. Food Chem.* **2008**, *56*, 2825–2830.
106. Shao, Y.; Bao, J. Polyphenols in whole rice grain: Genetic diversity and health benefits. *Food Chem.* **2015**, *180*, 86–97. [CrossRef] [PubMed]
107. Sakamoto, S.; Hayashi, T.; Hayashi, K.; Murai, F.; Hori, M.; Kimoto, K.; Murakami, K. Pre-germinated brown rice could enhance maternal mental health and immunity during lactation. *Eur. J. Nutr.* **2007**, *46*, 391–396. [CrossRef] [PubMed]
108. Wunjuntuk, K.; Kettawan, A.; Rungruang, T.; Charoenkiatkul, S. Anti-fibrotic and anti-inflammatory effects of parboiled germinated brown rice (*Oryza sativa* 'KDML 105') in rats with induced liver fibrosis. *J. Funct. Foods* **2016**, *26*, 363–372. [CrossRef]
109. Zhang, H.; Ma, Z.F.; Luo, X.; Li, X. Effect of mulberry fruit (*Morus alba* L.) consumption on health outcomes: A mini-review. *Antioxidants* **2018**, *7*, 69. [CrossRef]

6

Vitamin E as a Treatment for Nonalcoholic Fatty Liver Disease: Reality or Myth?

Hamza El Hadi, Roberto Vettor and Marco Rossato *

Internal Medicine 3, Department of Medicine—DIMED, University of Padova, Via Giustiniani 2, 35128 Padova, Italy; dr.hamza.elhadi@gmail.com (H.E.H.); roberto.vettor@unipd.it (R.V.)

* Correspondence: marco.rossato@unipd.it

Abstract: Obesity is one of the major epidemics of this millennium, and its incidence is growing worldwide. Following the epidemics of obesity, nonalcoholic fatty liver disease (NAFLD) has become a disease of increasing prevalence and a leading cause of morbidity and mortality closely related to cardiovascular disease, malignancies, and cirrhosis. It is believed that oxidative stress is a main player in the development and progression of NAFLD. Currently, a pharmacological approach has become necessary in NAFLD because of a failure to modify lifestyle and dietary habits in most patients. Vitamin E is a potent antioxidant that has been shown to reduce oxidative stress in NAFLD. This review summarizes the biological activities of vitamin E, with a primary focus on its therapeutic efficacy in NAFLD.

Keywords: vitamin E; nonalcoholic fatty liver disease; obesity; oxidative stress

---

1. Introduction

Nonalcoholic fatty liver disease (NAFLD) is defined as the accumulation of excessive fat in the liver, as demonstrated by imaging or by histology, in the setting of no significant alcohol consumptionand the absence of any secondary cause [1].

NAFLD encompasses a broad pathological spectrum of phenotypes ranging from isolated hepatic steatosis (IHS) to nonalcoholic steatohepatitis (NASH)—the progressive form of fatty liver disease associated with inflammation and cellular injury, which can lead to NASH-related cirrhosis and hepatocellular carcinoma [2]. This pathology is now regarded as a leading cause of chronic liver diseases and liver transplantation in most countries [3]. In addition, NAFLD has been also linked to extra-hepatic morbidity, including systemic metabolic complications, chronic kidney and cardiovascular disease, and malignancies, which all contribute to a higher mortality observed in NASH patients [4].

NAFLD is strongly associated with obesity and related metabolic disorders such as insulin resistance and dyslipidemia. In the last decades, adult and childhood obesity has reached epidemic levels, and as a consequence the global prevalence of NAFLD has increased significantly. According to a recent report, prevalence estimates in the general population of Europe and the Middle East are 20–30%, with higher prevalence in Western countries' populations with obesity or diabetes (75%) and with morbid obesity (90–95%) [5].

It is acknowledged that vitamin E is the major lipid-soluble chain-breaking antioxidant found in the human body. In addition to its anti-oxidative properties, molecules of the vitamin E family exertanti-atherogenicand anti-inflammatory activities [6]. Although the pathogenesis of NAFLD and its progression to fibrosis needs to be fully clarified, it is believed that oxidative stress plays a crucial role in producing the lethal hepatocyte injury associated with NAFLD.

Therefore, by targeting oxidative stress components, vitamin E appears as a promising therapeutic approach in NASH patients.

The present review briefly discusses the biological activities of vitamin E, focusing on its potential as a treatment for NAFLD/NASH. To this aim, we also highlight the role of oxidative stress in the pathogenesis of NAFLD.

2. Vitamin E: Brief Overview of Structure, Metabolism and Function

2.1. Structural Perspectives

The discovery of vitamin E dates back to 1922 due to the observations of Herbert Evans and his associate Bishop who isolated an as-yet uncharacterized fat-soluble compound from green leafy vegetables which is required for reproduction in rats [7]. Upon isolating this dietary compound, it was termed as tocopherol (Greek: tocos—child birth; pheros—to bear; ol—alcohol). Today the term "vitamin E" encompasses a group of eight lipophilic molecules that are synthesized by plants starting from homogentisic acid. It includes four tocopherols and four tocotrienols. Tocopherols and tocotrienols are subdivided into alpha (α), beta (β), gamma (γ), and delta (ε) forms based on the methyl and hydroxyl substitution in their phenolic rings [8] (Figure 1). The tocopherols are saturated forms of vitamin E, whereas the tocotrienols are unsaturated and possess an isoprenoid side chain [8]. α-Tocopherol is considered the most abundant form in nature, and is consequently the most widely studied. Common food oils including corn, peanut, and soybean oil contain largely α-tocopherol. In contrast, tocotrienols are relatively rarer in food sources and prevail in rice bran, barley, oats, and palm oil [9].

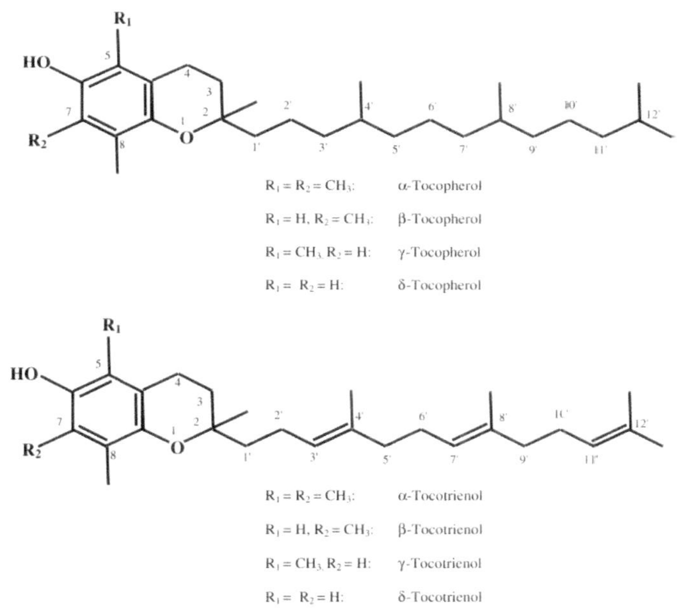

Figure 1. Structure of tocopherols and tocotrienols (with permission from reference [8]).

Currently, synthetic forms of vitamin E consist mainly of α-tocopherol, whichwas first synthesized in 1938 [10]. Unlike naturally-occurring d-RRR-α-tocopherol, synthesized α-tocopherol consists of a racemic mixture of eight stereoisomers named the all-racemic or (2RS, 4′RS, 8′RS) product [11].

2.2. Insight into Metabolism

Like other fat-soluble vitamins, the bioavailability of vitamin E depends on pancreatic function, biliary secretion, micellar formation, and penetration across intestinal membranes. After being cleaved by the enzyme esterase located in the stomach lining and partly processed enzymatically in the stomach by gastric lipase, vitamin E isoforms reach the basolateral side of enterocytes [12,13]. In the intestinal lumen, dietary tocopherols and tocotrienols appear to be similarly absorbed along with dietary fat, and are secreted in chylomicron particles together with triacylglycerol, phospholipids, and cholesterol [12,13]. The chylomicron-bound vitamin E isoforms are then transferred to peripheral tissues such as adipose tissues, bones, brain, lung, muscle, and skin via the lymphatic system. During their transport, chylomicrons are catabolized in the circulation by the endothelial-bound enzyme, which hydrolyzes triglycerides, releasing free fatty acids (FFAs) [12,13]. The resulting chylomicron remnants containing absorbed vitamin E are subsequently taken up by the liver, probably by a receptor-mediated process, and then preferentially incorporated within very low density lipoprotein (VLDL) and high-density lipoprotein (HDL) into the bloodstream [12]. After hepatic uptake, the α-tocopherol form of vitamin E is preferentially re-excreted into the circulation. α-Tocopherol transfer protein (α-TTP), a small cytoplasmic hepatic protein with differential affinity for various vitamin E forms, is responsible for the biodiscriminating process underlying the selective resecretion of α-tocopherol from the liver into plasma [14].

While α-TTP has a high affinity for α-tocopherol (100%), it has a lower affinity for other vitamin E isoforms: approximately 50% for β-tocopherol, 10–30% for γ-tocopherol, and 1% for δ-tocopherol [12]. In the liver, isoforms not bound to α-TTP will be susceptible to catabolization via cytochrome P450 (CYP4F2)-initiated ω-hydroxylation and oxidation by ω-hydroxylase, and thus vitamin E isoforms are metabolized to carboxychromanols, hydroxycarboxychromanol, and carboxyethylhydroxychroman derivatives [15]. Besides catabolism, it was estimated that metabolized vitamin E isoforms are also discarded via biliary excretion [16].

2.3. *Biological Activity of Vitamin E*

2.3.1. Antioxidant Activity

Oxidative stress is defined as the imbalance between the generation of reactive species and antioxidant defense, and leads to the damage of DNA and disturbances in cellular biology [17]. Vitamin E is widely accepted as one of the most potent antioxidants in nature [18]. The antioxidant property is attributed to the hydroxyl group from the aromatic ring of tocochromanols, which donates hydrogen to neutralize free radicals or reactive oxygen species (ROS). The antioxidant activity of α-, β-, γ-isoforms of tocotrienols and tocopherols is similar, but the γ-isoform showed weaker activity when tested in pyrogallolsulfonphthalein and 2,7-dichlorodihydrofluorescein diacetate methods [18,19].

In the same context, the antioxidant efficacy of vitamin E on reactive nitrogen species (RNS) has been gaining more attention recently. RNS include nitric oxide (NO), nitrogen dioxide (NO_2), and peroxynitrite ($ONOO^-$) [20–22].

On the other hand, in vitro studies have shown that vitamin E can alternatively switch to a pro-oxidant action under certain circumstances, such as a constant low-level flux of initiator free radicals and the absence of co-antioxidants as such as vitamin C [23]. In addition, current evidence from in vivo studies showed that vitamin E may produce pro-oxidant effects at high doses [24] or in cigarette smokers consuming a high polyunsaturated fat diet [25].

2.3.2. Beyond Vitamin E Antioxidant Activity

Vitamin E biological activity is not limited to antioxidant properties. In fact, vitamin E forms are involved in the regulation of inflammatory response, gene expression, membrane-bound enzymes, modulation of cellular signaling, and cell proliferation.

Over the last two decades, vitamin E has been shown to have direct and indirect effects on several enzymes involved in signal transduction, such as protein kinase C (PKC), protein phosphatase 2A (PP2A), protein tyrosine phosphatase (PTP), protein tyrosine kinase (PTK), diacylglycerol kinase (DAGK), 5-, 12- and 15-lipoxygenases (5-, 12-, and 15-LOX), phospholipase A2 (PLA2), cyclooxygenase-2 (COX-2), and the mitogen activated protein kinase (MAPK) signal transduction pathway [26,27].

The first evidence that vitamin E can modulate enzymes involved in signal transduction came from studies with PKC when α-tocopherol exerted an inhibitory effect unrelated to antioxidant action [28]. PKC inhibition by α-tocopherol is mainly correlated with the reduction of cell proliferation in many different cell types, including vascular smooth muscle cells, monocytes/macrophages, neutrophils, fibroblasts, mesangial cells, as well as various cancer cell lines [29]. In addition to interference with cell proliferation, the inhibition of PKC by α-tocopherol inhibited NADPH-oxidase assembly in monocytes, leading to lower superoxide production [30]. Additionally, PKC inhibition mediated by α-tocopherol and not by β-tocopherol suppressed endothelin secretion in endothelial cells [31].

Another evidence of a non-antioxidant function of α-tocopherol is related to its role in regulating the expression of specific genes not only coupled to oxidative stress but also involved in cholesterol homeostasis, inflammatory pathways, and cellular trafficking [32,33]. These genes include those encoding for proteins involved in inflammation and cell adhesion (such as E-selectin, intercellular adhesion molecule-1, vascular cell adhesion molecule [VCAM]-1, integrin, interleukin [IL]-1b, IL-2, IL-4, and transforming growth factor [TGF]-β), extracellular matrix formation and degradation (tropomyosin, glycoprotein IIb, collagen A1, matrix metalloproteinase [MMP]-1, MMP-19 and connective tissue growth factor), cell cycle regulation (cyclin D1, cyclin E1, and p27), transcriptional control lipoprotein (peroxisome proliferator-activated receptor [PPAR]-γ), receptors (CD36, scavenger receptor class B type 1, low density lipoprotein receptor), and metabolism (Cytochrome P450 3A4 [CYP3A4] and HMG-CoA reductase) [32,33].

3. Vitamin E and NAFLD

3.1. NAFLD/NASH Pathogenesis

NAFLD is a complex disease trait where inter-patient genetic and epigenetic variations and environmental factors are combined to define development and disease progression [34] (Figure 2).

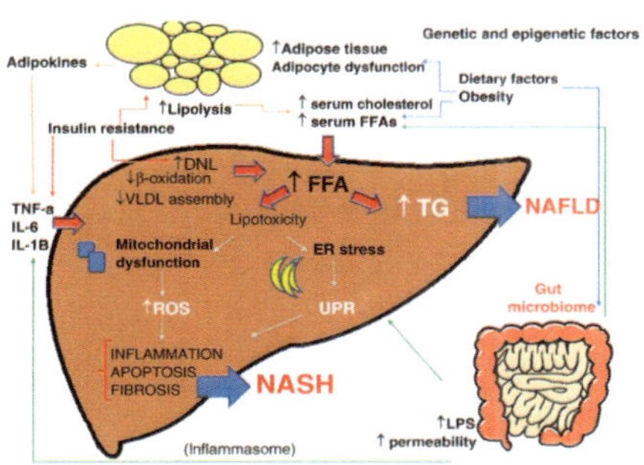

Figure 2. Multiple parallel-hit hypothesis of nonalcoholic fatty liver disease (NAFLD). Obesity together with dietary habits and environmental factors can lead to raised serum levels of free fatty acids (FFAs) and cholesterol, development of insulin resistance, adipocyte proliferation, and dysfunction in the intestinal microbiome. Insulin resistance acts on adipose tissue, worsening adipocyte dysfunction, induces hepatic de novo lipogenesis (DNL) and release of proinflammatory adipokines such as interleukin (IL)-6, IL-1β, and tumor necrosis factor (TNF)-α, which also exacerbates the insulin resistance state. The increased hepatic FFAs flux which derives from the above processes and from an altered activity of the gut microbiome leads to accumulation of triglycerides (TGs) and "toxic"levels of FFAs, free cholesterol, and other lipid metabolites which cause mitochondrial dysfunction, oxidative stress with the production of reactive oxygen species (ROS), and endoplasmic reticulum (ER) stress with the activation of the unfolded protein response (UPR), all leading to hepatic inflammation and fibrogenesis (nonalcoholic steatohepatitis, NASH). Increased intestinal permeability of gut-derived microbial products such as lipopolysaccharides (LPS) contributes to the activation of the inflammasome, ER stress, and activation of inflammatory cascades. Epigenetic factors are also involved in progression to NASH or persistence in a stable stage of disease (with permission from [34]). VLDL: very low density lipoprotein.

The generally accepted dogma in the pathogenesis of NAFLD is that insulin resistance—commonly associated with obesity—leads to the hepatic accumulation of triglycerides, a process that usually results from increased FFAs flux from adipose tissue to the liver, dietary fat via chylomicron metabolism, and increased de novo lipogenesis [35–37]. Obesity generates a state of low-grade inflammation characterized by the accumulation of immune cells in adipose tissue (particularly macrophages), and the production of proinflammatory cytokines by adipocytes contributes to the development of systemic and hepatic insulin resistance [35–37]. However, multiple pathways (multiple hits) are involved in the development of NASH and fibrosis. "Hits" that may contribute include oxidative stress, endotoxins, changes in the gut–liver axis, and mitochondrial dysfunction [34].

Oxidative stress and mitochondrial dysfunction were proposed as main triggers for the progression of steatosis to steatohepatitis [38]. FFAs catabolism in the liver takes place mainly via mitochondrial β-oxidation—a process that can lead to the generation of ROS, including superoxide, hydrogen peroxide, and hydroxyl radicals, in the case of increased FFAs delivery [38].

In the same context, impaired mitochondrial activity in NASH patients due to reduced enzymatic activities of mitochondrial electron transport chain and excessive in FA oxidation results in hepatic ATP depletion and may cause structural mitochondrial abnormalities consisting of enlargement (megamitochondria), paracrystalline inclusions, and loss of cristae [39,40].

In NAFLD, enhanced cytochrome P450 2E1 (CYP2E1) expression and activity seem to be an important source of ROS which trigger oxidative stress and perpetuate the hepatic mitochondrial dysfunction [41]. Moreover, it has been reported that upregulated microsomal CYP4A enzymes ω-hydroxylate fatty acids into dicarboxylic acids that are then preferentially oxidized by peroxisomes, thus promoting ROS production in NAFLD [42]. The ablation of a homolog of human CYP4A gene (CYP4A14) in animal models of steatohepatitis has shown to attenuate hepatic inflammation and fibrosis [43]. The abundant production of ROS induces the peroxidation of hepatic triglycerides with the release of reactive aldehydes such as 4-hydroxynonenal (4-HNE) and malondialdehyde (MDA) which can damage mitochondrial components [44].

Accumulating data have implicated the disruption of endoplasmic reticulum (ER) homeostasis (i.e., ER stress) in the development of NASH [45]. Factors that disturb ER folding capacity (e.g., excessive protein synthesis, mitochondrial dysfunction, oxidative stress) will lead to the activation of a physiologic mechanism called the "unfolded protein response" (UPR) in hepatocytes. This adaptive mechanism aims to increase the folding capacity of the ER, thus bringing the organelle and the cell into a state of equilibrium. When the activation of the UPR fails to promote cell survival, the cell is taken down the pro-apoptotic ER stress response pathway, which can ultimately lead to apoptotic cell death, inflammation, and/or fat accumulation [45].

Several studies have suggested a role of gut microbiome in NASH pathogenesis [46]. Intestinal barrier alterations cause increased intestinal permeability of bacteria, viruses, or microbial products such as lipopolysaccharide (LPS). These pathogens are recognized through specialized recognition receptors that include toll-like receptors (TLRs) and inflammasomes, inducing a signaling cascade leading to the production of inflammatory cytokines [46].

3.2. Vitamin E and NAFLD: Experimental Studies

The methionine and choline deficient (MCD) diet is a widely employed diet in NASH animal studies. The MCD diet is high in sucrose and fat (40% sucrose, 10% fat), and is deficient in methionine and choline, which are essential for hepatic beta-oxidation and the production of VLDL [47].

A trial carried out with rats fed with an MCD-diet showed that vitamin E significantly reduces the oxidative stress. In the control group, the authors observed a depletion in the liver glutathione stores and a notable increase in hepatic fibrosis, whereas vitamin E supplementation repleted hepatic glutathione, reduced steatosis, inflammation, hepatic stellate cell activation, and collagen mRNA expression, and ameliorated fibrosis [48].

In another animal NASH model, the combination of MCD diet and vitamin E significantly lowered serum transaminase levels and ameliorated hepatic steatosis and necroinflammation. These effects were associated with suppressed expression of the fibrotic genes TGF-β and MMP-2, inflammatory factor COX-2, and pro-apoptotic genes (Bax). In addition, vitamin E enhanced the activity of hepatic superoxide dismutase (SOD) and inhibited that of nuclear factor kappa B (NFkB) [49].

Similar effects were reported in arecent mouse model for NAFLD in which vitamin E therapy after partial hepatectomy significantly reduced the oxidative stress level and attenuated the progression of NAFLD [50].

In an obese (ob/ob) mouse model, α- or γ-tocopherol exerted a hepatoprotective role in alipopolysaccharide-induced NASH, as shown by suppressing hepatic malondialdehyde (MDA), tumor necrosis factor-α, and serum alanine aminotransferase levels [51].

Moreover, chickens fed ahigh-oxidant diet with the supplementation of vitamin E were able to normalize elevated hepatic transaminase levels [52]. In addition to the role of being an antioxidant, some studies have also proposed that vitamin E improves the liver integrity by down-regulating hepatic cluster of differentiation 36 protein (CD36)—a membrane transporter responsible for the uptake of fatty acids into the liver [53].

3.3. Vitamin E and NAFLD: Human Studies

Vitamin E has been used in monotherapy or with other agents in multiple clinical trials to treat NAFLD or NASH, with reported improvement in liver biochemistries and histology [54–68]. These trials varied in duration (24 weeks to >2 years) and dose (100–1200 IU/day) of vitamin E used. Long-term studies (≥2 years) are summarized in Table 1.

Treatment with vitamin E combined with vitamin C and atorvastatin was demonstrated to be effective in reducing the odds of having hepatic steatosis in individuals with computed tomography (CT)-diagnosed NAFLD after 4 years of active therapy [63].

The combination of ursodeoxycholic acid (UDCA) with vitamin E has been evaluated in a small sample size compared with UDCA alone or placebo. Improvement in steatosis and transaminases level were observed only in the group who received combination therapy with UDCA and vitamin E [64]. By evaluating the long-term (>2 years) efficacy of a similar combination (UDCA with vitamin E) in patients with NASH, Piettu et al.demonstrated an improvement in histological lesions in the majority of patients [62].

Nobili et al.studied 90 children with NAFLD who were given calorie-restricted diet and exercise. Patients were randomized to treatment with vitamin E (600 IU/day) in combination with ascorbic acid (500 mg/daily; n = 45) or placebo (n = 45) [65]. At the end of 24 months, both groups had significant improvement in steatosis, lobular inflammation, hepatocyte ballooning. However, the addition of α-tocopherol and ascorbic acid was not associated with a greater histological or biochemical improvement as compared to placebo [65,66].

Clinical trials with vitamin E supplementation in NASH patients yielded promising results. In the PIVENS (Pioglitazone, Vitamin E or Placebo for Nonalcoholic Steatohepatitis) trial, vitamin E was evaluated as a treatment for NASH. The rate of achievement of the primary outcome was higher in patients treated with high-dose vitamin E (800 IU/day) for 96 weeks compared to placebo (43% vs. 19%, p = 0.001), while pioglitazone did not reach statistical significance. The histological analysis showed a reduction in hepatocyte ballooning (50% vs. 29%, p = 0.005) and lobular inflammation (54% vs. 35%, p = 0.02), thus reflecting its expected effect as an antioxidant leading to a decrease of oxidative stress-mediated injury. Interestingly, it significantly reduced liver steatosis and alanine aminotransferase (ALT), but had no significant changes on fibrosis [60].

Table 1. Effects of Vitamin E administration in patients with NAFLD.

Author	Study Design	Duration	Vitamin E Dosage	Effect of Vitamin E on NAFLD/NASH Histology and Biochemistry Compared to Placebo				
				ALT	Steatosis	Inflammation	Hepatocytes Ballooning	Fibrosis
Dufour et al., 2006 [64]	48 NASH patients randomized to vitamin E plus UDCA, UDCA versus placebo	2 years	400 IU twice daily	↓	↓	ns	NA	ns
Nobili et al., 2008 [66]	53 NAFLD patients randomized to vitamin E plus ascorbic and life style intervention versus placebo	2 years	600 IU/day	ns	ns	ns	ns	ns
Sanyal et al., 2010 [60]	247 NASH patients randomized to vitamin E, pioglitazone versus placebo	96 weeks	800 IU daily	↓		↓	↓	ns
Foster et al., 2011 [63]	1005 randomized to vitamin E combined with ascorbic acid and atorvastatin versus placebo. At baseline 80 had CT-diagnosed NAFLD	4 years	1000 IU daily	ns	↓ (Based on abdominal CT scan)	NA	NA	NA
Lavine et al., 2011 [61]	173 NAFLD patients randomized to vitamin E, metformin versus placebo	96 weeks	400 IU twice daily	ns	ns	ns	↓	ns
Pietu et al., 2012 [62]	101 patients treated with a combination of vitamin E with UDCA. 10 patients had a second liver biopsy during follow-up	4 years	500 IU daily	↓	↓ 3/10 ↑ 1/10 patients	↓ 3/10 ↑ 2/10 patients	↓ 3/10 ↑ 1/10patients	↓ 4/10 ↑ 1/10 patients

ALT: alanine aminotransferase; CT: computed tomography; NAFLD: nonalcoholic fatty liver disease; NASH: nonalcoholic steatohepatitis; ns: no significant statistical difference versus placebo; NA: not available; UDCA: ursodeoxycholic acid; ↑: worsening; ↓: improvement.

Following those studies, Lavine et al. conducted a multicenter, double-blind, double-placebo, randomized clinical trial in pediatric patients. The TONIC (Treatment of NAFLD in Children) trial involved 173 children and adolescents witha mean age of 13 years that received metformin (500 mg twice daily), vitamin E (400 IU twice daily), or placebo twice daily for 96 weeks. The primary outcome was sustained reduction in ALT level (defined as ≤50% baseline or ≤40 U/L from 48 weeks to 96 weeks of treatment). The only histologic feature of NASH that improved after treatment with both medications was the hepatocellular ballooning. Disappointingly, neither vitamin E nor metformin were superior to placebo in achieving sustained ALT reduction or in improving steatosis, lobular inflammation, or fibrosis scores [61].

In the light of these observations, today the European Association for the Study of the Liver (EASL) and the American Association for the Study of Liver Diseases (AASLD) (Alexandria, VA, USA) guidelines consider vitamin E as a potential short-term treatment for non-diabetic adults with biopsy-proven NASH [69]. Until further data supporting its effectiveness is available, vitamin E is not recommended to treat NASH in diabetic patients, NAFLD without liver biopsy, NASH cirrhosis, or cryptogenic cirrhosis [1,69].

3.4. Vitamin E: Safety Concerns

Long-term safety should be carefully discussed with NASH patients before starting therapy with vitamin E.A meta-analysis has suggested that high-dosage (≥400 IU/day) vitamin E supplements may increase all-cause mortality [70]. However, this meta-analysis has been criticized because several studies with low mortality were excluded and concomitant vitamin A and the administration of other drugs as well as common factors such as smoking were not considered. Another meta-analysis where new clinical trials and updated results of mortality were included suggested that the higher mortality can be explained by a higher proportion of male patients that were included in these trials and not due to the higher dose of vitamin E supplementation [71]. On the other hand, large meta-analysis that included 57 trials showed that vitamin E supplementation appears to have no effect on all-cause mortality at doses up to 5500 IU/day [72].

Finally, a meta-analysis investigating the effect of vitamin E on the incidence of stroke reported an increase in the relative risk of hemorrhagic stroke by 22%, while the risk of ischemic stroke was reduced by 10% [73]. Another concern about vitamin E use is related to its association with a modest increase in the risk of prostate cancer [74].

Thus, patients chosen for treatment with vitamin E should be aware of these risks or be considered for alternative treatments.

4. Conclusions

Despite its high prevalence and the intensive research in the field, the treatment of NAFLD remains an unmet medical need. To date, no definite pharmacological treatment has been approved for NAFLD, and patients are often advised to engage in physical activity and lose weight, which is difficult to achieve and more difficult to maintain. However, policies to promote physical activity and the management of associated comorbidities (i.e., obesity and metabolic syndrome components) are expected to decrease both hepatic and cardiovascular-related morbidity and mortality in NASH patients.

Clinical trials for NAFLD or NASH showed a modest improvement in liver biochemistries and histology induced by vitamin E administration. However, some limitations of these trials should be noted. The duration of therapy may be not long enough to detect long-term histological change complications. Moreover, the number of randomized trials included was limited, and the number of participants in the trials was low. An additional reason for the lack of efficacy of vitamin E could be related to the use of oral preparations of varied dosage, which may not always guarantee an adequate bioavailability in patients with liver disease.

In this context, further monotherapy clinical trials and pharmacological evaluations are still needed to elucidate the underlying molecular mechanisms of prevention or therapy and possible adverse outcomes. This may also help to identify the optimal daily intake of vitamin E in both pediatric and adult patients.

In addition, more research is needed to seek novel biological activities of vitamin Emetabolites in the liver of NAFLD patients that may differ from those of parent compounds.

Finally, a better understanding of the pathophysiology of NAFLD/NASH will provide the opportunity to create trials of combination therapies that achieve high rates of therapeutic responses.

Author Contributions: Hamza El Hadi, Roberto Vettor and Marco Rossato designed the concept and wrote the manuscript.

Conflicts of Interest: The authors declare no conflict of interest.

References

1. Chalasani, N.; Younoss, Z.; Lavine, J.E.; Diehl, A.M.; Brunt, E.M.; Cusi, K.; Charlton, M.; Sanyal, A.J. The diagnosis and management of non-alcoholic fatty liver disease: Practice Guideline by the American Association for the Study of Liver Diseases, American College of Gastroenterology, and the American Gastroenterological Association. *Hepatology* **2012**, *55*, 2005–2023. [CrossRef] [PubMed]
2. Polyzos, S.A.; Kountouras, J.; Zavos, C. Nonalcoholic fatty liver disease: The pathogenetic roles of insulin resistance and adipocytokines. *Curr. Mol. Med.* **2009**, *72*, 299–314. [CrossRef]
3. Khan, R.S.; Newsome, P.N. Non-alcoholic fatty liver disease and liver transplantation. *Metabolism* **2016**, *65*, 1208–1223. [CrossRef] [PubMed]
4. Rinella, M.E. Nonalcoholic fatty liver disease: A systematic review. *JAMA* **2015**, *313*, 2263–2273. [CrossRef] [PubMed]
5. Review, T.; LaBrecque, D.R.; Abbas, Z.; Anania, F.; Ferenci, P.; Khan, A.G.; Goh, K.L.; Hamid, S.S.; Isakov, V.; Lizarzabal, M.; et al. World Gastroenterology Organisation global guidelines: Nonalcoholic fatty liver disease and nonalcoholic steatohepatitis. *J. Clin. Gastroenterol.* **2014**, *48*, 467–473.
6. El Hadi, H.; Vettor, R.; Rossato, M. Congenital Vitamin E deficiency. In *Handbook of Famine, Starvation, and Nutrient Deprivation*; Preedy, V.R., Patel, V.B., Eds.; Springer International Publishing AG: Basel, Switzerland, 2018; pp. 1–18, ISBN 978-3-319-40007-5.
7. Evans, H.M.; Bishop, K.S. On the existence of a hitherto unrecognized dietary factor essential for reproduction. *Science* **1922**, *56*, 650–651. [CrossRef] [PubMed]
8. Gee, P.T. Unleashing the untold and misunderstood observations on vitamin E. *Genes Nutr.* **2011**, *6*, 5–16. [CrossRef] [PubMed]
9. Sheppard, A.J.; Pennington, J.A.T.; Weihrauch, J.L. Analysis and distribution of vitamin E in vegetable oils and foods. In *Vitamin E in Health and Disease*; Packer, L., Fuchs, J., Eds.; Marcel Dekker Inc.: New York, NY, USA, 1993; pp. 9–31.
10. Karrer, P.; Fritzsche, H.; Ringier, B.; Salomon, H. Synthesis of alpha-tocopherol (vitamin E). *Nature* **1938**, *141*, 1057. [CrossRef]
11. Jensen, S.K.; Lauridsen, C. Alpha-tocopherol stereoisomers. *Vitam. Horm.* **2007**, *76*, 281–308. [PubMed]
12. Traber, M.G. Vitamin E regulatory mechanisms. *Annu. Rev. Nutr.* **2007**, *27*, 347–362. [CrossRef] [PubMed]
13. Kayden, H.J.; Traber, M.G. Absorption, lipoprotein transport, and regulation of plasma concentrations of vitamin E in humans. *J. Lipid Res.* **1993**, *34*, 343–358. [PubMed]
14. Kaempf-Rotzoll, D.E.; Traber, M.G.; Arai, H. Vitamin E and transfer proteins. *Curr. Opin. Lipidol.* **2003**, *14*, 249–254. [CrossRef] [PubMed]
15. Jiang, Q. Natural forms of vitamin E: Metabolism, antioxidant, and anti-inflammatory activities and their role in disease prevention and therapy. *Free Radic. Biol. Med.* **2014**, *72*, 76–90. [CrossRef] [PubMed]
16. Bardowell, S.A.; Duan, F.; Manor, D.; Swanson, J.E.; Parker, R.S. Disruption of mouse cytochrome p4504f14 (Cyp4f14 gene) causes severe perturbations in vitamin E metabolism. *J. Biol. Chem.* **2012**, *287*, 26077–26086. [CrossRef] [PubMed]

17. Birben, E.; Sahiner, U.M.; Sackesen, C.; Erzurum, S.; Kalayci, O. Oxidative stress and antioxidant defense. *World Allergy Organ J.* **2012**, *5*, 9–19. [CrossRef] [PubMed]
18. Peh, H.Y.; Tan, W.S.; Liao, W.; Wong, W.S. Vitamin E therapy beyond cancer: Tocopherol versus tocotrienol. *Pharmacol. Ther.* **2016**, *162*, 152–169. [CrossRef] [PubMed]
19. Yoshida, Y.; Saito, Y.; Jones, L.S.; Shigeri, Y. Chemical reactivities and physical effects in comparison between tocopherols and tocotrienols: Physiological significance and prospects as antioxidants. *J. Biosci. Bioeng.* **2007**, *104*, 439–445. [CrossRef] [PubMed]
20. Cooney, R.V.; Harwood, P.J.; Franke, A.A.; Narala, K.; Sundström, A.K.; Berggren, P.O.; Mordan, L.J. Products of gamma-tocopherol reaction with NO_2 and their formation in rat insulinoma (RINm5F) cells. *Free Radic. Biol. Med.* **1995**, *19*, 259–269. [CrossRef]
21. Christen, S.; Jiang, Q.; Shigenaga, M.K.; Ames, B.N. Analysis of plasma tocopherols α, γ, and 5-nitro-γ in rats with inflammation by HPLC coulometric detection. *J. Lipid Res.* **2002**, *43*, 1978–1985. [CrossRef] [PubMed]
22. Berbée, M.; Fu, Q.; Boerma, M.; Wang, J.; Kumar, K.S.; Hauer-Jensen, M. gamma-Tocotrienol ameliorates intestinal radiation injury and reduces vascular oxidative stress after total-body irradiation by an HMG-CoA reductase-dependent mechanism. *Radiat. Res.* **2009**, *171*, 596–605. [CrossRef] [PubMed]
23. Upston, J.M.; Terentis, A.C.; Stocker, R. Tocopherol-mediated peroxidation of lipoproteins: Implications for vitamin E as a potential antiatherogenic supplement. *FASEB J.* **1999**, *13*, 977–994. [PubMed]
24. Pearson, P.; Lewis, S.A.; Britton, J.; Young, I.S.; Fogarty, A. The pro-oxidant activity of high-dose vitamin E supplements in vivo. *BioDrugs* **2006**, *20*, 271–273. [CrossRef] [PubMed]
25. Weinberg, R.B.; VanderWerken, B.S.; Anderson, R.A.; Stegner, J.E.; Thomas, M.J. Pro-oxidant effect of vitamin E in cigarette smokers consuming a high polyunsaturated fat diet. *Arterioscler. Thromb. Vasc. Biol.* **2001**, *21*, 1029–1033. [CrossRef] [PubMed]
26. Zingg, J.M.; Azzi, A. Non-antioxidant activities of vitamin E. *Curr. Med. Chem.* **2004**, *11*, 1113–1133. [CrossRef] [PubMed]
27. Rimbach, G.; Minihane, A.M.; Majewicz, J.; Fischer, A.; Pallauf, J.; Virgli, F.; Weinberg, P.D. Regulation of cell signalling by vitamin E. *Proc. Nutr. Soc.* **2002**, *61*, 415–425. [CrossRef] [PubMed]
28. Boscoboinik, D.; Szewczyk, A.; Hensey, C.; Azzi, A. Inhibition of cell proliferation by alpha-tocopherol. Role of protein kinase C. *J. Biol. Chem.* **1991**, *266*, 6188–6194. [PubMed]
29. Cook-Mills, J.M. Isoforms of Vitamin E Differentially Regulate PKC α and Inflammation: A Review. *J. Clin. Cell. Immunol.* **2013**, *4*, 1000137. [CrossRef] [PubMed]
30. Venugopal, S.K.; Devaraj, S.; Yang, T.; Jialal, I. Alpha-tocopherol decreases superoxide anion release in human monocytes under hyperglycemic conditions via inhibition of protein kinase C-alpha. *Diabetes* **2002**, *51*, 3049–3054. [CrossRef] [PubMed]
31. Martin-Nizard, F.; Boullier, A.; Fruchart, J.C.; Duriez, P. Alpha-tocopherol but not beta-tocopherol inhibits thrombin-induced PKC activation and endothelin secretion in endothelial cells. *J Cardiovasc. Risk* **1998**, *5*, 339–345. [CrossRef] [PubMed]
32. Rimbach, G.; Moehring, J.; Huebbe, P.; Lodge, J.K. Gene-regulatory activity of alpha-tocopherol. *Molecules* **2010**, *15*, 1746–1761. [CrossRef] [PubMed]
33. Ahsan, H.; Ahad, A.; Iqbal, J.; Siddiqui, W.A. Pharmacological potential of tocotrienols: A review. *Nutr. Metab.* **2014**, *11*, 52. [CrossRef] [PubMed]
34. Buzzetti, E.; Pinzani, M.; Tsochatzis, E.A. The multiple-hit pathogenesis of non-alcoholic fatty liver disease (NAFLD). *Metabolism* **2016**, *65*, 1038–1048. [CrossRef] [PubMed]
35. Hassan, K.; Bhalla, V.; El Regal, M.E.; A-Kader, H.H. Nonalcoholic fatty liver disease: A comprehensive review of a growing epidemic. *World J. Gastroenterol.* **2014**, *20*, 12082–12101. [CrossRef] [PubMed]
36. Fabbrini, E.; Mohammed, B.S.; Magkos, F.; Korenblat, K.M.; Patterson, B.W.; Klein, S. Alterations in adipose tissue and hepatic lipid kinetics in obese men and women with nonalcoholic fatty liver disease. *Gastroenterology* **2008**, *134*, 424–431. [CrossRef] [PubMed]
37. Sanyal, A.J.; Campbell-Sargent, C.; Mirshahi, F.; Rizzo, W.B.; Contos, M.J.; Sterling, R.K.; Luketic, V.A.; Shiffman, M.L.; Clore, J.N. Nonalcoholic steatohepatitis: Association of insulin resistance and mitochondrial abnormalities. *Gastroenterology* **2001**, *120*, 1183–1192. [CrossRef] [PubMed]

38. Hardwick, R.N.; Fisher, C.D.; Canet, M.J.; Lake, A.D.; Cherrington, N.J. Diversity in antioxidant response enzymes in progressive stages of human nonalcoholic fatty liver disease. *Drug Metab. Dispos.* **2010**, *38*, 2293–2301. [CrossRef] [PubMed]
39. Day, C.P. Pathogenesis of steatohepatitis. *Best Prac. Res. Clin. Gastroenterol.* **2002**, *16*, 663–678. [CrossRef]
40. Caldwell, S.H.; Chang, C.Y.; Nakamoto, R.K.; Krugner-Higby, L. Mitochondria in nonalcoholic fatty liver disease. *Clin. Liver Dis.* **2004**, *8*, 595–617. [CrossRef] [PubMed]
41. Aubert, J.; Begriche, K.; Knockaert, L.; Robin, M.A.; Fromenty, B. Increased expression of cytochrome P450 2E1 in nonalcoholic fatty liver disease: Mechanisms and pathophysiological role. *Clin. Res. Hepatol. Gastroenterol.* **2011**, *35*, 630–637. [CrossRef] [PubMed]
42. Leclercq, I.A.; Farrell, G.C.; Field, J.; Bell, D.R.; Gonzalez, F.J.; Robertson, G.R. CYP2E1 and CYP4A as microsomal catalysts of lipid peroxides in murine nonalcoholic steatohepatitis. *J. Clin. Investig.* **2000**, *105*, 1067–1075. [CrossRef] [PubMed]
43. Zhang, X.; Li, S.; Zhou, Y.; Su, W.; Ruan, X.; Wang, B.; Zheng, F.; Warner, M.; Gustafsson, J.Å.; Guan, Y. Ablation of cytochrome P450 omega-hydroxylase 4A14 gene attenuates hepatic steatosis and fibrosis. *Proc. Natl. Acad. Sci. USA* **2017**, *114*, 3181–3185. [CrossRef] [PubMed]
44. Demeilliers, C.; Maisonneuve, C.; Grodet, A.; Mansouri, A.; Nguyen, R.; Tinel, M.; Lettéron, P.; Degott, C.; Feldmann, G.; Pessayre, D.; et al. Impaired adaptive resynthesis and prolonged depletion of hepatic mitochondrial DNA after repeated alcohol binges in mice. *Gastroenterology* **2002**, *123*, 1278–1290. [CrossRef] [PubMed]
45. Dara, L.; Ji, C.; Kaplowitz, N. The contribution of endoplasmic reticulum stress to liver diseases. *Hepatology* **2011**, *53*, 1752–1763. [CrossRef] [PubMed]
46. Marra, F.; Svegliati-Baroni, G. Lipotoxicity and the gut-liver axis in NASH pathogenesis. *J. Hepatol.* **2017**. [CrossRef] [PubMed]
47. Larter, C.Z.; Yeh, M.M.; Williams, J.; Bell-Anderson, K.S.; Farrell, G.C. MCD-induced steatohepatitis is associated with hepatic adiponectin resistance and adipogenic transformation of hepatocytes. *J. Hepatol.* **2008**, *49*, 407–416. [CrossRef] [PubMed]
48. Phung, N.; Pera, N.; Farrell, G.; Leclercq, I.; Hou, J.Y.; George, J. Pro-oxidant-mediated hepatic fibrosis and effects of antioxidant intervention in murine dietary steatohepatitis. *Int. J. Mol. Med.* **2009**, *24*, 171–180. [PubMed]
49. Nan, Y.M.; Wu, W.J.; Fu, N.; Liang, B.L.; Wang, R.Q.; Li, L.X.; Zhao, S.X.; Zhao, J.M.; Yu, J. Antioxidants vitamin E and 1-aminobenzotriazole prevent experimental non-alcoholic steatohepatitis in mice. *Scand. J. Gastroenterol.* **2009**, *44*, 1121–1131. [CrossRef] [PubMed]
50. Karimian, G.; Kirschbaum, M.; Veldhuis, Z.J.; Bomfati, F.; Porte, R.J.; Lisman, T. Vitamin E Attenuates the Progression of Non-Alcoholic Fatty Liver Disease Caused by Partial Hepatectomy in Mice. *PLoS ONE* **2015**, *10*, e0143121. [CrossRef] [PubMed]
51. Chung, M.Y.; Yeung, S.F.; Park, H.J.; Volek, J.S.; Bruno, R.S. Dietary α- and γ-tocopherol supplementation attenuates lipopolysaccharide-induced oxidative stress and inflammatory-related responses in an obese mouse model of nonalcoholic steatohepatitis. *J. Nutr. Biochem.* **2010**, *21*, 1200–1206. [CrossRef] [PubMed]
52. Lu, T.; Harper, A.F.; Zhao, J.; Corl, B.A.; LeRoith, T.; Dalloul, R.A. Effects of a dietary antioxidant blend and vitamin E on fatty acid profile, liver function, and inflammatory response in broiler chickens fed a diet high in oxidants. *Poult. Sci.* **2014**, *93*, 1658–1666. [CrossRef] [PubMed]
53. Podszun, M.C.; Grebenstein, N.; Spruss, A.; Schlueter, T.; Kremoser, C.; Bergheim, I.; Frank, J. Dietary alpha-tocopherol and atorvastatin reduce high-fat-induced lipid accumulation and down-regulate CD36 protein in the liver of guinea pigs. *J. Nutr. Biochem.* **2014**, *25*, 573–579. [CrossRef] [PubMed]
54. Lavine, J.E. Vitamin E treatment of nonalcoholic steatohepatitis in children: A pilot study. *J. Pediatr.* **2000**, *136*, 734–738. [CrossRef]
55. Hasegawa, T.; Yoneda, M.; Nakamura, K.; Makino, I.; Terano, A. Plasma transforming growth factor-beta1 level and efficacy of alpha-tocopherol in patients with non-alcoholic steatohepatitis: A pilot study. *Aliment. Pharmacol. Ther.* **2001**, *15*, 1667–1672. [CrossRef] [PubMed]
56. Kugelmas, M.; Hill, D.B.; Vivian, B.; Marsano, L.; McClain, C.J. Cytokines and NASH: A pilot study of the effects of lifestyle modification and vitamin E. *Hepatology* **2003**, *38*, 413–419. [CrossRef] [PubMed]

57. Yakaryilmaz, F.; Guliter, S.; Savas, B.; Erdem, O.; Ersoy, R.; Erden, E.; Akyol, G.; Bozkaya, H.; Ozenirler, S. Effects of vitamin E treatment on peroxisome proliferator-activated receptor-alpha expression and insulin resistance in patients with non-alcoholic steatohepatitis: Results of a pilot study. *Intern. Med. J.* **2007**, *37*, 229–235. [CrossRef] [PubMed]

58. Bugianesi, E.; Gentilcore, E.; Manini, R.; Natale, S.; Vanni, E.; Villanova, N.; David, E.; Rizzetto, M.; Marchesini, G. A randomized controlled trial of metformin versus vitamin E or prescriptive diet in nonalcoholic fatty liver disease. *Am. J. Gastroenterol.* **2005**, *100*, 1082–1090. [CrossRef] [PubMed]

59. Vajro, P.; Mandato, C.; Franzese, A.; Ciccimarra, E.; Lucariello, S.; Savoia, M.; Capuano, G.; Migliaro, F. Vitamin E treatment in pediatric obesity-related liver disease: A randomized study. *J. Pediatr. Gastroenterol. Nutr.* **2004**, *38*, 48–55. [CrossRef] [PubMed]

60. Sanyal, A.J.; Chalasani, N.; Kowdley, K.V.; McCullough, A.; Diehl, A.M.; Bass, N.M.; Neuschwander-Tetri, B.A.; Lavine, J.E.; Tonascia, J.; Unalp, A.; et al. Pioglitazone, vitamin E, or placebo for nonalcoholic steatohepatitis. *N. Engl. J. Med.* **2010**, *362*, 1675–1685. [CrossRef] [PubMed]

61. Lavine, J.E.; Schwimmer, J.B.; Van Natta, M.L.; Molleston, J.P.; Murray, K.F.; Rosenthal, P.; Abrams, S.H.; Scheimann, A.O.; Sanyal, A.J.; Chalasani, N.; et al. Effect of vitamin E or metformin for treatment of nonalcoholic fatty liver disease in children and adolescents: The TONIC randomized controlled trial. *JAMA* **2011**, *305*, 1659–1668. [CrossRef] [PubMed]

62. Pietu, F.; Guillaud, O.; Walter, T.; Vallin, M.; Hervieu, V.; Scoazec, J.Y.; Dumortier, J. Ursodeoxycholic acid with vitamin E in patients with nonalcoholic steatohepatitis: Long-term results. *Clin. Res. Hepatol. Gastroenterol.* **2012**, *36*, 146–155. [CrossRef] [PubMed]

63. Foster, T.; Budoff, M.J.; Saab, S.; Ahmadi, N.; Gordon, C.; Guerci, A.D. Atorvastatin and antioxidants for the treatment of nonalcoholic fatty liver disease: The St Francis Heart Study randomized clinical trial. *Am. J. Gastroenterol.* **2011**, *106*, 71–77. [CrossRef] [PubMed]

64. Dufour, J.F.; Oneta, C.M.; Gonvers, J.J.; Bihl, F.; Cerny, A.; Cereda, J.M.; Zala, J.F.; Helbling, B.; Steuerwald, M.; Zimmermann, A. Swiss Association for the Study of the Liver. Randomized placebo-controlled trial of ursodeoxycholic acid with vitamin E in nonalcoholic steatohepatitis. *Clin. Gastroenterol. Hepatol.* **2006**, *4*, 1537–1543. [CrossRef] [PubMed]

65. Nobili, V.; Manco, M.; Devito, R.; Ciampalini, P.; Piemonte, F.; Marcellini, M. Effect of vitamin E on aminotransferase levels and insulin resistance in children with non-alcoholic fatty liver disease. *Aliment. Pharmacol. Ther.* **2006**, *24*, 1553–1561. [CrossRef] [PubMed]

66. Nobili, V.; Manco, M.; Devito, R.; Di Ciommo, V.; Comparcola, D.; Sartorelli, M.R.; Piemonte, F.; Marcellini, M.; Angulo, P. Lifestyle intervention and antioxidant therapy in children with nonalcoholic fatty liver disease: A randomized, controlled trial. *Hepatology* **2008**, *48*, 119–128. [CrossRef] [PubMed]

67. Sanyal, A.J.; Mofrad, P.S.; Contos, M.J.; Sargeant, C.; Luketic, V.A.; Sterling, R.K.; Stravitz, R.T.; Shiffman, M.L.; Clore, J.; Mills, A.S. A pilot study of vitamin E versus vitamin E and pioglitazone for the treatment of nonalcoholic steatohepatitis. *Clin. Gastroenterol. Hepatol.* **2004**, *2*, 1107–1115. [CrossRef]

68. Harrison, S.A.; Torgerson, S.; Hayashi, P.; Ward, J.; Schenker, S. Vitamin E and vitamin C treatment improves fibrosis in patients with nonalcoholic steatohepatitis. *Am. J. Gastroenterol.* **2003**, *98*, 2485–2490. [CrossRef] [PubMed]

69. European Association for the Study of the Liver (EASL); European Association for the Study of Diabetes (EASD); European Association for the Study of Obesity (EASO). EASL-EASD-EASO Clinical Practice Guidelines for the management of non-alcoholic fatty liver disease. *J. Hepatol.* **2016**, *64*, 1388–1402.

70. Miller, E.R.; Pastor-Barriuso, R.; Dalal, D.; Riemersma, R.A.; Appel, L.J.; Guallar, E. Meta-analysis: High-dosage vitamin E supplementation may increase all-cause mortality. *Ann. Intern. Med.* **2005**, *142*, 37–46. [CrossRef] [PubMed]

71. Gerss, J.; Köpcke, W. The questionable association of vitamin E supplementation and mortality–inconsistent results of different meta-analytic approaches. *Cell. Mol. Biol.* **2009**, *55* (Suppl. OL), 1111–1120.

72. Abner, E.L.; Schmitt, F.A.; Mendiondo, M.S.; Marcum, J.L.; Kryscio, R.J. Vitamin E and all-cause mortality: A meta-analysis. *Curr. Aging Sci.* **2011**, *4*, 158–170. [CrossRef] [PubMed]

73. Schurks, M.; Glynn, R.J.; Rist, P.M.; Tzourio, C.; Kurth, T. Effects of vitamin E on stroke subtypes: Meta-analysis of randomised controlled trials. *BMJ* **2010**, *341*, c5702. [CrossRef] [PubMed]
74. Klein, E.A.; Thompson, I.M.; Tangen, C.M.; Crowley, J.J.; Lucia, M.S.; Goodman, P.J.; Minasian, L.M.; Ford, L.G.; Parnes, H.L.; Gaziano, J.M.; et al. Vitamin E and the risk of prostate cancer: The Selenium and Vitamin E Cancer Prevention Trial (SELECT). *JAMA* **2011**, *306*, 1549–1556. [CrossRef] [PubMed]

7

Reactive Oxygen and Nitrogen Species Regulate Key Metabolic, Anabolic, and Catabolic Pathways in Skeletal Muscle

Roland Nemes [1], Erika Koltai [2], Albert W. Taylor [3], Katsuhiko Suzuki [4], Ferenc Gyori [5] and Zsolt Radak [2,5,*]

1 Faculty of Sports and Health Studies, Hosei University, Tokyo 194-0298, Japan; nem_roland@hosei.ac.jp
2 Research Institute of Sport Science, University of Physical Education, Alkotas u. 44, H-1123 Budapest, Hungary; koltaie@gmail.com
3 Faculty of Health Sciences, The University of Western Ontario, London, ON N6G 1H1, Canada; ataylor2@uwo.ca
4 Faculty of Sport Sciences, Waseda University, Saitama 359-1192, Japan; katsu.suzu@waseda.jp
5 Institute of Sport Science, University of Szeged, H-6726 Szeged, Hungary; gyori@jgypk.szte.hu
* Correspondence: radak@tf.hu

Abstract: Reactive oxygen and nitrogen species (RONS) are important cellular regulators of key physiological processes in skeletal muscle. In this review, we explain how RONS regulate muscle contraction and signaling, and why they are important for membrane remodeling, protein turnover, gene expression, and epigenetic adaptation. We discuss how RONS regulate carbohydrate uptake and metabolism of skeletal muscle, and how they indirectly regulate fat metabolism through silent mating type information regulation 2 homolog 3 (SIRT3). RONS are causative/associative signaling molecules, which cause sarcopenia or muscle hypertrophy. Regular exercise influences redox biology, metabolism, and anabolic/catabolic pathways in skeletal muscle in an intensity dependent manner.

Keywords: training; skeletal muscle adaptation; oxidative stress

1. Introduction

Regular physical exercise results in systemic adaptation(s) of the whole body, alongside varied perturbations in blood flow and metabolism among different organs. The main adaptive effects, such as decreased levels of oxidative damage, increased activities of enzymatic antioxidants, enhanced mitochondrial efficiency, and more efficient physiological functions are, however, observed in the skeletal muscle, heart, brain, liver, kidneys, and testes, alongside other organs. Since skeletal muscle is the largest organ in the human body, and the main organ responsible for physical exercise, the present review focuses on exercise-associated adaptation of skeletal muscle, and reactive oxygen and nitrogen species (RONS).

2. Muscle Contraction and Reactive Oxygen and Nitrogen Species

Davies and co-workers [1] showed for the first time that after an exhaustive bout of exercise, a significant increase in reactive oxygen species (ROS) production occurs in the skeletal muscle, as measured by electron spin resonance. At that time, it was widely accepted that ROS were a so called "by-product" of aerobic metabolism that jeopardized the structure and function of muscle cells. However, an intriguing study was later published in which it was observed that whilst contracting skeletal muscle generates ROS, ex vivo exposure to the antioxidant enzymes, catalase and superoxide dismutase (SOD), decreased force generation [2]. This work was the first to show that

ROS could positively affect the function of skeletal muscle by facilitating muscle contraction at certain concentrations. In a previous study, the same research group showed that during muscle fatigue the concentration of ROS increased, which eventually led to a decreased force production, which could be delayed with the administration of exogenous antioxidants [2–4]. Therefore, this finding suggests that contracting skeletal muscle is producing ROS, which further facilitates the strength of the muscle contraction. However, if the ROS concentration exceeds a certain level, it reduces the force generation and causes fatigue. This phenomenon nicely demonstrates that ROS could have a positive or negative effect, depending on the concentration, and is a phenomenon that can be described by the hormesis curve [5–8]. Up-to a concentration, ROS and muscle force generation capacity increase together, but after reaching a point, greater levels of ROS decrease the force generation of skeletal muscle, and, therefore, the relationship between ROS and force generation of skeletal muscle has a bell-shaped dose-response curve.

It is known that mitochondrial electron transport chain is one main ROS generator found in skeletal muscle [9]. During high intensity exercise, ROS, mainly generated by Complex I and III with pyruvate/malate and succinate substrates, were increased by 187% and 138%, respectively [10]. Experimental data revealed that mitochondria isolated from skeletal muscle after contraction showed significantly increased levels of hydrogen peroxide (H_2O_2) generation [11] (Figure 1). H_2O_2 is the main signaling molecule because it can cross membranes and activate redox sensitive proteins, modulating cell signaling.

It has been shown that Complex I is the major ROS generator in skeletal muscle of ultra-endurance runners [12]. However, it must be noted that the earlier estimations of about 1–5% of the oxygen that entering the mitochondria being released as ROS [13] could be highly overestimated, with the real value being more than an order of magnitude lower [14]. However, the findings of Austin et al. [15] suggest that mitochondria might be important sources of ROS at Complex I and III, through peroxisome proliferator-activated receptor-γ coactivator alpha (PGC-1α).

Indeed, the iron-sulfur clusters, flavoprotein and oxidoreductase, at Complex I, and Q10 semiquinones at Complex III are thought to be the main sites of ROS generation [14,16]. In addition to mitochondria, 5-lipoxygenase, cyclooxygenase, sarcolemmal and leukocyte nicotinamide adenine dinucleotide phosphate-oxidase (NADPH), and xanthine oxidase (XO) have also been implicated in superoxide generation in skeletal muscle [9,17–19].

It has also been suggested that the basal level of intracellular H_2O_2 in skeletal muscle is between 10–100 nM, which increased to 100–200 nM with heavy muscle contraction [20]. Although the level of XO in skeletal muscle is very low, it is present to a significant degree in the endothelium, and, hence, it is a potential source of extracellular superoxide generation. High intensity exercise results in the generation of hypoxanthine [21,22], and a linear relationship has been observed between the levels of circulating lactic acid and XO. Interestingly, we could detect increased XO activity in the liver one day after exhaustive acute exercise [23], but administration of SOD derivatives identified endothelium associated with XO as one source of ROS generation during intense exercise [21]. However, the contribution of XO in ROS production during aerobic exercise is a real puzzle. A number of papers suggest that allopurinol administration can attenuate ROS production during aerobic exercise, and, moreover, allopurinol can even prevent the ROS associated adaptive responses to exercise [24].

Contraction of skeletal muscle results in ROS generation associated with phospholipase A (PLA_2). Indeed, ROS production decreased when various PLA_2 inhibitors were administered to a contracting diaphragm, suggesting that PLA_2 plays a critical role in modulating ROS formation during muscle contraction [25] (Figure 1). Furthermore, it has been suggested that, in the skeletal muscles of patients suffering from Duchenne muscular dystrophy, elevated intracellular calcium levels caused by altered regulation of calcium channels activate PLA_2, causing ROS production and increased membrane permeability [26]. In Duchenne muscular dystrophy, dystrophin is absent, and sarcolemmal neuronal nitric oxide synthase (nNOS) is lost because it is anchored to dystrophin. The absence of nNOS-generated NO could be one of the reasons for increased ROS generation by skeletal muscle of patients with this atrophy. Indeed, when nNOS is knocked out, higher levels of intrinsic hydrogen peroxidase activity were demonstrated in the extensor digitorum longus (EDL) of nNOS-knockout mice, when compared to C57 control mice [27]. Therefore, nNOS-generated NO could have an important scavenging role in the detoxification of superoxide. Interestingly, Ca^{2+}-independent ($iPLA_2$) beta is involved in membrane repair; suggesting that the interaction between ROS and membrane lipids not only disrupts the cellular milieu and jeopardizes the fate of the cell, but could also be important for the continuous remodeling requirements of cell membranes [28].

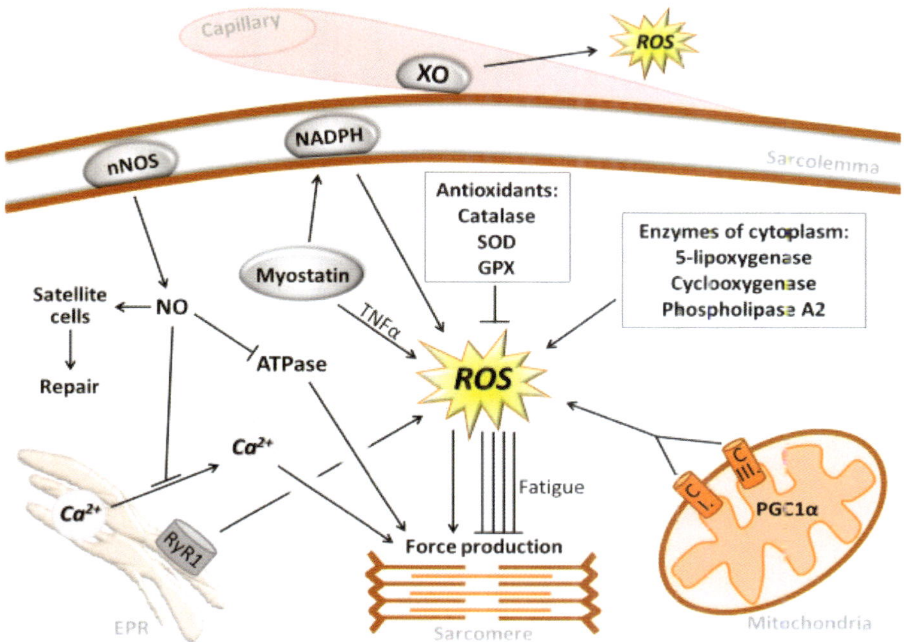

Figure 1. Sources of reactive oxygen species. Summarized potential sources of reactive oxygen species (ROS) in skeletal muscle. H_2O_2 up to a certain concentration enhance the force production of skeletal muscle, while in large concentrations, ROS causes fatigue and suppresses force generation.

Recently, myostatin emerged as a potential ROS-inducing factor, especially during sarcopenia [29]. It has been demonstrated that knocking out the myostatin gene resulted in attenuated loss of muscle mass with aging, and that myostatin can induce ROS production through tumor necrosis factor-α (TNF-α) and NADPH oxidase [29]. However, the role of exercise in myostatin-mediated redox signaling is still unclear and further research is warranted on this topic. Activation of ryanodine receptor 1 (RyR1) in the sarcoplasmic reticulum of skeletal muscle is necessary for Ca^{2+} release and the subsequent generation of cross-bridge-related force production. With the aging of skeletal muscle, a continuous Ca^{2+} leak is observed in RyR1 channels, which is associated with a decreased force production capacity and increased ROS production. Pharmacological intervention to normalize RyR1 function by stabilizing the binding of calstabin1 to RyR1 significantly reduced Ca^{2+} leakage and increased endurance capacity [30].

It has been shown that single and regular bouts of exercise differentially modulate ROS production in neutrophils. During acute exercise the adaptive response is limited, and, indeed, it has been shown that a single bout of exercise results in a loss of mitochondrial membrane potential, e [31]. Marathon running, which is a severe form of exercise, caused cytokines and neutrophil activation markers (myeloperoxidase (MPO) and lactoferrin (LTF), and priming neutrophils and monocytes were secreted and functional after exhaustive exercise [32]. These responses seemed to be overwhelming, inducing antioxidant and anti-inflammatory defenses systems, and preventing exercise-induced oxidative stress [32]. Therefore, it is quite clear that a single bout of exhaustive exercise induces inflammation [33,34] which can readily lead to oxidative stress.

Muscle contraction generates heat, which has been shown to enhance ROS production [35]. However, ROS production is an essential physiological process for muscle contraction, where it is estimated that H_2O_2 concentrations can increase by 100 nM during contractions [20]. Indeed, whilst it is known that low levels of exogenous H_2O_2 treatment increase force production, e.g., in the diaphragm, the addition of catalase decreases diaphragm force production [2]. This response has been associated with H_2O_2 modulating muscle contraction via Ca^{++} channels [36].

Moreover, it appears that not only Ca^{2+} sensitivity, but also the release of Ca^{2+} is altered by oxidants [37]. On the other hand, it is also known that Ca^{2+}-ATP-ase activity of the sarcoplasmic reticulum is easily depressed by H_2O_2 [38]. Whilst not completely clear, current information suggests that the physiological regulatory role of H_2O_2 is more significant than that of superoxide or hydroxyl radical due to the very shot half-life of the latter two [39]. Furthermore, H_2O_2 can cross the cell membrane, while superoxide ($O\bullet^{-}{}_2$) and hydroxyl radicals (•OH) apparently cannot.

NO could also affect the function of skeletal muscle. The synthesis of NO is catalyzed by the enzyme, NOS. NOS converts arginine and molecular oxygen to NO and citrulline in a reaction that requires NADPH, flavin adenine dinucleotide, flavin mononucleotide, and tetrahydrobiopterin as cofactors. The predominant NOS isoform in skeletal muscle is neuronal NOS (nNOS), although skeletal muscle also expresses endothelial NOS (eNOS) and inducible NOS (iNOS). The nNOS is present in the sarcolemma of both extra- and intra-fusal muscle fibers. In addition, nNOS is concentrated at the postsynaptic surface of the mammalian neuromuscular junction of all fibers. Also, whilst eNOS is abundant in skeletal muscle vasculature, iNOS is present at low levels in rodent and human skeletal muscles, and is localized to the sarcolemma through caveolin-3. NO could influence neuromuscular transmission and act as a retrograde signal to modify pre-synaptic function [40]. The effect of NO on contractile function is better known and studied than its role in neuromuscular transmission. However, observations have revealed that NO decreases isometric force, and, in general, decreases force production in skeletal muscle [41]. One of the reasons behind this phenomenon could be that actomyosin ATP-ase activity is reduced by nitrosylation, which is mediated by NO, and results in a decreased force production [42]. Moreover, NO can inhibit Ca^{2+} release from the sarcoplasmic reticulum [43], resulting in a decreased force production. Whilst muscle soreness is associated with marked decreases in maximal force generation, we have shown that NO could be one of the factors that is responsible for this. Significant increases have been shown in NO content with muscle soreness, which correlates with a decreased maximal force production [44]. We hypothesized that an increased NO level with muscle soreness could be a protective mechanism that does not allow high force production, which, due to high muscular tension, can lead to the development of micro-injuries. In addition, elevated levels of NO during muscle contraction could also be responsible for pain. This is a result of NO activating nociceptors that host the calcitonin gene-related peptide (CGRP) receptor, which is activated by NO, thus, causing pain. Moreover, it is well known that muscle soreness causes damage to sarcomeres due to the unaccustomed tension. The damage must be repaired and it appears that NO is involved in the repair process by activating satellite cells [44]. NO induces satellite cell proliferation, which is a crucial process in muscle repair; a process which is absent in patients with Duchenne muscular dystrophy due to a lack of nNOS.

NO is able to significantly interfere with cellular metabolism by decreasing oxygen consumption [45], altering glucose uptake, and controlling vasodilation. With muscle injury and inflammation, NO is generated to a greater extent by macrophages, mostly through the iNOS process. Nuclear factor kappa B (NF-kB), which is one of the master regulators of inflammation by the regulation of transcription of a number of inflammatory proteins, could also regulate the expression of iNOS. NF-kB is a redox sensitive transcription factor, which, besides its role in inflammation, could also alter the transcription of manganese-SOD (MnSOD) [46].

3. RONS-Associated Oxidative Damage and Repair

RONS are very potent inducers of the enzymatic antioxidant system. The extent of oxidative damage reveals the efficiency of antioxidant and oxidative damage repair systems, although it is intriguing that the level of oxidative damage is never zero. This could indicate that the damage might have some physiological roles, such as signaling [46]. It is known that during DNA replication generated errors initiate the repair process, and similar phenomena could happen with the oxidant-generated damage to DNA. The study of skeletal muscle is limited with regards to the effects of RONS. Nonetheless, adequate literature is available to suggest that more studies should be carried out, especially within exercise models. For example, the activity of 8-oxoguanine-DNA glycosylase 1 (OGG1) increased in human rectus femoris muscle after a marathon race [47]. We suggested that the level of 8-oxodeoxyguanosine (8-oxodG) increased in the muscle because of the exercise, which was followed by the induction of the enzyme necessary to repair the mutagenic damage. We have also reported that aging results in an increased level of nuclear 8-oxodG in the skeletal muscle of rats. This increase was prevented by exercise training and the induction of OGG1 [48]. This result led to an interest in measuring the activity of OGG1 and uracil DNA glycosylase (UDG) in white and red portions of the quadriceps muscle [49] because Type I and Type II fibers differ greatly in metabolic rate, as well as in their levels of antioxidant capacity. We found that OGG1 activity increased in the nuclei of red fibers as was expected; but, surprisingly, OGG1 activity decreased in the mitochondria of both red and white fibers. We were puzzled by this phenomenon and, in a related study, found that the export of OGG1 to the mitochondria could be accelerated by exercise training [50]. In other words, a sedentary life-style and/or detraining impairs the transfer of OGG1 into the mitochondrial matrix [50]. We suggest that exercise training results in biogenesis of mitochondria, and provides more accessible membranes for proteins to be transferred into mitochondria after their synthesis in the ribosomes.

It is well demonstrated that red fibers with high oxidative capacity host a substantial enzymatic antioxidant system, and express increased resistance to oxidative stress; whereas white fibers do not. The activity of OGG1 is also higher in red fibers, but significant differences in the activity of UDG in different fiber types are not evident. DNA repair enzymes work as house-keeping enzymes and are designed to decrease the level of oxidative damage for the protection of cells, and to avoid apoptosis and necrosis, as well as mutation. Although DNA suffers a significant attack from ROS, the extent of protein damage is one-fold higher [51]. Oxidized proteins are not repaired in the same fashion as DNA, but, to prevent the aggregation and cross-folding of oxidized defective proteins, the proteasome system is the first line of defense. Again, skeletal muscle is not a very well monitored tissue in the case of the proteasome system. It has been suggested that aging, which results in a very significant loss of muscle mass, does not alter the activity of the proteasome system [52,53] or decrease its activity [51,54]. However, there are reports that caloric restriction and exercise training increase the activity of the proteasome system [48,55]. This suggestion could be important for remodeling the tissues and removing damaged proteins. The response of the proteasome system to exercise is dependent on the exercise loading and the time of sampling [56]. Therefore, the findings must be evaluated accordingly. For example, Sultan and his co-workers [57] have shown that chronic low-frequency electrical stimulation, which induces fast-to-slow transitions of muscle fibers, alters the proteasome system, once again demonstrating the plasticity of skeletal muscle. Lipid peroxidation is not repaired as efficiently as DNA damage (that damage repaired first, which most directly affects the fate of the cell), but $iPLA_2$ beta can repair lipid damage to a certain degree. We have suggested that the limited extent of DNA damage is an important stimulator of gene expression, protein damage, protein turn-over, and lipid damage, and could be important for membrane remodeling [28].

4. The Role of ROS in Exercise-Induced Metabolism

During muscle contraction, there is a significant change in intracellular redox levels, and H_2O_2 concentration is elevated to 100–200 nM. However, an intriguing question is whether this could help cover the energy cost of muscle contraction. An early study on L6 myotubes showed that H_2O_2 increased the mRNA levels of glucose transporter 1 (GLUT1) and the glucose uptake of these cells [58]. Further, a later study on mouse skeletal muscle showed that repeated contractions increased 2-deoxyglucose (2-DG) uptake roughly threefold in isolated EDL (fast-twitch) muscle. N-Acetylcysteine (NAC), a non-specific antioxidant, inhibited contraction-mediated 2-DG uptake by approximately 50% ($p < 0.05$) compared with control values), yet did not significantly affect basal 2-DG uptake [59]. This suggests that elevated levels of H_2O_2 stimulate glucose uptake of skeletal muscle during exercise [59]. A follow-up study on isolated rat EDL muscle revealed that H_2O_2 also resulted in a dose-dependent increase in 2-DG uptake in isolated EDL muscles, and the maximal increase was threefold over basal levels at a concentration of 600 μM/L H_2O_2. H_2O_2-stimulated 2-DG uptake was completely inhibited by the phosphatidylinositol 3-kinase (PI3K) inhibitor, wortmannin, indicating a crucial role of the PI3K pathway in H_2O_2-mediated glucose uptake during contractions [60]. In addition, it has been reported that H_2O_2 induces phosphorylation of nNOS at the same residue as insulin does, but also stimulates NO production and GLUT4 translocation. nNOS inhibition prevented H_2O_2-induced GLUT4 translocation [61] (Figure 2). Moreover, inhibition of AMP activated protein kinase (AMPK) prevented H_2O_2 activation and phosphorylation of nNOS, leading to a reduction in NO production and significantly attenuated GLUT4 translocation [61]. It is important to note that acute exposure to H_2O_2 or NO increases insulin sensitivity and glucose uptake, while chronic exposure suppresses it, and can easily lead to type 2 diabetes [62]. A significant feature of physical exercise is the cyclic change of adaptive resting periods and exercise periods, with enhanced metabolic processes and ROS production. This cyclic nature is an important part of preconditioning. With increasing exercise intensity, there is an increased dependence on carbohydrate metabolism, which parallels the increased generation of ROS. This is unlikely to be a coincidental phenomenon, based on the direct relationship between H_2O_2, NO levels and glucose uptake of skeletal muscle.

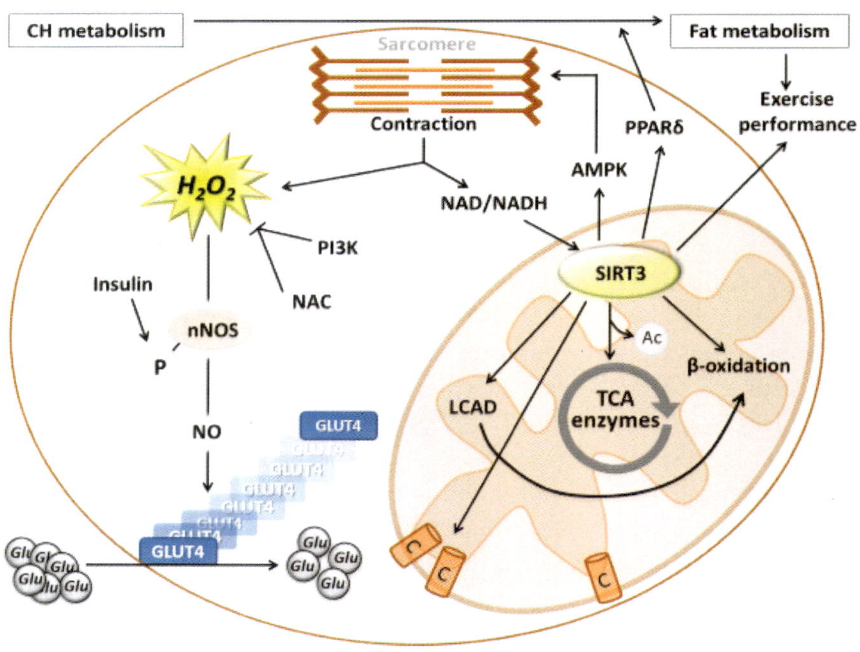

Figure 2. The role of reactive oxygen species on metabolism. H_2O_2 can stimulate cellular signaling pathways to dislocate GLUT4 to cellular membranes, which is crucial for glucose uptake. ROS levels influence the activity of SIRT3, which is an important regulator of fat metabolism.

On the other hand, a pertinent question regarding fat metabolism is whether ROS also regulate the availability of free fatty acids (FFA), and the metabolism of FFA in the TCA cycle. Data suggest that ROS can indirectly regulate the efficiency of fat metabolism through the enzyme silent mating type information regulation 2 homolog 3 (SIRT3), which is localized in the mitochondria, and NAD-dependent lysine deacetylase. In resting human muscle, total NAD^+ and NADH concentrations are estimated to be ~1.5–1.9 and ~0.08–0.20 mmol/kg dry weight of muscle, respectively [63]. Low intensity muscle contraction increases NAD/NADH concentration. However, the increase in the mitochondrial NAD^+/NADH ratio during the same absolute exercise seems lower in trained rats [64]. The NAD/NADH ratio reflects the redox state of cell or cellular compartments, which directly affects redox sensitive cellular processes, including metabolism, and particularly those enzymes that are dependent on the availability of NAD. SIRT3 is a NAD-dependent mitochondrial enzyme important for ATP production, since it deacetylates and activates a number of key enzymes in the TCA cycle. Indeed, when nicotinamide riboside, a precursor of NAD^+ biosynthesis, was supplemented, high fat, diet induced, nonalcoholic fatty liver disease was reverted, partly by the induction of hepatic β-oxidation and mitochondrial complex content and activity [65]. Moreover, when SIRT3 is knocked-out, there is a marked reduction of fatty acid metabolism due to the hyperacetylation of long-chain acyl coenzyme A dehydrogenase (LCAD) at lysine 42 [66]. These results suggest that SIRT3 is a potential regulator of fat metabolism. We, and others, have shown that exercise increases the level of SIRT3 in humans [67,68] and animals [69].

It has been demonstrated that transgenic mice with enhanced levels of SIRT3 in skeletal muscle exhibit 45% better running-based exercise performance than control animals [70]. In addition, these transgenic animals display a higher proportion of slow oxidative muscle fibers, increased muscle AMPK activation, and peroxisome proliferator-activated receptor delta (PPARδ) expression; both of which are known regulators promoting type I muscle fiber specification [70]. Up-regulation of PPARδ might be important because it can lead to a shift from glucose metabolism to fat metabolism, since PPARδ activation potently suppresses glucose catabolism, without affecting either muscle fiber type or mitochondrial content [71]. Higher levels of aerobic endurance capacity are associated with greater utilization of fatty acids. Indeed, it has been shown that mice with an overexpression of PPARδ had better endurance performance than control mice [71]. Overall, it is well demonstrated that redox sensitive SIRT3 activates the metabolism of fat, and, therefore, can influence exercise performance.

5. Role of ROS in Muscle Hypertrophy and Atrophy

The role of ROS in sarcopenia has seemingly been known for quite some time [72]. However, that role has recently been questioned. Transgenic mice expressing a proof-reading-deficient version of PolgA, the nucleus-encoded catalytic subunit of mitochondrial DNA polymerase, were generated [73]. These mice carried a three- to five-fold increase in the levels of point mutations, as well as increased amounts of deleted mitochondrial DNA [73]. As the consequence of genetic manipulation, PolG mice showed a premature onset of ageing-related phenotypes, such as weight loss, reduced subcutaneous fat, alopecia, kyphosis, osteoporosis, anaemia, reduced fertility, and heart enlargement [73]. However, PolG mice do not exhibit increased levels of mitochondrial ROS production [74], suggesting that in this transgenic model the premature aging is not a result of enhanced ROS production. On the other hand, when the gastrocnemius muscles of six month and 21 month-old rats were studied, it was shown that mitochondria obtained from aged muscle fibers show several functional abnormalities, explaining the enhancedproteolysis, ROS overproduction, and vulnerability to apoptosis exhibited by sarcopenic muscle [75]. In another transgenic mouse model where the Cu-ZnSOD was ablated, the aging process was accelerated in skeletal muscle, leading to a proposal that superoxide-induced neuromuscular junction degeneration and mitochondrial dysfunction are potential mechanisms of sarcopenia [76].

Systemic age-associated inflammation in the skeletal muscle has also been suggested to be one of the causative factors of loss of muscle strength and mass [77–79]. Massive involvement of ROS is suggested in sarcopenia-associated inflammation [78,80], with supporting data coming from a number of studies on aging [81–83]. One observed that inflammatory mediator angiopoietin-like protein 2 (ANGPTL2) increases in the skeletal muscle of aging mice, while exercise attenuates this elevation [84]. When we compared markers of anabolic and catabolic processes in the skeletal muscle of five month and twenty-eight month-old rats, we observed that aging resulted in decreased levels of follistatin/mTOR/Akt/Erk activation and increased myostatin/Murf1/2, proteasome subunits, and protein ubiquitination levels. In addition, the TNF-α, ROS, p53, and Bax levels were increased, while Bcl-2 levels were decreased in the skeletal muscle of aged rats [85]. We trained rats at an intensity of 60% of VO2max on a treadmill, and this running training attenuated age-associated increases in apoptotic and catabolic processes [85]. From a muscle hypertrophy perspective, it is difficult to cause muscle hypertrophy in laboratory animals. However, one of the most successful models is wing loading on birds. When young and aged Japanese quails were loaded for seven or 21 days to induce hypertrophy, data showed that H_2O_2 content was higher in muscles from aged birds following seven days of loading [86]. Moreover, it appears that loading suppresses pro-apoptotic signaling in quail muscle, but aging delays or attenuates these anti-apoptotic changes [86].

We have also studied muscle hypertrophy. Soleus and gastrocnemius muscles were ablated to cause compensatory hypertrophy on plantaris muscle [87]. Two weeks after the removal of soleus and gastrocnemius muscles we observed about a 40% increase in the muscle mass of plantaris muscle. This hypertrophy was associated with a significant increase in silent mating type information regulation 2 homologue 1 (SIRT1) content and activity ($p < 0.001$). SIRT1-regulated Akt, endothelial nitric oxide synthase, and GLUT4 levels. SIRT1 levels were correlated with muscle mass, paired box protein 7 (Pax7), proliferating cell nuclear antigen (PCNA), and nicotinamide phosphoribosyltransferase (Nampt) levels [87] (Figure 3). These data suggest that the redox state of the cells influences muscle growth, at least in this model. We also found that increased levels of K63 and muscle RING finger 2 (MuRF2) protein could also be important enhancers of muscle mass, and reported that the levels of microRNA (miR)1 and miR133a decrease in hypertrophy, and negatively correlate with muscle mass, SIRT1, and Nampt levels. These data suggest a strong correlation between SIRT1 and overload-induced hypertrophy [87].

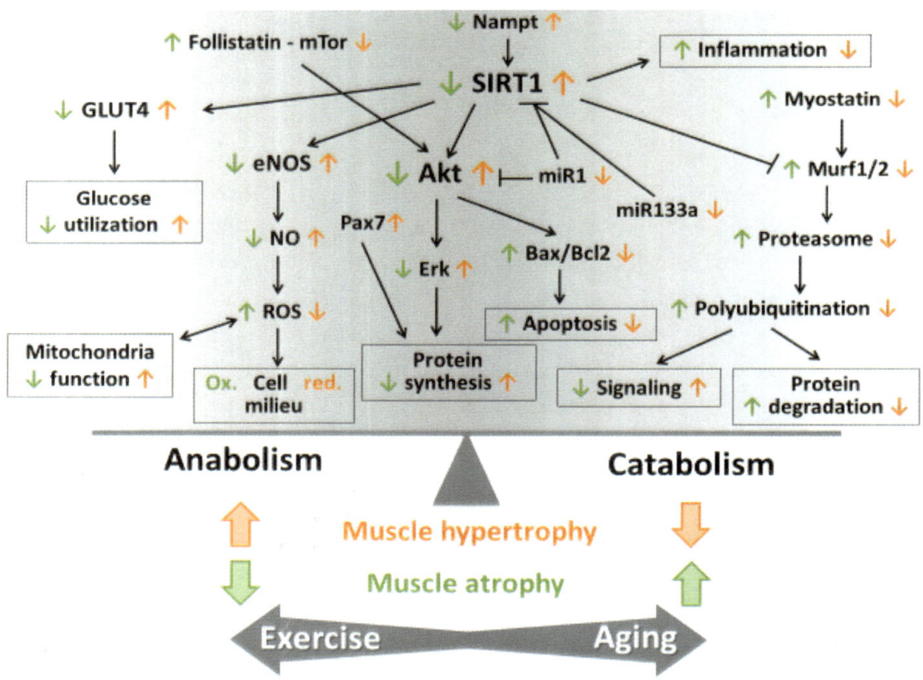

Figure 3. Schematic model of muscle hypertrophy and atrophy. The figure shows the schematic model, the molecular mechanisms of muscle hypertrophy, and age-associated muscle atrophy. SIRT1 is one of the key regulators of anabolic and catabolic processes in skeletal muscle.

6. Conclusions

Reactive oxygen species are continuously generated in contracting skeletal muscle, and their presence is obligatory for normal physiological function. Besides mitochondrial ROS production, XO and NADPH are the main sources of ROS. Moderate levels of ROS regulate metabolic processes in skeletal muscle, especially carbohydrate metabolism, and are also indirectly involved in fat metabolism through SIRT3. ROS-mediated structural changes of lipids, proteins, and DNA, to a degree, could be important for membrane remodeling, protein turnover, gene expression, or epigenetic regulation. Therefore, ROS are important causative or associative factors for sarcopenia and muscle hypertrophy.

Author Contributions: All author participated in reviewing the related literature and R.N., E.K., A.W.T., K.S., F.G., Z.R. wrote the paper.

Funding: This study was supported by OTKA (112810) and National Excellence Program (126823) grants awarded to Z.R.

Conflicts of Interest: Authors declare no conflict of interest.

References

1. Davies, K.J.; Quintanilha, A.T.; Brooks, G.A.; Packer, L. Free radicals and tissue damage produced by exercise. *Biochem. Biophys. Res. Commun.* **1982**, *107*, 1198–1205. [CrossRef]
2. Reid, M.B.; Khawli, F.A.; Moody, M.R. Reactive oxygen in skeletal muscle. III. Contractility of unfatigued muscle. *J. Appl. Physiol. (1985)* **1993**, *75*, 1081–1087. [CrossRef] [PubMed]
3. Reid, M.B.; Haack, K.E.; Franchek, K.M.; Valberg, P.A.; Kobzik, L.; West, M.S. Reactive oxygen in skeletal muscle. I. Intracellular oxidant kinetics and fatigue in vitro. *J. Appl. Physiol. (1985)* **1992**, *73*, 1797–1804. [CrossRef] [PubMed]
4. Reid, M.B.; Shoji, T.; Moody, M.R.; Entman, M.L. Reactive oxygen in skeletal muscle. II. Extracellular release of free radicals. *J. Appl. Physiol. (1985)* **1992**, *73*, 1805–1809. [CrossRef] [PubMed]
5. Goto, S.; Naito, H.; Kaneko, T.; Chung, H.Y.; Radak, Z. Hormetic effects of regular exercise in aging: Correlation with oxidative stress. *Appl. Physiol. Nutr. Metab.* **2007**, *32*, 948–953. [CrossRef] [PubMed]
6. Radak, Z.; Chung, H.Y.; Goto, S. Exercise and hormesis: Oxidative stress-related adaptation for successful aging. *Biogerontology* **2005**, *6*, 71–75. [CrossRef] [PubMed]
7. Radak, Z.; Chung, H.Y.; Goto, S. Systemic adaptation to oxidative challenge induced by regular exercise. *Free Radic. Biol. Med.* **2008**, *44*, 153–159. [CrossRef] [PubMed]
8. Radak, Z.; Chung, H.Y.; Koltai, E.; Taylor, A.W.; Goto, S. Exercise, oxidative stress and hormesis. *Ageing Res. Rev.* **2008**, *7*, 34–42. [CrossRef] [PubMed]
9. Powers, S.K.; Jackson, M.J. Exercise-induced oxidative stress: Cellular mechanisms and impact on muscle force production. *Physiol. Rev.* **2008**, *88*, 1243–1276. [CrossRef] [PubMed]
10. Saborido, A.; Naudi, A.; Portero-Otin, M.; Pamplona, R.; Megias, A. Stanozolol treatment decreases the mitochondrial ros generation and oxidative stress induced by acute exercise in rat skeletal muscle. *J. Appl. Physiol.* **2011**, *110*, 661–669. [CrossRef] [PubMed]
11. Vasilaki, A.; Mansouri, A.; Remmen, H.; van der Meulen, J.H.; Larkin, L.; Richardson, A.G.; McArdle, A.; Faulkner, J.A.; Jackson, M.J. Free radical generation by skeletal muscle of adult and old mice: Effect of contractile activity. *Aging Cell* **2006**, *5*, 109–117. [CrossRef] [PubMed]
12. Sahlin, K.; Shabalina, I.G.; Mattsson, C.M.; Bakkman, L.; Fernstrom, M.; Rozhdestvenskaya, Z.; Enqvist, J.K.; Nedergaard, J.; Ekblom, B.; Tonkonogi, M. Ultraendurance exercise increases the production of reactive oxygen species in isolated mitochondria from human skeletal muscle. *J. Appl. Physiol.* **2010**, *108*, 780–787. [CrossRef] [PubMed]
13. Boveris, A.; Chance, B. The mitochondrial generation of hydrogen peroxide. General properties and effect of hyperbaric oxygen. *Biochem. J.* **1973**, *134*, 707–716. [CrossRef] [PubMed]
14. St-Pierre, J.; Buckingham, J.A.; Roebuck, S.J.; Brand, M.D. Topology of superoxide production from different sites in the mitochondrial electron transport chain. *J. Biol. Chem.* **2002**, *277*, 44784–44790. [CrossRef] [PubMed]

15. Austin, S.; Klimcakova, E.; St-Pierre, J. Impact of pgc-1alpha on the topology and rate of superoxide production by the mitochondrial electron transport chain. *Free Radic. Biol. Med.* **2011**, *51*, 2243–2248. [CrossRef] [PubMed]
16. Muller, F.L.; Liu, Y.; Van Remmen, H. Complex III releases superoxide to both sides of the inner mitochondrial membrane. *J. Biol. Chem.* **2004**, *279*, 49064–49073. [CrossRef] [PubMed]
17. Ortenblad, N.; Young, J.F.; Oksbjerg, N.; Nielsen, J.H.; Lambert, I.H. Reactive oxygen species are important mediators of taurine release from skeletal muscle cells. *Am. J. Physiol. Cell Physiol.* **2003**, *284*, C1362–C1373. [CrossRef] [PubMed]
18. Bejma, J.; Ji, L.L. Aging and acute exercise enhance free radical generation in rat skeletal muscle. *J. Appl. Physiol.* **1999**, *87*, 465–470. [CrossRef] [PubMed]
19. Powers, S.K.; Nelson, W.B.; Hudson, M.B. Exercise-induced oxidative stress in humans: Cause and consequences. *Free Radic. Biol. Med.* **2011**, *51*, 942–950. [CrossRef] [PubMed]
20. Jackson, M.J. Control of reactive oxygen species production in contracting skeletal muscle. *Antioxid. Redox. Signal.* **2011**, *15*, 2477–2486. [CrossRef] [PubMed]
21. Radak, Z.; Asano, K.; Inoue, M.; Kizaki, T.; Oh-Ishi, S.; Suzuki, K.; Taniguchi, N.; Ohno, H. Superoxide dismutase derivative reduces oxidative damage in skeletal muscle of rats during exhaustive exercise. *J. Appl. Physiol.* **1995**, *79*, 129–135. [CrossRef] [PubMed]
22. Xia, Y.; Zweier, J.L. Substrate control of free radical generation from xanthine oxidase in the postischemic heart. *J. Biol. Chem.* **1995**, *270*, 18797–18803. [CrossRef] [PubMed]
23. Radak, Z.; Asano, K.; Inoue, M.; Kizaki, T.; Oh-Ishi, S.; Suzuki, K.; Taniguchi, N.; Ohno, H. Superoxide dismutase derivative prevents oxidative damage in liver and kidney of rats induced by exhausting exercise. *Eur. J. Appl. Physiol. Occup. Physiol.* **1996**, *72*, 189–194. [CrossRef] [PubMed]
24. Gomez-Cabrera, M.C.; Domenech, E.; Vina, J. Moderate exercise is an antioxidant: Upregulation of antioxidant genes by training. *Free Radic. Biol. Med.* **2008**, *44*, 126–131. [CrossRef] [PubMed]
25. Nethery, D.; Stofan, D.; Callahan, L.; DiMarco, A.; Supinski, G. Formation of reactive oxygen species by the contracting diaphragm is PLA_2 dependent. *J. Appl. Physiol (1985)* **1999**, *87*, 792–800. [CrossRef] [PubMed]
26. Allen, D.G.; Whitehead, N.P. Duchenne muscular dystrophy—What causes the increased membrane permeability in skeletal muscle? *Int. J. Biochem Cell Biol.* **2011**, *43*, 290–294. [CrossRef] [PubMed]
27. Da Silva-Azevedo, L.; Jahne, S.; Hoffmann, C.; Stalder, D.; Heller, M.; Pries, A.R.; Zakrzewicz, A.; Baum, O. Up-regulation of the peroxiredoxin-6 related metabolism of reactive oxygen species in skeletal muscle of mice lacking neuronal nitric oxide synthase. *J. Physiol.* **2009**, *587*, 655–668. [CrossRef] [PubMed]
28. Radak, Z.; Zhao, Z.; Goto, S.; Koltai, E. Age-associated neurodegeneration and oxidative damage to lipids, proteins and DNA. *Mol. Aspects Med.* **2011**, *32*, 305–315. [CrossRef] [PubMed]
29. Sriram, S.; Subramanian, S.; Sathiakumar, D.; Venkatesh, R.; Salerno, M.S.; McFarlane, C.D.; Kambadur, R.; Sharma, M. Modulation of reactive oxygen species in skeletal muscle by myostatin is mediated through nf-kappab. *Aging Cell* **2011**, *10*, 931–948. [CrossRef] [PubMed]
30. Andersson, D.C.; Betzenhauser, M.J.; Reiken, S.; Meli, A.C.; Umanskaya, A.; Xie, W.; Shiomi, T.; Zalk, R.; Lacampagne, A.; Marks, A.R. Ryanodine receptor oxidation causes intracellular calcium leak and muscle weakness in aging. *Cell Metab.* **2011**, *14*, 196–207. [CrossRef] [PubMed]
31. Syu, G.D.; Chen, H.I.; Jen, C.J. Severe exercise and exercise training exert opposite effects on human neutrophil apoptosis via altering the redox status. *PLoS ONE* **2011**, *6*, e24385. [CrossRef] [PubMed]
32. Suzuki, K.; Nakaji, S.; Yamada, M.; Liu, Q.; Kurakake, S.; Okamura, N.; Kumae, T.; Umeda, T.; Sugawara, K. Impact of a competitive marathon race on systemic cytokine and neutrophil responses. *Med. Sci. Sports Exerc.* **2003**, *35*, 348–355. [CrossRef] [PubMed]
33. Suzuki, K.; Totsuka, M.; Nakaji, S.; Yamada, M.; Kudoh, S.; Liu, Q.; Sugawara, K.; Yamaya, K.; Sato, K. Endurance exercise causes interaction among stress hormones, cytokines, neutrophil dynamics, and muscle damage. *J. Appl. Physiol. (1985)* **1999**, *87*, 1360–1367. [CrossRef] [PubMed]
34. Kawanishi, N.; Mizokami, T.; Niihara, H.; Yada, K.; Suzuki, K. Neutrophil depletion attenuates muscle injury after exhaustive exercise. *Med. Sci. Sports Exerc.* **2016**, *48*, 1917–1924. [CrossRef] [PubMed]
35. Zuo, L.; Christofi, F.L.; Wright, V.P.; Liu, C.Y.; Merola, A.J.; Berliner, L.J.; Clanton, T.L. Intra- and extracellular measurement of reactive oxygen species produced during heat stress in diaphragm muscle. *Am. J. Physiol. Cell Physiol.* **2000**, *279*, C1058–C1066. [CrossRef] [PubMed]

36. Andrade, F.H.; Reid, M.B.; Allen, D.G.; Westerblad, H. Effect of hydrogen peroxide and dithiothreitol on contractile function of single skeletal muscle fibres from the mouse. *J. Physiol.* **1998**, *509 Pt 2*, 565–575. [CrossRef] [PubMed]
37. Favero, T.G.; Zable, A.C.; Abramson, J.J. Hydrogen peroxide stimulates the Ca^{2+} release channel from skeletal muscle sarcoplasmic reticulum. *J. Biol. Chem.* **1995**, *270*, 25557–25563. [CrossRef] [PubMed]
38. Scherer, N.M.; Deamer, D.W. Oxidative stress impairs the function of sarcoplasmic reticulum by oxidation of sulfhydryl groups in the Ca^{2+}-atpase. *Arch. Biochem. Biophys.* **1986**, *246*, 589–601. [CrossRef]
39. Matsuo, M. Oxygen dependency of life-span in the nematode. *Comp. Biochem. Physiol. Comp. Physiol.* **1993**, *105*, 653–658. [CrossRef]
40. Zhu, X.; Heunks, L.M.; Ennen, L.; Machiels, H.A.; Van Der Heijden, H.F.; Dekhuijzen, P.N. Nitric oxide modulates neuromuscular transmission during hypoxia in rat diaphragm. *Muscle Nerve* **2006**, *33*, 104–112. [CrossRef] [PubMed]
41. King-Vanvlack, C.E.; Curtis, S.E.; Mewburn, J.D.; Cain, S.M.; Chapler, C.K. Role of endothelial factors in active hyperemic responses in contracting canine muscle. *J. Appl. Physiol. (1985)* **1995**, *79*, 107–112. [CrossRef] [PubMed]
42. Viner, R.I.; Ferrington, D.A.; Williams, T.D.; Bigelow, D.J.; Schoneich, C. Protein modification during biological aging: Selective tyrosine nitration of the SERCA2a isoform of the sarcoplasmic reticulum Ca^{2+}-atpase in skeletal muscle. *Biochem. J.* **1999**, *340 Pt 3*, 657–669. [CrossRef] [PubMed]
43. Meszaros, L.G.; Minarovic, I.; Zahradnikova, A. Inhibition of the skeletal muscle ryanodine receptor calcium release channel by nitric oxide. *FEBS Lett.* **1996**, *380*, 49–52. [CrossRef]
44. Radak, Z.; Pucsok, J.; Mecseki, S.; Csont, T.; Ferdinandy, P. Muscle soreness-induced reduction in force generation is accompanied by increased nitric oxide content and DNA damage in human skeletal muscle. *Free Radic. Biol. Med.* **1999**, *26*, 1059–1063. [CrossRef]
45. Wolin, M.S.; Hintze, T.H.; Shen, W.; Mohazzab, H.K.; Xie, Y.W. Involvement of reactive oxygen and nitrogen species in signalling mechanisms that control tissue respiration in muscle. *Biochem. Soc. Trans.* **1997**, *25*, 934–939. [CrossRef] [PubMed]
46. Rui, T.; Kvietys, P.R. NFκB and AP-1 differentially contribute to the induction of mn-sod and enos during the development of oxidant tolerance. *FASEB J.* **2005**, *19*, 1908–1910. [CrossRef] [PubMed]
47. Radak, Z.; Apor, P.; Pucsok, J.; Berkes, I.; Ogonovszky, H.; Pavlik, G.; Nakamoto, H.; Goto, S. Marathon running alters the DNA base excision repair in human skeletal muscle. *Life Sci.* **2003**, *72*, 1627–1633. [CrossRef]
48. Radak, Z.; Naito, H.; Kaneko, T.; Tahara, S.; Nakamoto, H.; Takahashi, R.; Cardozo-Pelaez, F.; Goto, S. Exercise training decreases DNA damage and increases DNA repair and resistance against oxidative stress of proteins in aged rat skeletal muscle. *Pflugers Arch.* **2002**, *445*, 273–278. [CrossRef] [PubMed]
49. Radak, Z.; Kumagai, S.; Nakamoto, H.; Goto, S. 8-Oxoguanosine and uracil repair of nuclear and mitochondrial DNA in red and white skeletal muscle of exercise-trained old rats. *J. Appl. Physiol. (1985)* **2007**, *102*, 1696–1701. [CrossRef] [PubMed]
50. Radak, Z.; Atalay, M.; Jakus, J.; Boldogh, I.; Davies, K.; Goto, S. Exercise improves import of 8-oxoguanine DNA glycosylase into the mitochondrial matrix of skeletal muscle and enhances the relative activity. *Free Radic. Biol. Med.* **2009**, *46*, 238–243. [CrossRef] [PubMed]
51. Radak, Z.; Takahashi, R.; Kumiyama, A.; Nakamoto, H.; Ohno, H.; Ookawara, T.; Goto, S. Effect of aging and late onset dietary restriction on antioxidant enzymes and proteasome activities, and protein carbonylation of rat skeletal muscle and tendon. *Exp. Gerontol.* **2002**, *37*, 1423–1430. [CrossRef]
52. Clavel, S.; Coldefy, A.S.; Kurkdjian, E.; Salles, J.; Margaritis, I.; Derijard, B. Atrophy-related ubiquitin ligases, atrogin-1 and MuRF1 are up-regulated in aged rat *Tibialis anterior* muscle. *Mech. Ageing Dev.* **2006**, *127*, 794–801. [CrossRef] [PubMed]
53. Raue, U.; Slivka, D.; Jemiolo, B.; Hollon, C.; Trappe, S. Proteolytic gene expression differs at rest and after resistance exercise between young and old women. *J. Gerontol. A Biol. Sci. Med. Sci.* **2007**, *62*, 1407–1412. [CrossRef] [PubMed]
54. Husom, A.D.; Peters, E.A.; Kolling, E.A.; Fugere, N.A.; Thompson, L.V.; Ferrington, D.A. Altered proteasome function and subunit composition in aged muscle. *Arch. Biochem. Biophys.* **2004**, *421*, 67–76. [CrossRef] [PubMed]

55. Radak, Z.; Kaneko, T.; Tahara, S.; Nakamoto, H.; Ohno, H.; Sasvari, M.; Nyakas, C.; Goto, S. The effect of exercise training on oxidative damage of lipids, proteins, and DNA in rat skeletal muscle: Evidence for beneficial outcomes. *Free Radic. Biol. Med.* **1999**, *27*, 69–74. [CrossRef]
56. Reid, M.B. Response of the ubiquitin-proteasome pathway to changes in muscle activity. *Am. J. Physiol. Regul. Integr. Comp. Physiol.* **2005**, *288*, R1423–R1431. [CrossRef] [PubMed]
57. Sultan, K.R.; Dittrich, B.T.; Leisner, E.; Paul, N.; Pette, D. Fiber type-specific expression of major proteolytic systems in fast- to slow-transforming rabbit muscle. *Am. J. Physiol. Cell Physiol.* **2001**, *280*, C239–C247. [CrossRef] [PubMed]
58. Kozlovsky, N.; Rudich, A.; Potashnik, R.; Bashan, N. Reactive oxygen species activate glucose transport in l6 myotubes. *Free Radic. Biol. Med.* **1997**, *23*, 859–869. [CrossRef]
59. Sandstrom, M.E.; Zhang, S.J.; Bruton, J.; Silva, J.P.; Reid, M.B.; Westerblad, H.; Katz, A. Role of reactive oxygen species in contraction-mediated glucose transport in mouse skeletal muscle. *J. Physiol.* **2006**, *575*, 251–262. [CrossRef] [PubMed]
60. Higaki, Y.; Mikami, T.; Fujii, N.; Hirshman, M.F.; Koyama, K.; Seino, T.; Tanaka, K.; Goodyear, L.J. Oxidative stress stimulates skeletal muscle glucose uptake through a phosphatidylinositol 3-kinase-dependent pathway. *Am. J. Physiol. Endocrinol. Metab.* **2008**, *294*, E889–E897. [CrossRef] [PubMed]
61. Kellogg, D.L., 3rd; McCammon, K.M.; Hinchee-Rodriguez, K.S.; Adamo, M.L.; Roman, L.J. Neuronal nitric oxide synthase mediates insulin- and oxidative stress-induced glucose uptake in skeletal muscle myotubes. *Free Radic. Biol. Med.* **2017**, *110*, 261–269. [CrossRef] [PubMed]
62. Ding, H.; Heng, B.; He, W.; Shi, L.; Lai, C.; Xiao, L.; Ren, H.; Mo, S.; Su, Z. Chronic reactive oxygen species exposure inhibits glucose uptake and causes insulin resistance in C2C12 myotubes. *Biochem. Biophys. Res. Commun.* **2016**, *478*, 798–803. [CrossRef] [PubMed]
63. White, A.T.; Schenk, S. NAD^+/NADH and skeletal muscle mitochondrial adaptations to exercise. *Am. J. Physiol. Endocrinol. Metab.* **2012**, *303*, E308–E321. [CrossRef] [PubMed]
64. Edington, D.W.; McCafferty, W.B. Mitochondrial size distribution analysis in the soleus muscle of trained and aged rats. *Experientia* **1973**, *29*, 692–693. [CrossRef] [PubMed]
65. Gariani, K.; Menzies, K.J.; Ryu, D.; Wegner, C.J.; Wang, X.; Ropelle, E.R.; Moullan, N.; Zhang, H.; Perino, A.; Lemos, V.; et al. Eliciting the mitochondrial unfolded protein response by nicotinamide adenine dinucleotide repletion reverses fatty liver disease in mice. *Hepatology* **2016**, *63*, 1190–1204. [CrossRef] [PubMed]
66. Hirschey, M.D.; Shimazu, T.; Goetzman, E.; Jing, E.; Schwer, B.; Lombard, D.B.; Grueter, C.A.; Harris, C.; Biddinger, S.; Ilkayeva, O.R.; et al. SIRT3 regulates mitochondrial fatty-acid oxidation by reversible enzyme deacetylation. *Nature* **2010**, *464*, 121–125. [CrossRef] [PubMed]
67. Radak, Z.; Bori, Z.; Koltai, E.; Fatouros, I.G.; Jamurtas, A.Z.; Douroudos, I.I.; Terzis, G.; Nikolaidis, M.G.; Chatzinikolaou, A.; Sovatzidis, A.; et al. Age-dependent changes in 8-oxoguanine-DNA glycosylase activity are modulated by adaptive responses to physical exercise in human skeletal muscle. *Free Radic. Biol. Med.* **2011**, *51*, 417–423. [CrossRef] [PubMed]
68. Vargas-Ortiz, K.; Perez-Vazquez, V.; Figueroa, A.; Diaz, F.J.; Montano-Ascencio, P.G.; Macias-Cervantes, M.H. Aerobic training but no resistance training increases SIRT3 in skeletal muscle of sedentary obese male adolescents. *Eur. J. Sport Sci.* **2018**, *18*, 226–234. [CrossRef] [PubMed]
69. Palacios, O.M.; Carmona, J.J.; Michan, S.; Chen, K.Y.; Manabe, Y.; Ward, J.L., 3rd; Goodyear, L.J.; Tong, Q. Diet and exercise signals regulate SIRT3 and activate AMPK and PGC-1α in skeletal muscle. *Aging (Albany N. Y.)* **2009**, *1*, 771–783. [CrossRef] [PubMed]
70. Lin, L.; Chen, K.; Abdel Khalek, W.; Ward, J.L., 3rd; Yang, H.; Chabi, B.; Wrutniak-Cabello, C.; Tong, Q. Regulation of skeletal muscle oxidative capacity and muscle mass by SIRT3. *PLoS ONE* **2014**, *9*, e85636. [CrossRef] [PubMed]
71. Fan, W.; Waizenegger, W.; Lin, C.S.; Sorrentino, V.; He, M.X.; Wall, C.E.; Li, H.; Liddle, C.; Yu, R.T.; Atkins, A.R.; et al. PPARδ promotes running endurance by preserving glucose. *Cell Metab.* **2017**, *25*, 1186–1193. [CrossRef] [PubMed]
72. Weindruch, R. Interventions based on the possibility that oxidative stress contributes to sarcopenia. *J. Gerontol. A Biol. Sci. Med. Sci.* **1995**, *50A*, 157–161.
73. Trifunovic, A.; Wredenberg, A.; Falkenberg, M.; Spelbrink, J.N.; Rovio, A.T.; Bruder, C.E.; Bohlooly, Y.M.; Gidlof, S.; Oldfors, A.; Wibom, R.; et al. Premature ageing in mice expressing defective mitochondrial DNA polymerase. *Nature* **2004**, *429*, 417–423. [CrossRef] [PubMed]

74. Hiona, A.; Sanz, A.; Kujoth, G.C.; Pamplona, R.; Seo, A.Y.; Hofer, T.; Someya, S.; Miyakawa, T.; Nakayama, C.; Samhan-Arias, A.K.; et al. Mitochondrial DNA mutations induce mitochondrial dysfunction, apoptosis and sarcopenia in skeletal muscle of mitochondrial DNA mutator mice. *PLoS ONE* **2010**, *5*, e11468. [CrossRef] [PubMed]
75. Martin, C.; Dubouchaud, H.; Mosoni, L.; Chardigny, J.M.; Oudot, A.; Fontaine, E.; Vergely, C.; Keriel, C.; Rochette, L.; Leverve, X.; et al. Abnormalities of mitochondrial functioning can partly explain the metabolic disorders encountered in sarcopenic gastrocnemius. *Aging Cell* **2007**, *6*, 165–177. [CrossRef] [PubMed]
76. Jang, Y.C.; Lustgarten, M.S.; Liu, Y.; Muller, F.L.; Bhattacharya, A.; Liang, H.; Salmon, A.B.; Brooks, S.V.; Larkin, L.; Hayworth, C.R.; et al. Increased superoxide in vivo accelerates age-associated muscle atrophy through mitochondrial dysfunction and neuromuscular junction degeneration. *FASEB J.* **2010**, *24*, 1376–1390. [CrossRef] [PubMed]
77. Degens, H. The role of systemic inflammation in age-related muscle weakness and wasting. *Scand. J. Med. Sci. Sports* **2010**, *20*, 28–38. [CrossRef] [PubMed]
78. Ji, L.L. Exercise at old age: Does it increase or alleviate oxidative stress? *Ann. N. Y. Acad. Sci.* **2001**, *928*, 236–247. [CrossRef] [PubMed]
79. McArdle, A.; Jackson, M.J. The role of attenuated redox and heat shock protein responses in the age-related decline in skeletal muscle mass and function. *Essays Biochem.* **2017**, *61*, 339–348. [CrossRef] [PubMed]
80. Marzetti, E.; Calvani, R.; Cesari, M.; Buford, T.W.; Lorenzi, M.; Behnke, B.J.; Leeuwenburgh, C. Mitochondrial dysfunction and sarcopenia of aging: From signaling pathways to clinical trials. *Int. J. Biochem. Cell Biol.* **2013**, *45*, 2288–2301. [CrossRef] [PubMed]
81. Rahman, M.; Halade, G.V.; El Jamali, A.; Fernandes, G. Conjugated linoleic acid (CLA) prevents age-associated skeletal muscle loss. *Biochem. Biophys. Res. Commun.* **2009**, *383*, 513–518. [CrossRef] [PubMed]
82. Beavers, K.M.; Beavers, D.P.; Serra, M.C.; Bowden, R.G.; Wilson, R.L. Low relative skeletal muscle mass indicative of sarcopenia is associated with elevations in serum uric acid levels: Findings from nhanes III. *J. Nutr. Health Aging* **2009**, *13*, 177–182. [CrossRef] [PubMed]
83. Lightfoot, A.P.; McCormick, R.; Nye, G.A.; McArdle, A. Mechanisms of skeletal muscle ageing; avenues for therapeutic intervention. *Curr. Opin. Pharmacol.* **2014**, *16*, 116–121. [CrossRef] [PubMed]
84. Zhao, J.; Tian, Z.; Kadomatsu, T.; Xie, P.; Miyata, K.; Sugizaki, T.; Endo, M.; Zhu, S.; Fan, H.; Horiguchi, H.; et al. Age-dependent increase in angiopoietin-like protein 2 accelerates skeletal muscle loss in mice. *J. Biol. Chem.* **2018**, *293*, 1596–1609. [CrossRef] [PubMed]
85. Ziaaldini, M.M.; Koltai, E.; Csende, Z.; Goto, S.; Boldogh, I.; Taylor, A.W.; Radak, Z. Exercise training increases anabolic and attenuates catabolic and apoptotic processes in aged skeletal muscle of male rats. *Exp. Gerontol.* **2015**, *67*, 9–14. [CrossRef] [PubMed]
86. Siu, P.M.; Alway, S.E. Aging alters the reduction of pro-apoptotic signaling in response to loading-induced hypertrophy. *Exp. Gerontol.* **2006**, *41*, 175–188. [CrossRef] [PubMed]
87. Koltai, E.; Bori, Z.; Chabert, C.; Dubouchaud, H.; Naito, H.; Machida, S.; Davies, K.J.; Murlasits, Z.; Fry, A.C.; Boldogh, I.; et al. SIRT1 may play a crucial role in overload-induced hypertrophy of skeletal muscle. *J. Physiol.* **2017**, *595*, 3361–3376. [CrossRef] [PubMed]

8

Selenium-Dependent Antioxidant Enzymes: Actions and Properties of Selenoproteins

Evangelos Zoidis [1,*], Isidoros Seremelis [2], Nikolaos Kontopoulos [2] and Georgios P. Danezis [2]

[1] Department of Nutritional Physiology and Feeding, Faculty of Animal Science and Aquaculture, Agricultural University of Athens, 75 Iera Odos, 11855 Athens, Greece

[2] Chemistry Laboratory, Department of Food Science and Human Nutrition, Agricultural University of Athens, 75 Iera Odos, 11855 Athens, Greece; iseremelis@gmail.com (I.S.); stud315044@aua.gr (N.K.); gdanezis@aua.gr (G.P.D.)

* Correspondence: ezoidis@aua.gr

Abstract: Unlike other essential trace elements that interact with proteins in the form of cofactors, selenium (Se) becomes co-translationally incorporated into the polypeptide chain as part of 21st naturally occurring amino acid, selenocysteine (Sec), encoded by the UGA codon. Any protein that includes Sec in its polypeptide chain is defined as selenoprotein. Members of the selenoproteins family exert various functions and their synthesis depends on specific cofactors and on dietary Se. The Se intake in productive animals such as chickens affect nutrient utilization, production performances, antioxidative status and responses of the immune system. Although several functions of selenoproteins are unknown, many disorders are related to alterations in selenoprotein expression or activity. Selenium insufficiency and polymorphisms or mutations in selenoproteins' genes and synthesis cofactors are involved in the pathophysiology of many diseases, including cardiovascular disorders, immune dysfunctions, cancer, muscle and bone disorders, endocrine functions and neurological disorders. Finally, heavy metal poisoning decreases mRNA levels of selenoproteins and increases mRNA levels of inflammatory factors, underlying the antagonistic effect of Se. This review is an update on Se dependent antioxidant enzymes, presenting the current state of the art and is focusing on results obtained mainly in chicken.

Keywords: antioxidant system; reactive oxygen species (ROS); selenium; selenocysteine; selenomethionine; selenoproteins

---

1. Introduction

Selenium (Se) is an essential trace element which is co-translationally incorporated into the polypeptide chain as part of the amino acid selenocysteine (Sec). Proteins that include Sec in their polypeptide chain are defined as selenoproteins and exist in all lineages of life (archaea, bacteria and eukarya) [1–6], however, some organisms do not have the ability to synthesize selenoproteins [7]. Selenoproteins have pivotal significance for optimal human and animal health mainly due to their antioxidant activity [8]. They have anti-inflammatory, chemo preventive and antiviral properties and are related with the improvement of immune responses [9,10]. The health-related properties of selenoproteins include among others protection against cancer [11,12], proper thyroid function [13] and protection against cardiovascular [14] and muscle disorders; however, the role of selenium supplementation in diseases of the thyroid gland is still subject to discussion [15–21].

There are 25 genes encoding for selenoproteins [22,23]. Selenoprotein family, in human, includes the following members: glutathione peroxidases (GPX1–GPX4 and GPX6), thioredoxin reductases (TXNRD1–2), thioredoxin-glutathione reductase (TXNRD3), iodothyronine deiodinases (DIO1–3), selenophosphate synthetase (SEPHS2), 15-kDa selenoprotein (SELENOF), selenoprotein H (SELENOH), selenoprotein I (SELENOI), selenoprotein K (SELENOK), selenoprotein M (SELENOM), selenoprotein N (SELENON), selenoprotein O (SELENOO), selenoprotein P (SELENOP), methionine sulfoxide reductase B1 (MSRB1), selenoprotein S (SELENOS), selenoprotein T (SELENOT), selenoprotein V (SELENOV) and selenoprotein W (SELENOW) [24,25]. Low dietary Se may result in selenoproteins deficiency leading to such human diseases as Keshan disease [26–28], Kashin-Beck disease [29], myxedematous endemic cretinism [30] and male infertility [31].

According to the Office of Dietary Supplements (ODS) of the National Institutes of Health (NIH, Bethesda, MD, USA), Recommended Daily Allowance (RDA) of Se is 55 μg/day for men of 31–50 years old up to 70 μg/day for women on lactation. Even though globally dietary Se intake is usually below 55 μg/day [8], European countries such as Greece [32], Poland [33], UK [34] and Spain [35] have an average Se intake below 40 μg/day and this appears to be the situation also for other parts of the world. For example, it has been estimated that the average Se intake for adult men and women in Argentina is 32 and 24 μg/day, respectively [36]. Further, a recent study carried out from German, Austrian and Swiss nutrition societies resulted in values of 70 μg/day for men and 60 μg/day for women using the reference body weights [37]. To help meeting the RDA, consumers could benefit from the use of Se-enriched functional foods. Production technology of Se-enriched eggs, milk and meat has been developed and successfully introduced. Actually, Se-enriched eggs can be obtained in more than 25 countries worldwide [36,38].

2. Synthesis of Selenoproteins from Dietary Selenium

Selenocysteine and selenomethionine (SeMet) are similar to cysteine and methionine except that the sulfur (S) atom is substituted by Se [39]. Yeast and plants do not incorporate Sec and, therefore, do not possess selenoproteins [40]. However, in a recent study, the analysis of cranberry mitochondrial genome revealed the presence of two copies of selenocysteine insertion sequence element (SECIS) and tRNA-Sec [41]. Plants absorb Se from the soil in the form of selenate or selenite and synthesize SeMet [42], which implies that in natural feed ingredients Se can be primarily found in the form of SeMet [43]. Vertebrates get dietary Se as SeMet and other Se-amino acids, including Sec and its methylated forms, depending on their contents in feed/food components. Moreover, presently, farm animal feeds are broadly supplemented with inorganic Se such as sodium-selenate and selenite as well as with organic sources of Se such as selenized yeast. There are major differences in the metabolism and absorption of these forms of Se. For example, sodium selenite is passively absorbed in the intestine and more efficiently in the ileum segment [44], while SeMet is actively absorbed and thus requires a transport mechanism to actually shift the molecules through the enterocyte cell membrane, by all segments of the intestine [45]. Absorption of Se compounds into cells is considered to occur via anion transporters [46–48]. Irrespective of the form that Se is received from the diet, it has to be metabolized into Sec to be incorporated into selenoproteins.

The incorporation of Se as Sec into a selenoprotein requires a specific mechanism to decode the UGA codon in mRNA, which normally operates in translation termination [49]. Initially, the oxidized forms of inorganic Se undergo reductive metabolism yielding hydrogen selenide (H_2Se) which is converted to Sec [50]. Organic sources of Se can also produce H_2Se. Selenomethionine can be trans-selenated into Sec, similarly to the trans-sulfuration pathway for methionine to cysteine, before lysis by β-lyase to H_2Se. Hydrogen selenide must be first transformed to Sec, which means that H_2Se has to be metabolized into selenophosphate after catalysis by the SEPHS2 [50]. Selenophosphate reacts with the tRNA specific for serine Ser-tRNASec via the enzyme Sec-tRNA synthase to give Sec bound tRNA (Sec-tRNASec), from which Sec is incorporated into selenoproteins by the Sec specific UGA codon [42,51–54]. Specific mutations in the coding sequence of the Sec-tRNA play a key role in the expression of particular selenoproteins but also in the progression and symptomatology of some diseases [55]. This incorporation of Sec into selenoproteins occurs when the mRNA contains a distinct hairpin mRNA sequence downstream of the UGA codon in its 3′-untranslated region (3′-UTR) called

Sec insertion sequence (SECIS) [56]. Sec insertion sequence prevents the termination of translation by competing for release factors that would otherwise lead to disassembly of the mRNA-ribosomal complex [53,57–60]. Biosynthesis of selenoproteins requires binding of SBP2 (SECIS-binding protein 2) to the SECIS element and recruitment of the Sec tRNA-specific elongation factor (EFsec), connected to tRNASec [61]. Namely, SECIS recruits SBP2 and binds the tRNASec-loaded EFSec, while several additional proteins bind to SECIS [62–64].

Selenium may also efficiently control UGA-Sec codon translation [65,66], regulate levels of Sec tRNASer(Sec) and control the ratio of the methylated and unmethylated Sec tRNA(Ser)Sec isoforms [67–70]. The methylated isoform is translationally active and Se-induced tRNA methylation is a mechanism of selenoprotein synthesis regulation. The methylated isoform has been shown to govern the synthesis of selenoproteins involved in the oxidative stress response such as GPX1 and GPX3, whereas the unmethylated form controls synthesis of housekeeping selenoproteins i.e., TXNRD1 and TXNRD3 [71].

It seems that all selenoproteins of eukaryotes require a form of the SECIS element for recoding UGA to the Sec codon [61]. However, there may be a SBP2 independent binding affinity for the Sec-tRNA. This must be clarified by further research [72]. Most of the selenoproteins can be classified into two groups according to the position of the Sec in the polypeptide chain. In the first group, Sec is located on the N-terminal while in the second group Sec is present on the C-terminal position of the function domain [73]. The first group includes all glutathione peroxidases and iodothyronine deiodinases, SEPHS2, SELENOF, SELENOH, SELENOM, SELENON, SELENOP, SELENOT, SELENOV, and SELENOW, while the second one includes thioredoxin reductases, SELENOS, MSRB1, SELENOO, SELENOI and SELENOK [50].

The first selenoenzyme identified—glutathione peroxidase (GPX)—catalyzes the oxidation of cytosolic glutathione (GSH) by H_2O_2 (Table 1). GPX1 was discovered in erythrocytes [74], where it removes H_2O_2 formed by dissociation of oxyhemoglobin into O_2 and methemoglobin [75]. The GPX1 gene codes for both the cytosolic and mitochondrial forms of the enzyme, which exist as a tetramer of four identical subunits, each containing a single Sec residue.

Table 1. Reactive oxygen and nitrogen species.

Radicals	Non-Radicals
$RO^{\bullet}$, Alkoxyl	H_2O_2, Hydrogen peroxide
$HOO^{\bullet}$, Hydroperoxyl	HOCl, Hypochlorous acid
$HO^{\bullet}$, Hydroxyl	O_3, Ozone
$ROO^{\bullet}$, Peroxyl	$^1O_2$, Singlet oxygen
$O_2^{\bullet -}$, Superoxide	$ONOO^-$, Peroxynitrite
$NO^{\bullet}$, Nitric oxide	NO^-, Nitroxyl anion
$NO_2^{\bullet}$, Nitrogen dioxide	HNO_2, Nitrous acid

3. Selenoproteins and the Antioxidant System

The lack of balance between generation of reactive oxygen/nitrogen species (ROS/RNS) and the action of protective antioxidant systems is defined as oxidative stress [76,77]. In normal conditions, a balance between generation of free radicals and antioxidant protection exists in the cell. However, increased ROS/RNS generation or impairment of the antioxidant protective ability leads to oxidative stress. Generation of ROS by a reduced coupling of oxidation and phosphorylation in the inner mitochondrial membrane results in an enhanced electron leakage and overproduction of superoxide radicals (Table 1).

Many pollutants, such as heavy metals (e.g., Cd and Pb), certain drugs and various radiations (ultra violet and γ rays), can induce high production of free radicals. When the generation of ROS surpasses the capacity of the antioxidant system to neutralize them, extensive peroxidation of lipids occurs and causes damage to the unsaturated lipids of the cellular membrane. As a result, the integrity of the cell is disturbed. In addition, disturbances of natural antioxidant and/or metallothionein

(MT) levels may cause peroxidation of lipids, which may result in ROS attacking and cleaving of double bonds. It is generally accepted that the susceptibility of polyunsaturated fatty acids (PUFA) to peroxidation corresponds to the number of double bounds in these molecules. In fact, arachidonic acid (AA, 20:4n-6) and docosahexaenoic acid (DHA, 22:6n-3) constitute the primary substrates of the peroxidation in the membrane. The same PUFA are mainly responsible for maintenance of physiologically crucial properties of the membrane including permeability and fluidity. In other words, both function and structure of biological membranes are compromised through lipid peroxidation [78]. This is correlated with reduced absorption of various nutrients and causes an imbalance of inorganic elements, amino acids, vitamins and other nutrients in the organism [79]. Thus, oxidative stress decreases productive and reproductive performances of organisms [80]. About 100,000 ROS hit rat cellular DNA each day [81–83]. DNA damage may occur via oxidation, methylation, deamination and depurination. Reactive oxygen species interaction with DNA is very complex and includes strand break, base modification, DNA-protein cross links and lesions in chromatin and sugars [84–86]. Organisms have evolutionary developed specific protective antioxidant mechanisms to defend against ROS/RNS. Consequently, it is the presence of natural antioxidants in living organisms that enables them to survive in an oxygen-rich environment [87].

Other major targets of two-electron oxidants and radicals in biological systems are proteins due to their rapid rates constants and abundance for reaction [88,89]. Protein oxidation by free radicals can occur in the protein backbone or at amino acid side chains [90]. Peroxides (protein peroxidation) and peroxyl radicals are formed under oxygen presence. They can oxidize both proteins and other targets. Protein modifications by oxidation, can include unstable intermediates formation, loss of the parent amino acid residue and also generation of stable products. Protein oxidation is linked with multiple human pathologies and aging [88,91–94]. Selenoproteins as wide range antioxidants also protect cell from damages caused by cellular proteins oxidation [95]. Further, selenium-containing compounds such as selenides (RSeR′), selenols (RSeH) and diselenides (RSeSeR′) react with peroxynitrite under raised rate constants [96].

The antioxidant system is mainly comprised of water-soluble antioxidants (uric acid, ascorbic acid, and taurine); natural fat-soluble antioxidants (carotenoids, vitamins A and E, and ubiquinones); antioxidant enzymes; the thioredoxin system (thioredoxin/thioredoxin peroxidase/thioredoxin reductases (TXNRDs)); and the thiol redox system (GSH/GSH reductase/glutaredoxin/GPXs) [97]. For maximum protection, the antioxidant system is located in various organelles, subcellular compartments as well as the extracellular space.

In vertebrates, GPXs have a single redox center and as redox-active residue the selenocystein. In contrast, non-vertebrate GPXs replace peroxidatic Sec by a cysteine (peroxidatic Cys) and work with a second redox center that contains a resolving cysteine [98].

Among the components of the thioredoxin and thiol redox systems, several enzymes contain Sec residues that are essential for enzyme function [99]. Nonetheless, most, if not all, of the currently known selenoproteins are also found as Cys-containing non-selenoprotein orthologs in other organisms, wherefore any potentially unique properties of selenoproteins are yet a matter of debate. The chemical rate enhancement obtained with Sec can have other consequences than those arising from a low redox potential of some Cys-dependent proteins, typically aiming at maintaining redox equilibria. Another unique aspect of Sec compared to Cys seems to be its efficient potency to support one-electron transfer reactions, which, however, has not yet been unequivocally shown as a Sec-dependent step during the natural catalysis of any known selenoprotein enzyme [100].

The antioxidant system of the cell includes three major levels of defense [101]. The first level (prevention) prevents the formation of free radical. It inactivates catalysts or removes precursors of free radicals and includes three antioxidant enzymes namely GPX, superoxide dismutase (SOD) and catalase (CAT) and metal-binding proteins such as transferrin, lactoferrin, haptoglobin, hemopexin, metallothionein, ceruloplasmin, ferritin, albumin and myoglobin. Thus, metal sequestration is an important part of extracellular antioxidant defense [80,102,103]. This first level of antioxidant defense is insufficient to fully impede generation of free radical in the cell. As a result, some radicals escape, initiating peroxidation of lipids and causing protein and DNA damages. However, lipids peroxidation can only be stopped by GPX4 and no other selenoprotein. Thus, a second level (interception) of antioxidant defense exists. It consists of chain-breaking antioxidants (vitamins A and E, ascorbic acid, uric acid, carotenoids, and ubiquinol) as well as other antioxidants. Thioredoxin and thiol redox systems play also an essential role in this second level of defense. Thioredoxin reductases use nicotinamide adenine dinucleotide phosphate to reduce oxidized thioredoxin and its homologs, which regulate many redox signaling events. Vitamin E cannot do the whole work in preventing peroxidation of lipids by scavenging free radicals and forming hydroperoxides [103]. Together with Se, they act in tandem; and even very high doses of dietary vitamin E cannot replace Se, which is indispensable to complete the second part of antioxidant defense. Thus, Se as an integral part of selenoproteins contribute both to the first and the second level of antioxidant defense [97].

Elemental Se and more often its compounds have been successfully used as stoichiometric reagents and catalysts for oxidation of different organic substrates. Selenium(IV) oxide, areneseleninic acids and their anhydrides are widely used as stoichiometric oxidants or as oxygen-transfer agents for oxygen donors, particularly hydrogen peroxide and tert-butyl hydroperoxide. The oxidation mechanisms depend on the substrate and oxidant or catalyst used. The electrophilic center localized on the selenium atom or the nucleophilic center localized on the oxygen atom of the selenahydroperoxide group are involved in the reaction mechanism [104].

While ROS are largely involved in causing cell damage, they also possess significant roles in several physiological aspects such as regulation of protein phosphorylation, intracellular signal transduction, regulation of the cytosolic Ca concentration, regulation of gene expression, intracellular killing of bacteria by neutrophils and macrophages and activation of certain transcription factors, such as nuclear factor-kappa B (NF-κB) and the activator protein 1 (AP-1) family factors [105–111]. Free radical reactions are part of normal human metabolism and can be induced by environmental sources [87,112].

Glutathione is the most abundant non-protein thiol in mammalian and avian cells, providing them with their reducing milieu [113,114]. Cellular GSH has an essential role in various biological processes including: synthesis of proteins and DNA [115,116], cell proliferation and growth [117], regulation of apoptosis and cancer growth [118], immune regulation (T cell growth and metabolic reprogramming) [119,120], xenobiotic metabolism, transport of amino acids and redox-sensitive signal transduction [121]. Moreover, GSH thiolic group may directly react with several ROS including hydroxyl radicals, hydroperoxides, alkoxyl radicals and superoxide anion (Table 1) [80,122,123]. Most importantly, GSH acts as scavenger of free radical, especially efficient against the hydroxyl radical, since there are no enzymatic defenses against this radical species [124]. Generally, reduced concentration of GSH in tissues is connected with increased peroxidation of lipids [101,125]. Moreover, in stress conditions, GSH prevents the loss of vitamin E and protein thiols [126] and acts as a key modulator of cell signaling [127]. Humans as well as animals can synthesize GSH. In this respect, eight GPX members have been discovered [97,128]. Apart from their specific functions, all of them exert antioxidant tasks, protecting cells against oxidation damage from free radicals and ROS [129].

Selenoproteins have the unique ability to trap H_2O_2 and use the resulting selenenic acid to form specific disulfide bonds in the presence of 10–20 mM GSH and are thus well suited for controlling the formation of disulfide bonds with specific Cys residues. Because of the rapid oxidation kinetics of selenols, H_2O_2 in the cytosol reacts completely with Sec-containing proteins to produce Sec selenenic acid before it can react with other potential targets. Thus, rapid consumption of H_2O_2 by selenoproteins acts to limit the duration of H_2O_2 signals and the distance over which those signals are transmitted by diffusion [130].

Nevertheless, even this second level of cell antioxidant defense (interception) is unable to hinder the deteriorating effects of ROS/RNS on DNA and proteins. In this case, the third level of antioxidant defense depends on systems that repair damaged molecules or eliminate them [131]. This level of defense consists of proteolytic (peptidases or proteases), lipolytic (lipases) and other enzymes (proteinases, phospholipases, nucleases, DNA repair enzymes, polymerases, ligases and diverse transferases). However, the enzymes of the third level of antioxidant defense cannot achieve total removal or repair of damaged DNA molecules and this may result to arrest of cell cycle and cell death [132]. In fact, the process of apoptosis (programmed cell death in multicellular organisms) is involved in maintenance of the genetic integrity by eliminating genetically altered cells [78].

4. Effects of Selenium Supplementation in Chicken

As already stated, the major role of Se is the protection against free radical detrimental effects via the action of selenoproteins. Many studies have shown that Se/vitamin E dietary deficiencies are related to presumed oxidative cell damage. It has been shown that selenoproteins impede nutritional muscular dystrophy (NMD) initiation in chicks via metabolism of peroxides and redox regulation mechanisms [133]. In addition, dietary Se deficiency has a negative impact in the mRNA expression of 23 selenoproteins in broiler immune organs (thymus, spleen and bursa). Additionally, at Se super-nutritional status, most selenoproteins were upregulated in chicken kidney [134–136]. Moreover, 24 selenoproteins and associated transcription factors were influenced by Se intake in chickens' pancreas. Selenium contributions to chicken development and regulation of blood sugar were associated with pancreatic redox homeostasis via a modulated selenotranscriptome [137]. Selenoprotein genes in spleen and thymus were down-regulated, inflammation-related genes were up-regulated due to supranutritional dietary Se status. Further, chickens' growth performances were depressed. Over high ambient temperature, Se enriched probiotics reduced the effects of Se deficiency on heart lesion. In addition, in chicken heart, upregulation of mRNA expression of GPX1 and GPX4 and downregulation of heat shock protein genes (HSP90, HSP70 and HSP60) were induced with Se enriched probiotics [138] and, similarly, in broilers exposed at high ambient temperature, prebiotics enriched with Se improved meat quality [139]. Notably, investigations have reported the protective role of selenoprotein W against H_2O_2 which means that an association of selenoprotein W mRNA expression, oxidative stress and metabolic status may exist. Moreover, selenoprotein W expression could be regulated by metabolic factors and Cd in fish [140].

Improved action of Se containing antioxidant enzymes, for instance TXNRD and GPX, decreased free radical-mediated peroxidation and regeneration of GSH was observed due to Se supplementation [141]. Thus, Se levels above nutritional requirements may be capable of maintaining optimal TXNRD and GPX activities and detoxifying Cd [142–144].

Many studies highlight the effectiveness of Se in preventing heavy metal poisoning. A recent study revealed Se-Cr (VI) interaction and other trace elements accumulation in chicken serum and brain. The results demonstrated that Se supplementation decreased accumulation of Cr both in chicken brain and serum and this interaction regulated the correlation and contents of Ca, Cu, Mn, Fe, Zn, and Mg in these tissues [145]. Another study investigated the effects of Se on the toxicity of Pb and the expressions of selenoproteins mRNA in chicken cartilage tissue. The results showed that reduced expression of GPX4, GPX2, GPX1, DIO1–2, TXNRD2–3, selenoprotein U, selenoprotein I, Sepx1, selenoprotein O, selenoprotein M, selenoprotein K, selenoprotein W, selenoprotein 15, Sepn1, selenoprotein T, and selenoprotein S in the meniscus cartilage, triggered by Pb exposure, might be alleviated by Se. In addition, in cartilage of sword fish, the reduction in the mRNA expression levels of GPX2–4, TXNRD1–2, DIO2–3, selenoprotein H, selenoprotein I, SEPHS2, MSRB1, selenoprotein W, selenoprotein K, selenoprotein M, selenoprotein O, selenoprotein 15, selenoprotein T, Sepn1 and selenoprotein Pb due to Pb exposure could be mitigated by Se [146].

Lead toxicity mitigative effect by Se has been investigated via expression analysis of 25 selenoproteins and 5 HSPs. The results indicated that Se declined the increase of HSPs mRNA expression and enhanced the diminished mRNA expression levels of all selenoproteins caused by Pb in chicken testes, pointing that HSP70 could be an indicator of Pb poisoning in this tissue [147]. Moreover, Pb exposure increased Pb content in serum, activated the NF-κB pathway, and increased the expression of selenoproteins in chicken neutrophils. Selenium supplements could reduce Pb concentration in serum, had a mitigative effect on the activation of the NF-κB pathway and further enhanced the upward trend of selenoproteins expression induced by Pb exposure [148]. Further studies investigated the antagonistic effect of Se on Pb-induced inflammation injury and the results showed that Pb poisoning enhanced mRNA levels of inflammation, reduced mRNA levels of selenoproteins, and induced histological modifications in chicken hearts. Except Pb, toxicity was also induced by Cd. Thus, studies aimed to evaluate potential cytoprotective mechanisms of Se and to examine the actions of Se in mitigating Cd induced toxicity in chicken heart. It seems that Cd can cause serious myocardial damage by inducing the necroptosis route, while Se could act in the prevention of Cd-induced myocardial damage via the activation of the adiponectin pathway [149]. In addition, Se supplementation in laying chickens seems to change pancreatic ions and profile decreasing Cd accumulation in chicken pancreas [150].

Furthermore, enhanced incorporation of Sec after Se treatment led to increased TXNRD and GPX activities [151]. DNA repair and integrity can be affected by organic forms of Se. For instance, diets supplemented with SeMet at 3 or 6 μg/kg body weight per day for seven months were provided to elderly male dogs and the results were compared to untreated controls. Dogs supplemented with Se presented lower expansion of DNA damage in peripheral blood lymphocytes and in prostate cells compared to controls [152]. Moreover, supplementation of supranutritional organic Se to chicken nutrition, at safe subtoxic levels, prevented the peroxidation of health-promoting long-chain PUFA, like eicosapentaenoic acid (EPA) and DHA, and protected meat quality from oxidation [153]. Another study [154] revealed that SeMet stimulated cell protection against DNA damage and DNA repair. The increased repair complex formation in SeMet-treated cells was indicated as a feasible mechanism for the DNA repair response. Kibriya et al. [155] found that many genes, after Se supplementation, were upregulated. Further, Whanger et al. [156] stated that Se counteracts the neurotoxicity of Cd, Hg, V and Pb through a mechanism that induces their accumulation in brain, probably via a non-toxic complex. Selenium preventing action against DNA damage is affected by the used dose. For instance, a study on exocrine pancreas cells proposed a faster repair of DNA single-strand breaks in hamsters fed with 2.5 ppm Se than those fed with 0.1 ppm Se [157]. Selenomethionine could initiate the p53 tumor suppressor protein via a redox mode of action which needs the redox factor Ref1 [158]. Further, SeMet could protect against biological effects caused by radiation, via enhancement of DNA repair mechanisms in radiated cells. Consequently, SeMet may exert a particular action on the DNA repair machinery preventing DNA damage. Interestingly, this outcome is not the case or may be even opposite if selenite is used instead [159,160].

5. Actions and Properties of Selenoproteins

The mechanism of Se insertion into cysteine and further to selenoproteins has been extensively studied [161,162]. Similarly, many homologs of selenoproteins are not considered as such since they contain cysteine and not Sec [163]. Presently, the essentiality of Se is undoubted and its effects on the development of several diseases have been extensively reviewed in the literature [25,164,165]. Selenoproteins are essential for life and several selenoproteins have been characterized as antioxidant enzymes, protecting from damage caused by free radicals as already stated.

Functions of endoplasmic reticulum (ER) such as protein folding, post-translational modification, and transport are assisted by selenoproteins located in ER [166]. Further, the abundant 15 kDa SELENOF protein seems to control the quality of glycoprotein folding by improving glucosyltransferase activity of UDP-glucose: glycoprotein glucosyltransferase via formation of stable heterodimeric complexes [167]. Selenoprotein F may also function as oxidoreductase due to its thioredoxin-like folding which is mediated by CGU redox motif [168]. In addition, SELENOM, which shares a 31% sequence identity with SELENOF, enhances the formation of disulfide bond in proteins [168]. On the other hand, SELENOS and SELENOK participate in the machinery of the ER-associated protein degradation (ERAD) [166]. They are upregulated under conditions promoting protein misfolding.

Furthermore, they are both single membrane-spanning parts of multi-protein complexes that transport misfolded proteins from the ER to the cytosol for degradation. Their exact way of action is elusive, though they probably act as chaperones for some ERAD substrates.

Identification of more than 50 selenoproteins has been performed since the discovery of Se incorporation in GPX [169]. Isolation and biochemical characterization of several of these proteins such as thioredoxin reductase, selenophosphate synthase, methionine-sulfoxide reductase and iodothyronine deiodinase has been achieved. Their significance for human health and physiology can be generally attributed to the special redox characteristics of the highly conserved active site Sec [170,171]. However, their mode of action is not known in detail. Localization of selenoproteins in various subcellular compartments is evidence of their critical function. For instance, almost one third of total human selenoproteins are located in the ER [166]. These include SELENOF, DIO2, SELENOM, SELENOK, SELENOS, SELENON and SELENOT. Type 2 deiodinase is important for thyroid hormone signaling [172] while redox regulation of calcium metabolism is connected with SELENOT and SELENON. Selenoprotein N is an in integral ER membrane protein that interacts with RyR an intracellular ryanodine receptor of Ca channel [173] and mutations that decrease the efficiency of selenocysteine-insertion lead to various muscle disorders.

6. Effects of Se Deficiency on mRNA Expression of Selenoproteins and Non-Selenoproteins

Selenium metabolism has been discussed in the literature with specific regard to the role of Se within the central nervous system [174]. There are also reviews on the action of Se on productive characteristics, antioxidative status, immune responses and nutrient utilization of poultry [175,176]. Members of this selenoproteome take part in diverse biological pathways and processes in chicken, such as in maintenance of the redox balance; interactions with metals and transport of Se. Six membrane-bound selenoproteins (selenoprotein I, selenoprotein K, selenoprotein S, selenoprotein T, DIO1 and DIO3) had pivotal roles in maintaining the membrane integrity. According to their ligand binding sites, chicken selenoproteins were classified as zinc-containing matrix metalloselenoproteins (selenoprotein 15, MSRB1, selenoprotein W and selenoprotein M), FAD-interacting selenoproteins (TXNRD1–3), prolyl oligopeptidase activity (POP)-containing selenoproteins (GPX1–4), secretory transport selenoproteins (GPX3 and selenoprotein Pa) and other selenoproteins [177].

The effects of Se deficiency on the induction of inflammation injury and oxidative damage to [178] chicken aorta vessels as well as on the deficiency of mRNA expression levels of selenoproteins, HSPs and immune functions in chicken have also been investigated. The results were linked with a downregulation of mRNA expression levels of 25 selenoproteins, upregulation of the mRNA expression of HSPs and immunosuppression [179,180]. Selenium deficiency can also lead to marked loss of selenoproteins activity, including GPXs, DIOs and TXNRDs [73].

The correlation of selenoproteins and Se deficiency causing apoptosis of chick embryonic vascular smooth muscle cells (VSMCs) has been examined [181]. Selenium deficiency led to higher cell apoptosis and decrease of cell viability. Selenium supplementation may mitigate these alterations. Moreover, at every level of Se supplementation, selenoprotein W1, selenoprotein 15, GPX1, GPX3, and GPX4 mRNAs were highly expressed in VSMCs [181]. An interesting work conducted in 55 days broilers with a Se-deficient diet (0.033 mg Se/kg) and a normal diet (0.2 mg/kg) showed that Se deficiency reduced HSP (HSP40, HSP60, and HSP90) and selenoprotein (selenoprotein K, GPX1, and selenoprotein H) mRNA expression, although the expression levels of selenoprotein Pb, selenoprotein I, selenoprotein N, MSRB1, HSP27, GPX2 and inflammatory factors (TNF-α, COX-2, HO-1 and iNOS) were upregulated. These results also indicated that selenoproteins play different roles in chicken testes [182]. Huang et al. [183] studied the effect of Se deficiency on selenoprotein expression levels in chicken muscular stomach and a correlation of muscular stomach injuries and selenoproteins was found. Selenium deficiency decreased the expression of 25 selenoprotein genes but raised the levels of mRNA expression of NF-κB, iNOS, TNF-α, COX-2, HO-1 and HSP27, HSP40, HSP60, HSP70 and HSP90. In other words, selenoproteins showed negative correlation with inflammation factors and HSPs. Therefore, the results showed that Se deficiency induced injuries in muscular stomach by reducing the levels of selenoproteins mRNA expression [183]. Selenium supplementation expedited and increased cell surface markers expression such as CD11c, CD40, CD86, and MHC II in a study investigating the impact of Se on chicken dendritic cells (DCs). Principal component analysis showed that the expression of selenoprotein W, selenoprotein K, DIO3, GPX1, GPX2, selenoprotein N, selenoprotein S, and selenoprotein H in chicken DCs was highly correlated, and selenoprotein W had highest correlation with the cell surface markers MHC II and CD11c [184]. Furthermore, Se-deficient, high energy diet in swine could cause oxidative stress, and downregulated the phagocytic dysfunction and the Nrf2 pathway in neutrophils.

The effect of Se deficiency on inflammatory factors and selenoprotein gene transcription in broiler kidneys was also studied. In the low Se diet group the expression of inflammation factors (TNF-α, COX-2, iNOS, and NF-κB) was raised, the mRNA expression level of 14 selenoprotein genes (GPX3, selenoprotein K, selenoprotein O, selenoprotein 15, selenoprotein H, selenoprotein P1, selenoprotein I, selenoprotein n1, selenoprotein W, selenoprotein T, selenoprotein U, selenoprotein S, DIO1 and DIO2) was reduced while the expression level of nine selenoprotein genes (selenoprotein M, selenoprotein SPS2, selenoprotein Pb, TXNRD1–3, and GPX1, GPX2, and GPX4) was elevated. The results indicated that Se deficiency caused changes in the expression of selenoprotein genes, kidney dysfunction and activation of the NF-κB pathway. In addition, Se supplementation can mitigate Pb toxicity effects via attenuation of apoptosis caused by Pb [185]. Finally, Se deficiency in chicken caused reduced tissue Se content as well as GPX and catalase activities, decreased the mRNA and protein expression of selenoprotein M and increased malondialdehyde (MDA) content in brain [186]. Under this contexts, recent transcriptional studies in chicken revealed that some selenoproteins, such as GPX4, are regulated at transcriptional level by high dietary Se. Supranutritional Se levels seem to down-regulate liver GPX4 mRNA levels, which means that reserves built by excess of Se may meet antioxidant requirements and no extra GPX4 transcription is required [187].

Other studies aimed to prove if chicken selenoprotein W has similar functions as mammal selenoprotein W and to examine its preventive action against H_2O_2 by affecting the expression of apoptosis and inflammation via developing a model of over-expressed or/and knocked down selenoprotein W in cultured chicken liver cells. Results revealed that after cell exposure to H_2O_2, levels of caspase-3, p53, Bak, Bax, prostaglandin E synthase (PTGEs, COX-2, TNF-α, NF-κB and iNOS were reduced in the selenoprotein W overexpressed cells but increased in the selenoprotein W knockdown cells in comparison to the H_2O_2-only treatment group. Levels of Bax, Bak, p53, COX-2, PTGEs, TNF-α, iNOS and NF-κB in the liver of Se-deficient chickens were highly increased compared to the control group [188]. Next, positive correlation has been reported in GPX1-4, DIO1, DIO3, selenoprotein S, selenoprotein N, selenoprotein T, selenoprotein W, selenoprotein 15, selenoprotein H, selenoprotein U and selenoprotein I with selenoprotein K, whereas selenoprotein P and DIO2 presented negative correlation with selenoprotein K. The above study was demonstrated by silencing selenoprotein K in chickens myoblasts [189].

In addition, studies have shown positive correlations between the mRNA expression of selenoprotein W and selenoprotein N genes and the quality (pH and muscle fiber diameter) of chicken muscle [190]. Cultured chicken liver cells exposed to H_2O_2 had lower levels of interleukin (IL)-1, IL-4, IL-6, IL-8, IL-10, IL-17 and interferon gamma (IFN-γ) in the selenoprotein W over-expressing cells but higher levels in the selenoprotein W knockdown cells compared to the H_2O_2 only control group. Besides, IL-1, IL-4, IL-6, IL-8, IL-10, IL-17 and IFN-γ in Se-deficient chicken serum and liver were much higher compared to the control group. Similar results have been shown in a study examining the effect of Se deficiency on the expression of selenoproteins and cytokines. The mRNA expression of 24 selenoproteins and seven cytokines (IL-2, IL-4, IL-8, IL-10, IL-12β, transforming growth factor (TGF)-β4, and IFN-γ) decreased, and the expression of three cytokines (IL-1γ, IL-6 and IL-7) increased in the Se-deficient group [191]. Selenoprotein W not only seemed to interfere with the destruction of H_2O_2 pathways, but also had a role in the immune system function. Studies have shown that inflammatory injury in immune tissues and cultured splenic lymphocytes can be influenced by Se in chicken, because it interacts with the expression levels of inflammatory factors (TNF-α, iNOS, NF-κB, COX-2 and PTGEs) and selenoprotein W. Further studies in selenoproteins' gene expression and cytokine content in the chicken thymus have shown that, significant decrease in the expression levels of selenoproteins could result in oxidative stress in chicken thymus [192].

Studies with Chinese egg-laying ducks have shown that Se requirement for daily egg production is 0.18 mg Se/kg for early-laying birds, 0.24 mg Se/kg for peak-laying birds while for optimal GPX unction in peak-laying ducks it is 0.37 mg Se/kg [193]. Similarly, today's minimum Se requirement in broilers is 0.15 μg Se/g diet and pancreas data indicate that the Se requirement should be raised to 0.2 μg Se/g diet [194]. Likewise, Turkey's dietary Se requirement today is 0.2 μg Se/g and should be raised to 0.3 μg Se/g [195].

Concerns about the impact of inorganic and different organic Se sources on tissues and serum Se content, antioxidant capacity, performance, and liver mRNA expression of selenoproteins in broilers were also examined. The results suggested that Se sources did not affect broiler growth performance and organic Se exhibited highest Se concentration in serum, liver, and kidney [196]. Zhao et al. [197] examined the regulation of Se speciation, selenoproteins and degradation-related genes expression and Sec biosynthesis, by three forms of Se in broiler tissues. It has been shown that SeO further raised concentrations of total Se and SeMet in the liver, pectoral muscle, and thigh by 13–37% and 43–87%, respectively, compared with Se-yeast. Compared with inorganic Se or Se-yeast, SeO showed the ability to enrich SeMet and total Se accumulation, to induce the early mRNA expression of selenoprotein S and MSRB1, and to enhance protein expression of GPX4, selenoprotein P, and selenoprotein U in broiler tissues [197].

Molecular biomarkers in contrast to conventional ones seem to be better predictors of physiological effects connected with high Se intake. Investigations regarding super-nutritional Se effects on transcription did not identify well-regulated molecular biomarkers of high Se status. Microarray studies in rodents identified 14–242 genes altered by a Se intake of 1.0 μg Se/g as compared to Se deficient diets. From all these genes, the ones that were consistently regulated were the selenoprotein genes. Furthermore, the Se-specific effects noted were caused primarily by Se deficiency and not high Se [198].

7. Ranking in the Hierarchy of Selenoproteins

Selenoprotein synthesis is regulated [199–202] and a hierarchy in the expression of selenoproteins during Se deprivation and repletion has been reported [199]. The lowest ranking selenoprotein in the hierarchy is GPX1. Hierarchy of selenoproteins denotes that selenoproteins are not evenly supplied with Se, specifically not when Se gets limiting. Some selenoproteins disappear rapidly while others remain stable until deficiency becomes more serious. Therefore, rapidly disappearing selenoproteins, rank low in the hierarchy, while those remaining stable rank high. Instability is usually caused by the degradation of respective mRNAs [128].

It has been shown that some tissues and organs are more effective in maintaining Se levels and in synthesizing certain selenoproteins during Se deprivation compared to others. This is indicatory of differences in the biologic roles and in the selenoproteins requirements in different tissues [199,203]. The hierarchy during Se deprivation and repletion reveals the importance of particular selenoproteins and in turn determines the priority of the mRNA level and protein expression [50]. In Se-deficient states, the activities of most selenoproteins in the kidney, liver and lung decrease while in the brain remain at levels similar to those during normal Se intake levels [50]. Furthermore, stability of mRNA may be regulated by Se level since in Se deficiency cases excessive susceptibility to the nonsense-mediated decay pathway (NMD) and consequently mRNA decay has been observed [204–206].

Selenium may also efficiently control UGA-Sec codon translation [65,66], regulate levels of Sec tRNASer(Sec) and control the ratio of the methylated and unmethylated Sec tRNA(Ser)Sec isoforms [67–70]. The methylated isoform is translationally active and Se-induced tRNA methylation is a mechanism of Sel synthesis regulation. The methylated isoform has been shown to govern the synthesis of selenoproteins involved in the oxidative stress response such as GPX1 and GPX3, whereas the unmethylated form controls synthesis of housekeeping selenoproteins, i.e., TXNRD1 and TXNRD3 [71].

Selenoproteins' hierarchy expression plays important role in Se metabolism into birds' central nervous system (CNS). Brain is the last affected tissue by nutritional Se deficiency. However, selenoprotein expression follows a hierarchy by altering Se content so that GPX2-4, selenoprotein K, selenoprotein N, selenoprotein O, selenoprotein T, selenoprotein U, selenoprotein W, selenoprotein P1-2 and selenoprotein 15 take more necessary function in the CNS of chicken [207]. In contrast, Se deficiency down regulates chicken selenoprotein U mRNA levels in heart, kidney, liver, lung, muscle and spleen. On the other hand, selenoprotein U mRNA levels in testes and brain are not affected [208]. However, in Turkeys, studies on the expression levels of selenoproteins showed that expression of GPX1 was high in kidney, expression of GPX3 was high in all tissues except kidney, expression of selenoprotein U was high in liver, and selenoprotein W1 expression was high in heart, gizzard and muscle [209].

8. Recent Findings and Main Characteristics of Major Selenoproteins

Glycoprotein selenoprotein N (SELENON) is localized within the endoplasmatic reticulum (ER). Multiminicore disease (in the classical form) and the rigid spine muscular dystrophy are straight linked with SELENON [210]. Regulation of redox-related Ca homeostasis and antioxidant activity in cell is one of the major functions of SELENON [211]. Regulation of Ca levels in ER occurs through Ca pump ATP2A2 (ATPase sarcoplasmic/endoplasmic reticulum Ca^{2+} transporting protein 2) protection against the oxidative damage caused by endoplasmic reticulum oxidoreductase 1 alpha (ERO1A). Activity of ERO1A increases H_2O_2 concentration in the ER and this causes attack on ATP2A2 luminal thiols that leads to cysteinyl sulfenic acid formation (–SOH), which is reduced to free thiol (–SH) by SELENON, and in this way brings back ATP2A2 action [212]. In addition, it acts as RyR activity modulator by RyR oxidation prevention due to elevated oxidative stress and RyR redox state direct control through regulation of the RyR-mediated Ca mobilization which is required for normal differentiation and muscle development [173,213–215]. Further, SELENON is essential part of satellite cell maintenance and muscle regeneration [216]. Moreover, it seems that SELENON is necessary for Se regulation in mice uterine smooth muscle contraction [217]. On the other hand, intracellular Ca concentration rise is caused by overexpression of selenoprotein T [218]. Selenoprotein T plays a role in Ca homeostasis regulation and via cAMP-stimulating trophic factor in the control of the neuroendocrine secretion response [218]. Selenoprotein T is a protein with oxidoreductase activity as thioredoxin reductase and it is important in dopaminergic neurons protection against oxidative stress and apoptosis [219]. It is involved in neuroendocrine secretion, ADCYAP1/PACAP-induced Ca mobilization and has a role in redox regulation and fibroblast anchorage. In addition, contraction processes of the gastric smooth muscle are modulated by SELENOT which controls the release of Ca and myosin light chain kinase (MYLK) activation. In pancreatic islets, it contributes to ADCYAP1/PACAP-induced prolonged insulin secretion and is implicated in the glucose homeostasis control [219]. Moreover, a selenide-sulfide bond is maybe located between Cys-46 and Sec-49 in SELENOT polypeptide chain, which is considered to serve as redox-active pair. Further, the protective role of SELENOT and other selenoproteins on dopaminergic neurons against oxidative stress and apoptosis has been revealed recently. Selenoprotein T participates in neuron protection against oxidative stress and in the prevention of onset and intensive movement impairment in Parkinson Disease animal models [219].

A role in apoptosis and control of chemopreventive implications of Se seems to be attributed to SELENOF or also named selenoprotein 15 [73], which may be involved in redox reactions associated with the formation of disulfide bonds and in the quality control of protein folding in the ER. It is located in the ER and is expressed in higher levels in prostate and thyroid gland [220,221]. Selenoprotein M is distantly related to SELENOF but, its exact function is still elusive. Its role in causality of cancer and in early initiation of Alzheimer's disease is under investigation. It has an oxidoreductase thiol-disulfide function which is involved in formation of disulfide bonds. By similarity, it is localized within the ER, but also within Golgi apparatus and perinuclear region [222].

Not only ER selenoproteins repair proteins. Methionine sulfoxide reductase B1 (MSRB1) is a selenoenzyme with wide distribution, which catalyzes the reduction of methionine (R)-sulfixide to methionine. Methionine oxidation is often a random effect induced by oxidative stress but it can also be a modification at post-translational stages which occurs on specific residue. Another MSRB1 function via methionine (R)-sulfoxide reduction is actin assembly and thereby stimulation of filament repolymerization. Besides, it contributes in innate immunity by reducing oxidized actin allowing repolymerization in macrophages. In vivo, immune response is controlled by MSRB1. Further, it promotes inflammatory cytokine gene expression in macrophages [223]. By similarity, to reverse random oxidation of methionine residues, MSRB1 exploits Sec [224] and, interestingly, it reduces more readily unfolded polypeptides than their folded counterparts, maybe due to better approach to otherwise hidden residues [225]. Therefore, cell protection from oxidative stress by methionine sulfoxide reductase enzymes can be explained by the recovery of unfolded proteins and oxidatively damaged nascent polypeptides. It has been recently shown that by regulating the oxidation state of two crucial methionine residues in actin monomer, MSRB1 controls mammalian actin assembly dynamics in collaboration with flavin-dependent monooxygenases (MICALs) [226]. Methionine stereoselective oxidation via MICALs causes disassembly of filaments and, on the other hand, reduction back to methionine via MSRB1 enhances filament assembly. Consequently, reversible sulfoxidation of methionine may serve as a general redox mechanism for protein folding/function regulation.

Selenoprotein K is essential for Ca flux in immune cells and in proliferation of T-cells and migration of neutrophils [166–168,227]. It is further implicated in ER-associated degradation (ERAD) of misfolded, soluble glycosylated proteins and Sec92 in SELENOK serves to stabilize the palmitoyl-DHHC6 intermediate by reducing hydrolyzation of the thioester bond until transfer of the palmitoyl group to the Cys residue on the target protein can occur [120]. Moreover, SELENOK is indispensable for CD36 cell surface expression and palmitoylation and contributes in foam cell formation and in low density lipoprotein (LDL) uptake by macrophages. In addition, selenoprotein K has been shown to protect cells from apoptosis induced by ER stress [121] and it preserves cells from oxidative stress when overexpressed in cardiomyocytes [122]. Further, a recent a study shows that the proliferation, migration, and invasion of human choriocarcinoma cells is mediated by SELENOK through negative regulation of human chorionic gonadotropin expression via p38 MAPK, Akt signaling and ERK pathways. In addition, SELENOK may act as suppressor of tumor in human choriocarcinoma cells by negatively regulating expression of β-human chorionic gonadotropin (β-hCG) via p38 MAPK, Akt and ERK signaling pathways [228].

Selenoprotein S contributes in the transfer of misfolded proteins from ER to the cytosol, for destruction by the proteasome in a ubiquitin-dependent manner. In addition, SELENOS is an efficient disulfide reductase [229]. SELENOS influences the activity and conformation of the ATPase complex VCP (vasolin-containing protein) which is involved in ubiquitination and translocation of misfolded proteins and DERL1 (degradation in endoplasmatic reticulum protein 1) which acts as a retro translocator into the cytosol [229]. Deprivation of glucose, together with tunicamycin and thapsigargin (stress inducers of ER), was shown to elevate gene and protein expression of SELENOS several-fold concomitantly with glucose-regulated protein 78. Moreover, SELENOS overexpression decreased Min6 cell oxidative stress-induced toxicity. These results indicate that SELENOS may be a member of the glucose-regulated protein family and a regulator of cellular redox balance [230]. Furthermore, the underling mechanism of SENELOS preventive role in atherosclerotic cardiovascular diseases was investigated [19,230]. Additionally, it may be implicated in the control of inflammation response [231]. The selenocysteine residue of SELENOS is localized in an essentially disordered region of the cytoplasmic C-terminal domain which interacts with VCP and DERL1 and indicates the formation of a DERL1-SELENOS membrane complex acting as VCP receptor. Furthermore, interaction has been shown with DERL2 and DERL3 as also with SELENOK gene which in turn interacts with VCP. In vitro studies showed that this residue provides high thioredoxin-dependent reductase activity [207,208] and that SELENOS may also act as a signaling molecule linking the unfolded protein response to the ERAD machinery

Eight homologs of GPX are found in mammals [232], five of which are selenoproteins, including GPXl (also known as cGPx), GPX2 (also known as GI-GPx), GPX3 (also known as pGPx), GPX4 (also known as PHGPx) and GPX6. More precisely, GPX family has a potent antioxidant function in cell cytosol (GPX1), gastrointestinal tract (GPX2), extracellular space and plasma (GPX3) and in cell membrane and sperm (GPX4). Glutathione peroxidase 5 is called epididymal GPX due to its exclusive localization in the epididymis [32]. Glutathione peroxidase 6, GPX7 and GPX8 where initially discovered via large-scale sequencing programs in mammals. The GPX6 is located in olfactory epithelium and in embryonic tissues [233,234]. Moreover, a study on β-cells in rats showed that antioxidant capacity of ER was improved by GPX7 or GPX8 without compromising production of insulin and the oxidative protein folding machinery [117].

As mentioned above, in the antioxidant system section, major functions of peroxidases are to remove and detoxificate H_2O_2 and hydroperoxides of lipids. Additionally, another important function is to preserve redox state of the cell. Apart from these, differentiation, signal transduction and pro-inflammatory cytokine synthesis regulation are also major physiological events where GPXs actively participate. In addition, GPXs have important roles in the antioxidant defense in spermiogenesis, in the maturation of spermatozoa and during embryonic development [235]. Glutathione peroxidases are involved in signaling cascades, e.g., GPX1 is involved in the molecular pathway of insulin signaling; GPX2 is involved in carcinogenesis; the membrane associated GPX3 has possibly peroxidative function in spite of low plasma concentrations of GSH; and GPX4 and GPX5 have major roles in apoptosis regulation, for full viability of mice and male fertility [236]. Though, the actions of GPX6 remain elusive [237]. However, applying SLIC (Sequence-and Ligation—Independent Cloning, a method for sequence-and ligation-independent cloning) [233] in a study on Huntington's disease, it has been identified that toxicity of huntingtin mutation is modulated via age-regulated GPX6 gene. Moreover, in a mouse model, molecular and behavioral phenotypes linked with Huntington's disease were drastically reduced after overexpression of GPX6 [234]. On the other hand, elucidation is awaited for GPX7 and GPX8 suggested involvement in protein folding [238,239]. The phospholipids-hydroperoxide glutathione peroxidase (GPX7 or NPGPx) which does not contain Sec residue is expressed in cancerous breast cells [240] and the name GPX8 has been proposed for a novel member of the GPX family, the existence of which was revealed via phylogenetic analysis in amphibians and mammals [241].

Three protein types with a variety of specific roles in thyroid metabolism are included in the iodothyronine deiodinase family. These 3 deiodinases (DIO1–3) are found in all vertebrates and have notable roles in activating thyroxine (T4) and inactivating both T3 and T4. Their importance resides in the fact that T4 must be activated by deiodination to the short-lived biologically active T3 for thyroid hormone action initiation [242]. Bioactive 3,5,3′-tri-iodothyronine (T3) is converted to thyroxin (T4) by DIO1 and DIO2. Thioredoxin reductases, deiodinases and glutathione peroxidases are all present in the thyroid gland and contribute in biosynthesis of thyroid hormone, redox control of thyrocytes, antioxidant defense and in the metabolism of thyroid hormone [243].

Other selenoproteins that may not be part of a family include, but are not restricted to, the selenophosphate synthetase 2 (SEPHS2), SELENOI, SELENOH, SELENOO, SELENOP, SELENOW, and SELENOV. Moreover, in eukaryotes, the selenoprotein family includes the Fep15, SELENOJ, SELENOU1, the plasmodium selenoprotein, SELENO1–SELENO4 and the protein disulfide isomerase (PDI) which is narrowly distributed in eukaryotes. While the role of some of them is still largely unknown, the role of others is clearly understood. The greater attention has been received by the selenoproteins in humans. More specifically, SEPHS2 is involved in selenophosphate formation intended for selenoprotein synthesis [244] and forms selenophosphate from selenide and ATP. Furthermore, it is located in the cytosol and binds ATP, nucleotides and Se.

Expression level regulation in de novo GSH synthesis relative genes and response to redox status phase II detoxification is regulated by SELENOH [245]. Overexpression of SELENOH gene in hippocampal neuronal cells has neuroprotective effects against ultra violet B (UVB)-induced cell death. In addition, SELENOH overexpression is involved in mitochondrial biogenesis and mitochondrial functional performance [246].

Selenoprotein I in *E. coli* catalyzes biosynthesis of phosphatidylethanolamine from cytidine diphosphate (CDP)-ethanolamine and it has a main role in vesicular membranes formation and maintenance. Selenoprotein I seems to be involved in the formation of phosphatidylethanolamine via "Kennedy" pathway (catalytic activity) [247,248]. However, until now, the function of selenoprotein I is largely elusive.

Selenoprotein O is a protein with wide distribution that has homologs in yeast, bacteria, animals and plants, although its function is still undiscovered [249,250]. It has high priority for Se supply and this is deduced by the slight Se effect on selenoprotein O gene expression. It may be a redox-active mitochondrial selenoprotein which interacts with a redox target protein.

Selenoprotein P is a glycoprotein with a high Sec content, which is abundant in extracellular environment. Its functions include endothelium located antioxidant defense, Se transport among tissues and Se homeostasis [251]. Additionally, it is the main selenoprotein in plasma and contains at least 40% of the whole amount of Se in plasma [252]. Moreover, SELENOP plasma level is a finer indicator of nutritional Se compared to the previously used GPX3 [73] because a greater Se intake is required for SELENOP than GPX3 full expression [253].

Selenoprotein V is about 37 kDa and is mainly produced in chicken testes. This selenoprotein contains specific amino acid sequence motives that predict a role in redox-regulation, although its exact function is unexplained [22]. On the other hand, selenoprotein W seems to be implicated in antioxidant protection of cardiac and skeletal muscle, protecting chicken embryonic myoblast cells against H_2O_2 mediated apoptosis. Selenoprotein W regulates also inflammation-related cytokines during H_2O_2 chicken liver damage [254,255]. Finally, regarding selenoprotein D, a recent study has been conducted using the TargeTron gene knockout system to explore the role of selenoproteins in *Clostridium difficile* nosocomial pathogen [256]. TargeTron insertion into selenoprotein D resulted in a significant growth deficiency and global loss of Se incorporation. Stickland metabolism could be a potential target for antibiotic therapies in the future.

9. Conclusions

Selenoproteins need for their synthesis several cofactors and depend mainly on Se intake through the diet. The organism pays a high cost of energy for the production and preservation of these cofactors for selenoprotein synthesis which consequently suggests the significance of this family of proteins to cell function. Notwithstanding, the functions of selenoproteins are fairly heterogeneous. Selenoproteins play essential roles in numerous conditions and diseases including neurodegeneration and endocrine disorders, cardiovascular disorders and cancer. On account of the various functions of selenoproteins, strategies targeting function and/or expression of specific selenoproteins could be considered for prevention and therapeutic treatment of disorders. Different forms of dietary Se may selectively increase synthesis of specific selenoproteins. Pharmaceuticals could also target factors involved in selenoprotein synthesis or specific selenoproteins. Nevertheless, the functions of many selenoproteins are still elusive, which is why understanding the function of each member of the selenoprotein protein family will be ssignificant for defining the health benefits of Se.

Author Contributions: All authors contributed equally to the completion of this paper. E.Z. and G.P.D. conceived the idea and contributed to manuscript writing, analysis and review. I.S., N.K. collected sources of information and contributed to the manuscript writing.

Conflicts of Interest: The authors declare no conflict of interest.

References

1. Mariotti, M.; Santesmasses, D.; Guigó, R. *Evolution of Selenophosphate Synthetase*; Springer: New York, NY, USA, 2016.
2. Hatfield, D.L.; Marla, J.B.; Vadim, N.; Gladyshev, V.N. *Selenium: Its Molecular Biology and Role in Human Health*; Springer Science & Business Media: Berlin, Germany, 2011.
3. Mariotti, M. Selenocysteine Extinctions in Insects. In *Short Views on Insect Genomics and Proteomics*; Springer: New York, NY, USA, 2016.
4. Mariotti, M.; Lobanov, A.V.; Manta, B.; Santesmasses, D.; Bofill, A.; Guigó, R.; Gabaldón, T.; Gladyshev, V.N. Lokiarchaeota marks the transition between the archaeal and eukaryotic selenocysteine encoding systems. *Mol. Biol. Evol.* **2016**, *33*, 2441–2453. [CrossRef] [PubMed]
5. Sarangi, K.G.; White, L.; Castellano, S. *Genetic Adaptation and Selenium Uptake in Vertebrates*; Wiley: Chichester, UK, 2017.
6. Peng, T.; Lin, J.; Xu, Y.-Z.; Zhang, Y. Comparative genomics reveals new evolutionary and ecological patterns of selenium utilization in bacteria. *ISME J.* **2016**, *10*, 2048–2059. [CrossRef] [PubMed]
7. Santesmasses, D.; Mariotti, M.; Guigó, R. Computational identification of the selenocysteine tRNA (tRNASec) in genomes. *PLoS Comput. Biol.* **2017**, *13*. [CrossRef] [PubMed]
8. European Food Safety Authority. Scientific opinion on dietary reference values for selenium. *EFSA J.* **2014**, *12*. [CrossRef]
9. Rayman, M.P. Selenium and human health. *Lancet* **2012**, *379*, 1256–1268. [CrossRef]
10. Steinbrenner, H.; Speckmann, B.; Sies, H. Toward understanding success and failures in the use of selenium for cancer prevention. *Antioxid. Redox Signal.* **2013**, *19*, 181–191. [CrossRef] [PubMed]
11. Méplan, C. Association of single nucleotide polymorphisms in selenoprotein genes with cancer risk. In *Selenoproteins*; Humana Press: New York, NY, USA, 2018.
12. Bertz, M.; Kühn, K.; Koeberle, S.C.; Müller, M.F.; Hoelzer, D.; Thies, K.; Deubel, S.; Thierbach, R.; Kipp, A.P. Selenoprotein H controls cell cycle progression and proliferation of human colorectal cancer cells. *Free Radic. Biol. Med.* **2018**, in press. [CrossRef] [PubMed]
13. Schomburg, L. Selenium, selenoproteins and the thyroid gland: Interactions in health and disease. *Nat. Rev. Endocrinol.* **2012**, *8*, 160–171. [CrossRef] [PubMed]
14. Handy, D.E.; Joseph, L. *Selenoproteins in Cardiovascular Redox Pathology*; Springer: Cham, Switzerland, 2016.
15. Pekar, J.; Skolarczyk, J.; Małecka-Massalska, T.; Skórzyńska-Dziduszko, K. Effect of selenium supplementation in thyroid gland diseases. *J. Elementol.* **2017**, *22*. [CrossRef]
16. Misu, H.; Takayama, H.; Saito, Y.; Mita, Y.; Kikuchi, A.; Ishii, K.-A.; Chikamoto, K.; Kanamori, T.; Tajima, N.; Lan, F. Deficiency of the hepatokine selenoprotein P increases responsiveness to exercise in mice through upregulation of reactive oxygen species and AMP-activated protein kinase in muscle. *Nat. Med.* **2017**, *23*, 508–516. [CrossRef] [PubMed]
17. Kikuchi, N.; Satoh, K.; Omura, J.; Satoh, T.; Kurosawa, R.; Nogi, M.; Otsuki, T.; Numano, K.; Kozu, K.; Suzuki, K. Selenoprotein P promotes vascular smooth muscle cell proliferation and pulmonary hypertension-a possible novel therapeutic target. *Am. Heart Assoc.* **2016**, *36*, A62.
18. Wright, C.R.; Allsopp, G.L.; Addinsall, A.B.; McRae, N.L.; Andrikopoulos, S.; Stupka, N. A Reduction in selenoprotein S amplifies the inflammatory profile of fast-twitch skeletal muscle in the mdx dystrophic mouse. *Med. Inflamm.* **2017**, *2017*. [CrossRef] [PubMed]
19. Ye, Y.; Fu, F.; Li, X.; Yang, J.; Liu, H. Selenoprotein s is highly expressed in the blood vessels and prevents vascular smooth muscle cells from apoptosis. *J. Cell. Biochem.* **2016**, *117*, 106–117. [CrossRef] [PubMed]
20. Yao, H.; Fan, R.; Zhao, X.; Zhao, W.; Liu, W.; Yang, J.; Sattar, H.; Zhao, J.; Zhang, Z.; Xu, S. Selenoprotein W redox-regulated Ca^{2+} channels correlate with selenium deficiency-induced muscles Ca^{2+} leak. *Oncotarget* **2016**, *7*, 57618–57632. [CrossRef] [PubMed]
21. Rocourt, C.R.; Cheng, W.-H. Selenium supranutrition: Are the potential benefits of chemoprevention outweighed by the promotion of diabetes and insulin resistance? *Nutrients* **2013**, *5*, 1349–1365. [CrossRef] [PubMed]
22. Kryukov, G.V.; Castellano, S.; Novoselov, S.V.; Lobanov, A.V.; Zehtab, O.; Guigó, R.; Gladyshev, V.N. Characterization of mammalian selenoproteomes. *Science* **2003**, *300*, 1439–1443. [CrossRef] [PubMed]

23. Gladyshev, V.N.; Arnér, E.S.; Berry, M.J.; Brigelius-Flohé, R.; Bruford, E.A.; Burk, R.F.; Carlson, B.A.; Castellano, S.; Chavatte, L.; Conrad, M. Selenoprotein gene nomenclature. *J. Biol. Chem.* **2016**, *291*, 24036–24040. [CrossRef] [PubMed]
24. Kumar, B.S.; Priyadarsini, K. Selenium nutrition: How important is it? *Biomed. Prev. Nutr.* **2014**, *4*, 333–341. [CrossRef]
25. Roman, M.; Jitaru, P.; Barbante, C. Selenium biochemistry and its role for human health. *Metallomics* **2014**, *6*, 25–54. [CrossRef] [PubMed]
26. Zhou, H.; Wang, T.; Li, Q.; Li, D. Prevention of keshan disease by selenium supplementation: A systematic review and meta-analysis. *Biol. Trace Elem. Res.* **2018**. [CrossRef] [PubMed]
27. Liu, H.; Yu, F.; Shao, W.; Ding, D.; Yu, Z.; Chen, F.; Geng, D.; Tan, X.; Lammi, M.J.; Guo, X. Associations between selenium content in hair and kashin-beck disease/keshan disease in children in northwestern china: A prospective cohort study. *Biol. Trace Elem. Res.* **2017**. [CrossRef] [PubMed]
28. Loscalzo, J. Keshan disease, selenium deficiency, and the selenoproteome. *N. Engl. J. Med.* **2014**, *370*, 1756–1760. [CrossRef] [PubMed]
29. Zhang, R. Polymorphism of antioxidant selenoprotein genes and kashin-beck disease susceptibility, a systematic review and meta-analysis. *Osteoarthr. Cartil.* **2017**, *25*, 213–214. [CrossRef]
30. Ventura, M.; Melo, M.; Carrilho, F. Selenium and thyroid disease: From pathophysiology to treatment. *Int. J. Endocrinol.* **2017**. [CrossRef] [PubMed]
31. Agarwal, A.; Majzoub, A. Role of antioxidants in male infertility. *BJUI Knowl.* **2016**, 1–9.
32. Pappa, E.C.; Pappas, A.C.; Surai, P.F. Selenium content in selected foods from the greek market and estimation of the daily intake. *Sci. Total Environ.* **2006**, *372*, 100–108. [CrossRef] [PubMed]
33. Wasowicz, W.; Gromadzinska, J.; Rydzynski, K.; Tomczak, J. Selenium status of low-selenium area residents: Polish experience. *Toxicol. Lett.* **2003**, *137*, 95–101. [CrossRef]
34. Barclay, M.N.I.; MacPherson, A.; Dixon, J. Selenium content of a range of UK foods. *J. Food Compos. Anal.* **1995**, *8*, 307–318. [CrossRef]
35. Diaz-Alarcon, J.; Navarro-Alarcón, M.; de la Serrana, H.L.-G.; Lopez-Martinez, M. Determination of selenium in cereals, legumes and dry fruits from southeastern spain for calculation of daily dietary intake. *Sci. Total Environ.* **1996**, *184*, 183–189. [CrossRef]
36. Sigrist, M.; Brusa, L.; Campagnoli, D.; Beldoménico, H. Determination of selenium in selected food samples from argentina and estimation of their contribution to the Se dietary intake. *Food Chem.* **2012**, *134*, 1932–1937. [CrossRef] [PubMed]
37. Kipp, A.P.; Strohm, D.; Brigelius-Flohé, R.; Schomburg, L.; Bechthold, A.; Leschik-Bonnet, E.; Heseker, H. German Nutrition Society (DGE). Revised reference values for selenium intake. *J. Trace Elem. Med. Biol.* **2015**, *32*, 195–199. [CrossRef] [PubMed]
38. Fisinin, V.I.; Papazyan, T.T.; Surai, P.F. Producing selenium-enriched eggs and meat to improve the selenium status of the general population. *Crit. Rev. Biotechnol.* **2009**, *29*, 18–28. [CrossRef] [PubMed]
39. Combs, G.; Combs, S. The nutritional biochemistry of selenium. *Annu. Rev. Nutr.* **1984**, *4*, 257–280. [CrossRef] [PubMed]
40. Heras, I.L.; Palomo, M.; Madrid, Y. Selenoproteins: The key factor in selenium essentiality. State of the art analytical techniques for selenoprotein studies. *Anal. Bioanal. Chem.* **2011**, *400*, 1717–1727. [CrossRef] [PubMed]
41. Fajardo, D.; Schlautman, B.; Steffan, S.; Polashock, J.; Vorsa, N.; Zalapa, J. The american cranberry mitochondrial genome reveals the presence of selenocysteine (tRNA-Sec and SECIS) insertion machinery in land plants. *Gene* **2014**, *536*, 336–343. [CrossRef] [PubMed]
42. Rayman, M.P. The use of high-selenium yeast to raise selenium status: How does it measure up? *Br. J. Nutr.* **2004**, *92*, 557–573. [CrossRef] [PubMed]
43. Combs, G.F. Selenium in global food systems. *Br. J. Nutr.* **2001**, *85*, 517–547. [CrossRef] [PubMed]
44. Pesti, G.; Combs, G., Jr. Studies on the enteric absorption of selenium in the chick using localized coccidial infections. *Poult. Sci.* **1976**, *55*, 2265–2274. [CrossRef] [PubMed]
45. Wolffram, S. Absorption and metabolism of selenium: Difference between organic and inorganic sources. In *Biotechnology in the Feed Industry*; Nottingham University Press: Nottingham, UK, 1999; Volume 15, pp. 547–566.

46. Würmli, R.; Wolffram, S.; Stingelin, Y.; Scharrer, E. Stimulation of mucosal uptake of selenium from selenite by L-cysteine in sheep small intestine. *Biol. Trace Elem. Res.* **1989**, *20*, 75–85. [CrossRef] [PubMed]
47. Huang, K.; Lauridsen, E.; Clausen, J. The uptake of Na-selenite in rat brain. *Biol. Trace Elem. Res.* **1994**, *46*, 91–102. [CrossRef] [PubMed]
48. Vendeland, S.; Deagen, J.; Butler, J.; Whanger, P. Uptake of selenite, selenomethionine and selenate by brush border membrane vesicles isolated from rat small intestine. *Biometals* **1994**, *7*, 305–312. [CrossRef] [PubMed]
49. Mariotti, M.; Guigó, R. Selenoprofiles: Profile-based scanning of eukaryotic genome sequences for selenoprotein genes. *Bioinformatics* **2010**, *26*, 2656–2663. [CrossRef] [PubMed]
50. Lu, J.; Holmgren, A. Selenoproteins. *J. Biol. Chem.* **2009**, *284*, 723–727. [CrossRef] [PubMed]
51. Rayman, M.P. The importance of selenium to human health. *Lancet* **2000**, *356*, 233–241. [CrossRef]
52. Carlson, B.A.; Lee, B.J.; Tsuji, P.A.; Copeland, P.R.; Schweizer, U.; Gladyshev, V.N.; Hatfield, D.L. Selenocysteine tRNA [Ser] Sec, the central component of selenoprotein biosynthesis: Isolation, identification, modification, and sequencing. In *Selenoproteins*; Humana Press: New York, NY, USA, 2018.
53. Böck, A. Biosynthesis of selenoproteins—An overview. *Biofactors* **2000**, *11*, 77–78. [CrossRef] [PubMed]
54. Lacourciere, G.M.; Stadtman, T.C. Utilization of selenocysteine as a source of selenium for selenophosphate biosynthesis. *Biofactors* **2001**, *14*, 69–74. [CrossRef] [PubMed]
55. Schoenmakers, E.; Carlson, B.; Agostini, M.; Moran, C.; Rajanayagam, O.; Bochukova, E.; Tobe, R.; Peat, R.; Gevers, E.; Muntoni, F. Mutation in human selenocysteine transfer RNA selectively disrupts selenoprotein synthesis. *J. Clin. Investig.* **2016**, *126*, 992–996. [CrossRef] [PubMed]
56. Gribling-Burrer, A.-S.; Leichter, M.; Wurth, L.; Huttin, A.; Schlotter, F.; Troffer-Charlier, N.; Cura, V.; Barkats, M.; Cavarelli, J.; Massenet, S. SECIS-binding protein 2 interacts with the SMN complex and the methylosome for selenoprotein mRNP assembly and translation. *Nucleic Acids Res.* **2017**, *45*, 5399–5413. [CrossRef] [PubMed]
57. Chambers, I.; Frampton, J.; Goldfarb, P.; Affara, N.; McBain, W.; Harrison, P.R. The structure of the mouse glutathione peroxidase gene: The selenocysteine in the active site is encoded by the 'termination' codon, TGA. *EMBO J.* **1986**, *5*, 1221–1227. [PubMed]
58. Copeland, P.R.; Driscoll, D.M. RNA binding proteins and selenocysteine. *Biofactors* **2001**, *14*, 11–16. [CrossRef] [PubMed]
59. Shen, J.-R.; Burnap, R.L.; Inoue, Y. An independent role of cytochrome c-550 in cyanobacterial photosystem II as revealed by double-deletion mutagenesis of the psbO and psbV genes in *Synechocystis* sp. PCC 6803. *Biochemistry* **1995**, *34*, 12661–12668. [CrossRef] [PubMed]
60. Low, S.C.; Berry, M.J. Knowing when not to stop: Selenocysteine incorporation in eukaryotes. *Trends Biochem. Sci.* **1996**, *21*, 203–208. [CrossRef]
61. Bellinger, F.P.; Raman, A.V.; Reeves, M.A.; Berry, M.J. Regulation and function of selenoproteins in human disease. *Biochem. J.* **2009**, *422*, 11–22. [CrossRef] [PubMed]
62. Copeland, P.R.; Fletcher, J.E.; Carlson, B.A.; Hatfield, D.L.; Driscoll, D.M. A novel RNA binding protein, SBP2, is required for the translation of mammalian selenoprotein mRNAs. *EMBO J.* **2000**, *19*, 306–314. [CrossRef] [PubMed]
63. Schomburg, L.; Schweizer, U.; Köhrle, J. Selenium and selenoproteins in mammals: Extraordinary, essential, enigmatic. *Cell. Mol. Life Sci.* **2004**, *61*, 1988–1995. [CrossRef] [PubMed]
64. Fujiwara, T.; Busch, K.; Gross, H.J.; Mizutani, T. A SECIS binding protein (SBP) is distinct from selenocysteyl-tRNA protecting factor (SePF). *Biochimie* **1999**, *81*, 213–218. [CrossRef]
65. Fletcher, J.E.; Copeland, P.R.; Driscoll, D.M. Polysome distribution of phospholipid hydroperoxide glutathione peroxidase mRNA: Evidence for a block in elongation at the UGA/selenocysteine codon. *RNA* **2000**, *6*, 1573–1584. [CrossRef] [PubMed]
66. Martin, G.W., III; Berry, M.J. Selenocysteine codons decrease polysome association on endogenous selenoprotein mRNAs. *Genes Cells* **2001**, *6*, 121–129. [CrossRef] [PubMed]
67. Hatfield, D.; Lee, B.J.; Hampton, L.; Diamond, A.M. Selenium induces changes in the selenocysteine tRNA [Ser] Sec population in mammalian cells. *Nucleic Acids Res.* **1991**, *19*, 939–943. [CrossRef] [PubMed]
68. Chittum, H.S.; Baek, H.J.; Diamond, A.M.; Fernandez-Salguero, P.; Gonzalez, F.; Ohama, T.; Hatfield, D.L.; Kuehn, M.; Lee, B.J. Selenocysteine tRNA [Ser] Sec levels and selenium-dependent glutathione peroxidase activity in mouse embryonic stem cells heterozygous for a targeted mutation in the tRNA [Ser] Sec gene. *Biochemistry* **1997**, *36*, 8634–8639. [CrossRef] [PubMed]

69. Jameson, R.R.; Carlson, B.A.; Butz, M.; Esser, K.; Hatfield, D.L.; Diamond, A.M. Selenium influences the turnover of selenocysteine tRNA [Ser] Sec in chinese hamster ovary cells. *J. Nutr.* **2002**, *132*, 1830–1835. [CrossRef] [PubMed]
70. Carlson, B.A.; Xu, X.-M.; Gladyshev, V.N.; Hatfield, D.L. Selective rescue of selenoprotein expression in mice lacking a highly specialized methyl group in selenocysteine tRNA. *J. Biol. Chem.* **2005**, *280*, 5542–5548. [CrossRef] [PubMed]
71. Jameson, R.R.; Diamond, A.M. A regulatory role for sec tRNA [Ser] Sec in selenoprotein synthesis. *RNA* **2004**, *10*, 1142–1152. [CrossRef] [PubMed]
72. Seeher, S.; Atassi, T.; Mahdi, Y.; Carlson, B.A.; Braun, D.; Wirth, E.K.; Klein, M.O.; Reix, N.; Miniard, A.C.; Schomburg, L. Secisbp2 is essential for embryonic development and enhances selenoprotein expression. *Antioxid. Redox Signal.* **2014**, *21*, 835–849. [CrossRef] [PubMed]
73. Papp, L.V.; Lu, J.; Holmgren, A.; Khanna, K.K. From selenium to selenoproteins: Synthesis, identity, and their role in human health. *Antioxid. Redox Signal.* **2007**, *9*, 775–806. [CrossRef] [PubMed]
74. Mills, G.C. The purification and properties of glutathione peroxidase of erythrocytes. *J. Biol. Chem.* **1959**, *234*, 502–506. [PubMed]
75. Schacter, L. Generation of superoxide anion and hydrogen peroxide by erythrocytes from individuals with sickle trait or normal haemoglobin. *Eur. J. Clin. Investig.* **1986**, *16*, 204–210. [CrossRef]
76. Persson, T.; Popescu, B.O.; Cedazo-Minguez, A. Oxidative stress in alzheimer's disease: Why did antioxidant therapy fail? *Oxid. Med. Cell. Longev.* **2014**. [CrossRef] [PubMed]
77. Ramoutar, R.R.; Brumaghim, J.L. Antioxidant and anticancer properties and mechanisms of inorganic selenium, oxo-sulfur, and oxo-selenium compounds. *Cell Biochem. Biophys.* **2010**, *58*, 1–23. [CrossRef] [PubMed]
78. Surai, P.F. *Selenium in Nutrition and Health*; Nottingham University Press: Nottingham, UK, 2006.
79. Ayala, A.; Muñoz, M.F.; Argüelles, S. Lipid peroxidation: Production, metabolism, and signaling mechanisms of malondialdehyde and 4-hydroxy-2-nonenal. *Oxid. Med. Cell. Longev.* **2014**. [CrossRef] [PubMed]
80. Surai, P.F. *Vitamin e in Avian Reproduction*; FAO: Rome, Italy, 1999.
81. Ames, B.N.; Gold, L.S. The causes and prevention of cancer: Gaining perspective. *Environ. Health Perspect.* **1997**, *105*, 865–873. [CrossRef] [PubMed]
82. Helbock, H.J.; Beckman, K.B.; Shigenaga, M.K.; Walter, P.B.; Woodall, A.A.; Yeo, H.C.; Ames, B.N. DNA oxidation matters: The HPLC-electrochemical detection assay of 8-oxo-deoxyguanosine and 8-oxo-guanine. *Proc. Natl. Acad. Sci. USA* **1998**, *95*, 288–293. [CrossRef] [PubMed]
83. Ames, B.N. An enthusiasm for metabolism. *J. Biol. Chem.* **2003**, *278*, 4369–4380. [CrossRef] [PubMed]
84. Lobo, V.; Patil, A.; Phatak, A.; Chandra, N. Free radicals, antioxidants and functional foods: Impact on human health. *Pharmacogn. Rev.* **2010**, *4*, 118–126. [CrossRef] [PubMed]
85. Lagouge, M.; Larsson, N.G. The role of mitochondrial DNA mutations and free radicals in disease and ageing. *J. Intern. Med.* **2013**, *273*, 529–543. [CrossRef] [PubMed]
86. Diplock, A. *Antioxidants and Disease Prevention Molecular Aspects of Medicine*; Pergamon Press: Oxford, UK, 1994.
87. Halliwell, B. Free radicals and antioxidants: A personal view. *Nutr. Rev.* **1994**, *52*, 253–265. [CrossRef] [PubMed]
88. Davies, M.J. Protein oxidation and peroxidation. *Biochem. J.* **2016**, *473*, 805–825. [CrossRef] [PubMed]
89. Hawkins, C.L.; Morgan, P.E.; Davies, M.J. Quantification of protein modification by oxidants. *Free Radic. Biol. Med.* **2009**, *46*, 965–988. [CrossRef] [PubMed]
90. Berlett, B.S.; Stadtman, E.R. Protein oxidation in aging, disease, and oxidative stress. *J. Biol. Chem.* **1997**, *272*, 20313–20316. [CrossRef] [PubMed]
91. Tramutola, A.; Lanzillotta, C.; Perluigi, M.; Butterfield, D.A. Oxidative stress, protein modification and alzheimer disease. *Brain Res. Bull.* **2017**, *133*, 88–96. [CrossRef] [PubMed]
92. Stadtman, E.R. Protein oxidation and aging. *Science* **1992**, *257*, 1220–1224. [CrossRef] [PubMed]
93. Stadtman, E.R.; Levine, R.L. Protein oxidation. *Ann. N. Y. Acad. Sci.* **2000**, *899*, 191–208. [CrossRef] [PubMed]
94. Sultana, R.; Perluigi, M.; Butterfield, D.A. Protein oxidation and lipid peroxidation in brain of subjects with alzheimer's disease: Insights into mechanism of neurodegeneration from redox proteomics. *Antioxid. Redox Signal.* **2006**, *8*, 2021–2037. [CrossRef] [PubMed]
95. Steinbrenner, H.; Speckmann, B.; Klotz, L.-O. Selenoproteins: Antioxidant selenoenzymes and beyond. *Arch. Biochem. Biophys.* **2016**, *595*, 113–119. [CrossRef] [PubMed]

96. Storkey, C.; Pattison, D.I.; Ignasiak, M.T.; Schiesser, C.H.; Davies, M.J. Kinetics of reaction of peroxynitrite with selenium-and sulfur-containing compounds: Absolute rate constants and assessment of biological significance. *Free Radic. Biol. Med.* **2015**, *89*, 1049–1056. [CrossRef] [PubMed]
97. Pappas, A.; Zoidis, E.; Surai, P.; Zervas, G. Selenoproteins and maternal nutrition. *Comp. Biochem. Physiol. B* **2008**, *151*, 361–372. [CrossRef] [PubMed]
98. Toppo, S.; Flohé, L.; Ursini, F.; Vanin, S.; Maiorino, M. Catalytic mechanisms and specificities of glutathione peroxidases: Variations of a basic scheme. *BBA-Gen. Subj.* **2009**, *1790*, 1486–1500. [CrossRef] [PubMed]
99. Sun, Q.-A.; Kirnarsky, L.; Sherman, S.; Gladyshev, V.N. Selenoprotein oxidoreductase with specificity for thioredoxin and glutathione systems. *Proc. Natl. Acad. Sci. USA* **2001**, *98*, 3673–3678. [CrossRef] [PubMed]
100. Arnér, E.S. Selenoproteins—What unique properties can arise with selenocysteine in place of cysteine? *Exp. Cell Res.* **2010**, *316*, 1296–1303. [CrossRef] [PubMed]
101. Brzezińska-Ślebodzińska, E.; Ślebodziński, A.B.; Pietras, B.; Wieczorek, G. Antioxidant effect of vitamin E and glutathione on lipid peroxidation in boar semen plasma. *Biol. Trace Elem. Res.* **1995**, *47*, 69–74. [CrossRef]
102. Kagan, V.; Nohl, H.; Quinn, P.; Cadenas, E.; Packer, L. *Handbook of Antioxidants*; Marcel Dekker: New York, NY, USA, 1996.
103. Surai, P.F. *Natural Antioxidants in Avian Nutrition and Reproduction*; Nottingham University Press: Nottingham, UK, 2002.
104. Młochowski, J.; Brząszcz, M.; Giurg, M.; Palus, J.; Wójtowicz, H. Selenium-promoted oxidation of organic compounds: Reactions and mechanisms. *Eur. J. Org. Chem.* **2003**, *2003*, 4329–4339. [CrossRef]
105. Bowie, A.; O'Neill, L.A. Oxidative stress and nuclear factor-κb activation: A reassessment of the evidence in the light of recent discoveries. *Biochem. Pharmacol.* **2000**, *59*, 13–23. [CrossRef]
106. Thundathil, J.; de Lamirande, E.; Gagnon, C. Nitric oxide regulates the phosphorylation of the threonine-glutamine-tyrosine motif in proteins of human spermatozoa during capacitation. *Biol. Reprod.* **2003**, *68*, 1291–1298. [CrossRef] [PubMed]
107. Halliwell, B.; Gutteridge, J.M. *Free Radicals in Biology and Medicine*; Oxford University Press: Oxford, UK, 2015.
108. McCord, J.M. The evolution of free radicals and oxidative stress. *Am. J. Med.* **2000**, *108*, 652–659. [CrossRef]
109. Dröge, W. Free radicals in the physiological control of cell function. *Physiol. Rev.* **2002**, *82*, 47–95. [CrossRef] [PubMed]
110. Yoon, S.-O.; Yun, C.-H.; Chung, A.-S. Dose effect of oxidative stress on signal transduction in aging. *Mech. Ageing Dev.* **2002**, *123*, 1597–1604. [CrossRef]
111. Seifried, H.E.; Anderson, D.E.; Fisher, E.I.; Milner, J.A. A review of the interaction among dietary antioxidants and reactive oxygen species. *J. Nutr. Biochem.* **2007**, *18*, 567–579. [CrossRef] [PubMed]
112. Steinbrenner, H.; Sies, H. Protection against reactive oxygen species by selenoproteins. *Biochim. Biophys. Acta* **2009**, *1790*, 1478–1485. [CrossRef] [PubMed]
113. Zhang, H.; Limphong, P.; Pieper, J.; Liu, Q.; Rodesch, C.K.; Christians, E.; Benjamin, I.J. Glutathione-dependent reductive stress triggers mitochondrial oxidation and cytotoxicity. *FASEB J.* **2012**, *26*, 1442–1451. [CrossRef] [PubMed]
114. Meister, A. On the antioxidant effects of ascorbic acid and glutathione. *Biochem. Pharmacol.* **1992**, *44*, 1905–1915. [CrossRef]
115. Dannenmann, B.; Lehle, S.; Hildebrand, D.G.; Kübler, A.; Grondona, P.; Schmid, V.; Holzer, K.; Fröschl, M.; Essmann, F.; Rothfuss, O.; et al. High glutathione and glutathione peroxidase-2 levels mediate cell-type-specific DNA damage protection in human induced pluripotent stem cells. *Stem Cell Rep.* **2015**, *4*, 886–898.
116. Kanwal, R.; Pandey, M.; Bhaskaran, N.; MacLennan, G.T.; Fu, P.; Ponsky, L.E.; Gupta, S. Protection against oxidative DNA damage and stress in human prostate by glutathione S-transferase P1. *Mol. Carcinog.* **2014**, *53*, 8–18. [CrossRef] [PubMed]
117. Diaz-Vivancos, P.; de Simone, A.; Kiddle, G.; Foyer, C.H. Glutathione—Linking cell proliferation to oxidative stress. *Free Radic. Biol. Med.* **2015**, *89*, 1154–1164. [CrossRef] [PubMed]
118. Jin, L.; Li, D.; Alesi, G.N.; Fan, J.; Kang, H.-B.; Lu, Z.; Boggon, T.J.; Jin, P.; Yi, H.; Wright, E.R.; et al. Glutamate dehydrogenase 1 signals through antioxidant glutathione peroxidase 1 to regulate redox homeostasis and tumor growth. *Cancer Cell* **2015**, *27*, 257–270. [CrossRef] [PubMed]
119. Geltink, R.I.K.; O'Sullivan, D.; Pearce, E.L. Caught in the crossfire: GSH controls T cell metabolic reprogramming. *Immunity* **2017**, *46*, 525–527. [CrossRef] [PubMed]

120. Mak, T.W.; Grusdat, M.; Duncan, G.S.; Dostert, C.; Nonnenmacher, Y.; Cox, M.; Binsfeld, C.; Hao, Z.; Brüstle, A.; Itsumi, M. Glutathione primes T cell metabolism for inflammation. *Immunity* **2017**, *46*, 675–689. [CrossRef] [PubMed]
121. Sen, C.K.; Packer, L. Thiol homeostasis and supplements in physical exercise. *Am. J. Clin. Nutr.* **2000**, *72*, 653s–669s. [CrossRef] [PubMed]
122. Lenzi, A.; Gandini, L.; Picardo, M.; Tramer, F.; Sandri, G.; Panfili, E. Lipoperoxidation damage of spermatozoa polyunsaturated fatty acids (PUFA): Scavenger mechanisms and possible scavenger therapies. *Front. Biosci.* **2000**, *5*, 1–15.
123. Meister, A.; Anderson, M.E. Glutathione. *Annu. Rev. Biochem.* **1983**, *52*, 711–760. [CrossRef] [PubMed]
124. Bains, J.S.; Shaw, C.A. Neurodegenerative disorders in humans: The role of glutathione in oxidative stress-mediated neuronal death. *Brain Res. Rev.* **1997**, *25*, 335–358. [CrossRef]
125. Thompson, K.H.; Godin, D.V.; Lee, M. Tissue antioxidant status in streptozotocin-induced diabetes in rats. *Biol. Trace Elem. Res.* **1992**, *35*, 213–224. [CrossRef] [PubMed]
126. Palamanda, J.R.; Kehrer, J.P. Involvement of vitamin E and protein thiols in the inhibition of microsomal lipid peroxidation by glutathione. *Lipids* **1993**, *28*, 427–431. [CrossRef] [PubMed]
127. Elliott, S.J.; Koliwad, S.K. Redox control of ion channel activity in vascular endothelial cells by glutathione. *Microcirculation* **1997**, *4*, 341–347. [CrossRef] [PubMed]
128. Brigelius-Flohé, R.; Maiorino, M. Glutathione peroxidases. *BBA-Gen. Subj.* **2013**, *1830*, 3289–3303. [CrossRef] [PubMed]
129. Pedrero, Z.; Madrid, Y. Novel approaches for selenium speciation in foodstuffs and biological specimens: A review. *Anal. Chim. Acta* **2009**, *634*, 135–152. [CrossRef] [PubMed]
130. Winterbourn, C.C.; Hampton, M.B. Thiol chemistry and specificity in redox signaling. *Free Radic. Biol. Med.* **2008**, *45*, 549–561. [CrossRef] [PubMed]
131. Sies, H. Strategies of antioxidant defense. *Eur. J. Biochem.* **1993**, *215*, 213–219. [CrossRef] [PubMed]
132. Buttke, T.M.; Sandstrom, P.A. Oxidative stress as a mediator of apoptosis. *Immunol. Today* **1994**, *15*, 7–10. [CrossRef]
133. Huang, J.-Q.; Ren, F.-Z.; Jiang, Y.-Y.; Xiao, C.; Lei, X.G. Selenoproteins protect against avian nutritional muscular dystrophy by metabolizing peroxides and regulating redox/apoptotic signaling. *Free Radic. Biol. Med.* **2015**, *83*, 129–138. [CrossRef] [PubMed]
134. Yang, Z.; Liu, C.; Liu, C.; Teng, X.; Li, S. Selenium deficiency mainly influences antioxidant selenoproteins expression in broiler immune organs. *Biol. Trace Elem. Res.* **2016**, *172*, 209–221. [CrossRef] [PubMed]
135. Xu, J.-X.; Zhang, C.; Cao, C.-Y.; Zhu, S.-Y.; Li, H.; Sun, Y.-C.; Li, J.-L. Dietary selenium status regulates the transcriptions of selenoproteome and activities of selenoenzymes in chicken kidney at low or super-nutritional levels. *Biol. Trace Elem. Res.* **2016**, *170*, 438–448. [CrossRef] [PubMed]
136. Tang, J.; Huang, X.; Wang, L.; Li, Q.; Xu, J.; Jia, G.; Liu, G.; Chen, X.; Shang, H.; Zhao, H. Supranutritional dietary selenium depressed expression of selenoprotein genes in three immune organs of broilers. *Anim. Sci. J.* **2017**, *88*, 331–338. [CrossRef] [PubMed]
137. Xiang, L.-R.; Li, W.; Wang, L.-L.; Cao, C.-Y.; Li, N.; Li, X.-N.; Jiang, X.-Q.; Li, J.-L. The supranutritional selenium status alters blood glucose and pancreatic redox homeostasis via a modulated selenotranscriptome in chickens (*Gallus gallus*). *RSC Adv.* **2017**, *7*, 24438–24445. [CrossRef]
138. Khan, A.Z.; Kumbhar, S.; Hamid, M.; Afzal, S.; Parveen, F.; Liu, Y.; Shu, H.; Mengistu, B.M.; Huang, K. Effects of selenium-enriched probiotics on heart lesions by influencing the mRNA expressions of selenoproteins and heat shock proteins in heat stressed broiler chickens. *Pak. Vet. J.* **2016**, *36*, 460–464.
139. Khan, A.Z.; Kumbhar, S.; Liu, Y.; Hamid, M.; Pan, C.; Nido, S.A.; Parveen, F.; Huang, K. Dietary supplementation of selenium-enriched probiotics enhances meat quality of broiler chickens (*Gallus gallus domesticus*) raised under high ambient temperature. *Biol. Trace Elem. Res.* **2018**, *182*, 328–338. [CrossRef] [PubMed]
140. Chen, W.; Zhang, Z.; Dong, H.; Jiang, X. Molecular cloning and sequence analysis of selenoprotein W gene and its mRNA expression patterns in response to metabolic status and cadmium exposure in goldfish, carassius auratus. *Comp. Biochem. Physiol. B* **2015**, *184*, 1–9. [CrossRef] [PubMed]
141. Gan, L.; Liu, Q.; Xu, H.-B.; Zhu, Y.-S.; Yang, X.-L. Effects of selenium overexposure on glutathione peroxidase and thioredoxin reductase gene expressions and activities. *Biol. Trace Elem. Res.* **2002**, *89*, 165–175. [CrossRef]

142. El-Sharaky, A.; Newairy, A.; Badreldeen, M.; Eweda, S.; Sheweita, S. Protective role of selenium against renal toxicity induced by cadmium in rats. *Toxicology* **2007**, *235*, 185–193. [CrossRef] [PubMed]
143. Jamba, L.; Nehru, B.; Bansal, M. Effect of selenium supplementation on the influence of cadmium on glutathione and glutathione peroxidase system in mouse liver. *J. Trace Elem. Exp. Med.* **2000**, *13*, 299–304. [CrossRef]
144. Al-Waeli, A.; Zoidis, E.; Pappas, A.; Demiris, N.; Zervas, G.; Fegeros, K. The role of organic selenium in cadmium toxicity: Effects on broiler performance and health status. *Animal* **2013**, *7*, 386–393. [CrossRef] [PubMed]
145. Zhu, Y.; Chen, P.; Wan, H.; Wang, Y.; Hao, P.; Liu, Y.; Liu, J. Selenium–chromium (VI) interaction regulates the contents and correlations of trace elements in chicken brain and serum. *Biol. Trace Elem. Res.* **2018**, *181*, 154–163. [CrossRef] [PubMed]
146. Gao, H.; Liu, C.; Song, S.; Fu, J. Effects of dietary selenium against lead toxicity on mRNA levels of 25 selenoprotein genes in the cartilage tissue of broiler chicken. *Biol. Trace Elem. Res.* **2016**, *172*, 234–241. [CrossRef] [PubMed]
147. Huang, H.; Wang, Y.; An, Y.; Tian, Y.; Li, S.; Teng, X. Selenium for the mitigation of toxicity induced by lead in chicken testes through regulating mRNA expressions of HSPs and selenoproteins. *Environ. Sci. Pollut. Res.* **2017**, *24*, 14312–14321. [CrossRef] [PubMed]
148. Li, X.; Xing, M.; Chen, M.; Zhao, J.; Fan, R.; Zhao, X.; Cao, C.; Yang, J.; Zhang, Z.; Xu, S. Effects of selenium-lead interaction on the gene expression of inflammatory factors and selenoproteins in chicken neutrophils. *Ecotoxicol. Environ. Saf.* **2017**, *139*, 447–453. [CrossRef] [PubMed]
149. Cai, J.; Zhang, Y.; Yang, J.; Liu, Q.; Zhao, R.; Hamid, S.; Wang, H.; Xu, S.; Zhang, Z. Antagonistic effects of selenium against necroptosis injury via adiponectin-necrotic pathway induced by cadmium in heart of chicken. *RSC Adv.* **2017**, *7*, 44438–44446. [CrossRef]
150. Bao, R.; Wang, X.; Zheng, S.; Zhang, Q.; Lin, H.; Li, S. Selenium supplementation changes the ion profile in the pancreas of chickens treated with cadmium. *Biol. Trace Elem. Res.* **2018**, *181*, 133–141. [CrossRef] [PubMed]
151. Berggren, M.M.; Mangin, J.F.; Gasdaska, J.R.; Powis, G. Effect of selenium on rat thioredoxin reductase activity: Increase by supranutritional selenium and decrease by selenium deficiency. *Biochem. Pharmacol.* **1999**, *57*, 187–193. [CrossRef]
152. Rayman, M.P. Selenium in cancer prevention: A review of the evidence and mechanism of action. *Proc. Nutr. Soc.* **2005**, *64*, 527–542. [CrossRef] [PubMed]
153. Pappas, A.; Zoidis, E.; Papadomichelakis, G.; Fegeros, K. Supranutritional selenium level affects fatty acid composition and oxidative stability of chicken breast muscle tissue. *J. Anim. Physiol. Anim. Nutr.* **2012**, *96*, 385–394. [CrossRef] [PubMed]
154. Seo, Y.R.; Kelley, M.R.; Smith, M.L. Selenomethionine regulation of p53 by a ref1-dependent redox mechanism. *Proc. Natl. Acad. Sci. USA* **2002**, *99*, 14548–14553. [CrossRef] [PubMed]
155. Kibriya, M.G.; Jasmine, F.; Argos, M.; Verret, W.J.; Rakibuz-Zaman, M.; Ahmed, A.; Parvez, F.; Ahsan, H. Changes in gene expression profiles in response to selenium supplementation among individuals with arsenic-induced pre-malignant skin lesions. *Toxicol. Lett.* **2007**, *169*, 162–176. [CrossRef] [PubMed]
156. Whanger, P.D. Selenium and the brain: A review. *Nutr. Neurosci.* **2001**, *4*, 81–97. [CrossRef] [PubMed]
157. Birt, D.F.; Julius, A.D.; Runice, C.E.; White, L.T.; Lawson, T.; Pour, P.M. Enhancement of bop-induced pancreatic carcinogenesis in selenium-fed syrian golden hamsters under specific dietary conditions. *Nutr. Cancer* **1988**, *11*, 21–33. [CrossRef] [PubMed]
158. Seo, Y.R.; Sweeney, C.; Smith, M.L. Selenomethionine induction of DNA repair response in human fibroblasts. *Oncogene* **2002**, *21*, 3663–3669. [CrossRef] [PubMed]
159. Christmann, M.; Tomicic, M.T.; Roos, W.P.; Kaina, B. Mechanisms of human DNA repair: An update. *Toxicology* **2003**, *193*, 3–34. [CrossRef]
160. Kennedy, A.R.; Ware, J.H.; Guan, J.; Donahue, J.J.; Biaglow, J.E.; Zhou, Z.; Stewart, J.; Vazquez, M.; Wan, X.S. Selenomethionine protects against adverse biological effects induced by space radiation. *Free Radic. Biol. Med.* **2004**, *36*, 259–266. [CrossRef] [PubMed]
161. Turanov, A.A.; Xu, X.-M.; Carlson, B.A.; Yoo, M.-H.; Gladyshev, V.N.; Hatfield, D.L. Biosynthesis of selenocysteine, the 21st amino acid in the genetic code, and a novel pathway for cysteine biosynthesis. *Adv. Nutr.* **2011**, *2*, 122–128. [CrossRef] [PubMed]

162. Araiso, Y.; Palioura, S.; Ishitani, R.; Sherrer, R.L.; O'Donoghue, P.; Yuan, J.; Oshikane, H.; Domae, N.; DeFranco, J.; Söll, D. Structural insights into RNA-dependent eukaryal and archaeal selenocysteine formation. *Nucl. Acids Res.* **2007**, *36*, 1187–1199. [CrossRef] [PubMed]
163. Fairweather-Tait, S.J.; Collings, R.; Hurst, R. Selenium bioavailability: Current knowledge and future research requirements. *Am. J. Clin. Nutr.* **2010**, *91*, 1484S–1491S. [CrossRef] [PubMed]
164. Short, S.P.; Williams, C.S. Selenoproteins in tumorigenesis and cancer progression. In *Advances in Cancer Research*; Academic Press Inc.: Cambridge, MA, USA, 2017.
165. Schomburg, L. Dietary selenium and human health. *Nutrients* **2017**, *9*. [CrossRef] [PubMed]
166. Shchedrina, V.A.; Zhang, Y.; Labunskyy, V.M.; Hatfield, D.L.; Gladyshev, V.N. Structure–function relations, physiological roles, and evolution of mammalian er-resident selenoproteins. *Antioxid. Redox Signal.* **2010**, *12*, 839–849. [CrossRef] [PubMed]
167. Labunskyy, V.M.; Yoo, M.-H.; Hatfield, D.L.; Gladyshev, V.N. Sep15, a thioredoxin-like selenoprotein, is involved in the unfolded protein response and differentially regulated by adaptive and acute ER stresses. *Biochemistry* **2009**, *48*, 8458–8465. [CrossRef] [PubMed]
168. Ferguson, A.D.; Labunskyy, V.M.; Fomenko, D.E.; Araç, D.; Chelliah, Y.; Amezcua, C.A.; Rizo, J.; Gladyshev, V.N.; Deisenhofer, J. NMR structures of the selenoproteins Sep15 and SelM reveal redox activity of a new thioredoxin-like family. *J. Biol. Chem.* **2006**, *281*, 3536–3543. [CrossRef] [PubMed]
169. Metanis, N.; Hilvert, D. Natural and synthetic selenoproteins. *Curr. Opin. Chem. Biol.* **2014**, *22*, 27–34. [CrossRef] [PubMed]
170. Gromer, S.; Johansson, L.; Bauer, H.; Arscott, L.D.; Rauch, S.; Ballou, D.P.; Williams, C.H.; Schirmer, R.H.; Arnér, E.S. Active sites of thioredoxin reductases: Why selenoproteins? *Proc. Natl. Acad. Sci. USA* **2003**, *100*, 12618–12623. [CrossRef] [PubMed]
171. Ishizaki, A. Onitai-itai (ouch-ouch) disease. *Asian Med. J.* **1971**, *14*, 421–436.
172. Bianco, A.C.; Larsen, P.R. Cellular and structural biology of the deiodinases. *Thyroid* **2005**, *15*, 777–786. [CrossRef] [PubMed]
173. Jurynec, M.J.; Xia, R.; Mackrill, J.J.; Gunther, D.; Crawford, T.; Flanigan, K.M.; Abramson, J.J.; Howard, M.T.; Grunwald, D.J. Selenoprotein N is required for ryanodine receptor calcium release channel activity in human and zebrafish muscle. *Proc. Natl. Acad. Sci. USA* **2008**, *105*, 12485–12490. [CrossRef] [PubMed]
174. Cardoso, B.R.; Roberts, B.R.; Bush, A.I.; Hare, D.J. Selenium, selenoproteins and neurodegenerative diseases. *Metallomics* **2015**, *7*, 1213–1228. [CrossRef] [PubMed]
175. Habibian, M.; Sadeghi, G.; Ghazi, S.; Moeini, M.M. Selenium as a feed supplement for heat-stressed poultry: A review. *Biol. Trace Elem. Res.* **2015**, *165*, 183–193. [CrossRef] [PubMed]
176. Dalgaard, T.S.; Briens, M.; Engberg, R.M.; Lauridsen, C. The influence of selenium and selenoproteins on immune responses of poultry and pigs. *Anim. Feed Sci. Technol.* **2018**, *238*, 73–83. [CrossRef]
177. Zhu, S.-Y.; Li, X.-N.; Sun, X.-C.; Lin, J.; Li, W.; Zhang, C.; Li, J.-L. Biochemical characterization of the selenoproteome in gallus gallus via bioinformatics analysis: Structure–function relationships and interactions of binding molecules. *Metallomics* **2017**, *9*, 124–131. [CrossRef] [PubMed]
178. Reeg, S.; Grune, T. Protein oxidation in aging: Does it play a role in aging progression? *Antioxid. Redox Signal.* **2015**, *23*, 239–255. [CrossRef] [PubMed]
179. Khoso, P.A.; Yang, Z.; Liu, C.; Li, S. Selenoproteins and heat shock proteins play important roles in immunosuppression in the bursa of fabricius of chickens with selenium deficiency. *Cell Stress Chaperones* **2015**, *20*, 967–978. [CrossRef] [PubMed]
180. Du, Q.; Yao, H.; Yao, L.; Zhang, Z.; Lei, X.; Xu, S. Selenium deficiency influences the expression of selenoproteins and inflammatory cytokines in chicken aorta vessels. *Biol. Trace Elem. Res.* **2016**, *173*, 501–513. [CrossRef] [PubMed]
181. Wang, Q.; Huang, J.; Zhang, H.; Lei, X.; Du, Z.; Xiao, C.; Chen, S.; Ren, F. Selenium deficiency-induced apoptosis of chick embryonic vascular smooth muscle cells and correlations with 25 selenoproteins. *Biol. Trace Elem. Res.* **2017**, *176*, 407–415. [CrossRef] [PubMed]
182. Gao, Y.; Zhang, J.; Huang, X.; Zhang, G. Glutathione peroxidase 1, selenoprotein K, and selenoprotein H may play important roles in chicken testes in response to selenium deficiency. *Biol. Trace Elem. Res.* **2017**, *179*, 1–6. [CrossRef] [PubMed]

183. Huang, X.; Sun, B.; Zhang, J.; Gao, Y.; Li, G.; Chang, Y. Selenium deficiency induced injury in chicken muscular stomach by downregulating selenoproteins. *Biol. Trace Elem. Res.* **2017**, *179*, 277–283. [CrossRef] [PubMed]
184. Sun, Z.; Liu, C.; Pan, T.; Yao, H.; Li, S. Selenium accelerates chicken dendritic cells differentiation and affects selenoproteins expression. *Dev. Comp. Immunol.* **2017**, *77*, 30–37. [CrossRef] [PubMed]
185. Wang, X.; An, Y.; Jiao, W.; Zhang, Z.; Han, H.; Gu, X.; Teng, X. Selenium protects against lead-induced apoptosis via endoplasmic reticulum stress in chicken kidneys. *Biol. Trace Elem. Res.* **2017**, *182*, 354–363. [CrossRef] [PubMed]
186. Huang, J.-Q.; Ren, F.-Z.; Jiang, Y.-Y.; Lei, X. Characterization of selenoprotein M and its response to selenium deficiency in chicken brain. *Biol. Trace Elem. Res.* **2016**, *170*, 449–458. [CrossRef] [PubMed]
187. Zoidis, E.; Pappas, A.; Georgiou, C.; Komaitis, E.; Feggeros, K. Selenium affects the expression of GPx4 and catalase in the liver of chicken. *Comp. Biochem. Physiol. B* **2010**, *155*, 294–300. [CrossRef] [PubMed]
188. Jiang, Z.-H.; Lin, H.-J.; Yao, H.-D.; Zhang, Z.-W.; Fu, J.; Xu, S.-W. Selw protects against H_2O_2-induced liver injury in chickens via inhibiting inflammation and apoptosis. *RSC Adv.* **2017**, *7*, 15158–15167. [CrossRef]
189. Fan, R.; Yao, H.; Zhao, X.; Cao, C.; Yang, T.; Luan, Y.; Zhang, Z.; Xu, S. Gene expression of selenoproteins can be regulated by selenoprotein k silencing in chicken myoblasts. *BioMetals* **2016**, *29*, 679–689. [CrossRef] [PubMed]
190. Huang, J.; Jiang, Y.; Guo, H.; Zhang, H.; Lei, X.; Ren, F. Association Analysis between Selenoprotein Genes (Selw and Seln) and Meat Quality Traits in Chicken. Available online: https://www.researchgate.net/publication/312119322_Association_analysis_between_selenoprotein_genes_Selw_and_Seln_and_meat_quality_traits_in_chicken (accessed on 23 March 2018).
191. Luan, Y.; Zhao, J.; Yao, H.; Zhao, X.; Fan, R.; Zhao, W.; Zhang, Z.; Xu, S. Selenium deficiency influences the mrna expression of selenoproteins and cytokines in chicken erythrocytes. *Biol. Trace Elem. Res.* **2016**, *171*, 427–436. [CrossRef] [PubMed]
192. Khoso, P.A.; Yang, Z.; Liu, C.; Li, S. Selenium deficiency downregulates selenoproteins and suppresses immune function in chicken thymus. *Biol. Trace Elem. Res.* **2015**, *167*, 48–55. [CrossRef] [PubMed]
193. Chen, W.; Zhang, H.; Wang, S.; Ruan, D.; Xie, X.; Yu, D.; Lin, Y. Estimation of dietary selenium requirement for chinese egg-laying ducks. *Anim. Prod. Sci.* **2015**, *55*, 1056–1063. [CrossRef]
194. Li, J.-L.; Sunde, R.A. Selenoprotein transcript level and enzyme activity as biomarkers for selenium status and selenium requirements of chickens (*Gallus gallus*). *PLoS ONE* **2016**, *11*. [CrossRef] [PubMed]
195. Taylor, R.M.; Sunde, R.A. Selenoprotein transcript level and enzyme activity as biomarkers for selenium status and selenium requirements in the turkey (*Meleagris gallopavo*). *PLoS ONE* **2016**, *11*. [CrossRef] [PubMed]
196. Dalia, A.; Loh, T.; Sazili, A.; Jahromi, M.; Samsudin, A. The effect of dietary bacterial organic selenium on growth performance, antioxidant capacity, and selenoproteins gene expression in broiler chickens. *BMC Vet. Res.* **2017**, *13*. [CrossRef] [PubMed]
197. Zhao, L.; Sun, L.-H.; Huang, J.-Q.; Briens, M.; Qi, D.-S.; Xu, S.-W.; Lei, X.G. A novel organic selenium compound exerts unique regulation of selenium speciation, selenogenome, and selenoproteins in broiler chicks. *J. Nutr.* **2017**, *147*, 789–797. [CrossRef] [PubMed]
198. Sunde, R.A.; Raines, A.M. Selenium regulation of the selenoprotein and nonselenoprotein transcriptomes in rodents. *Adv. Nutr.* **2011**, *2*, 138–150. [CrossRef] [PubMed]
199. Behne, D.; Kyriakopoulos, A. Mammalian selenium-containing proteins. *Annu. Rev. Nutr.* **2001**, *21*, 453–473. [CrossRef] [PubMed]
200. Hatfield, D.L.; Gladyshev, V.N. How selenium has altered our understanding of the genetic code. *Mol. Cell. Biol.* **2002**, *22*, 3565–3576. [CrossRef] [PubMed]
201. O'Driscoll, M.; Ruiz-Perez, V.L.; Woods, C.G.; Jeggo, P.A.; Goodship, J.A. A splicing mutation affecting expression of ataxia–telangiectasia and Rad3–related protein (ATR) results in Seckel syndrome. *Nat. Genet.* **2003**, *33*, 497–501. [CrossRef] [PubMed]
202. Schomburg, I.; Chang, A.; Ebeling, C.; Gremse, M.; Heldt, C.; Huhn, G.; Schomburg, D. Brenda, the enzyme database: Updates and major new developments. *Nucl. Acids Res.* **2004**, *32*, D431–D433. [CrossRef] [PubMed]
203. Brigelius-Flohe, R.; Traber, M.G. Vitamin e: Function and metabolism. *FASEB J.* **1999**, *13*, 1145–1155. [CrossRef] [PubMed]

204. Moriarty, P.M.; Reddy, C.C.; Maquat, L.E. Selenium deficiency reduces the abundance of mRNA for se-dependent glutathione peroxidase 1 by a UGA-dependent mechanism likely to be nonsense codon-mediated decay of cytoplasmic mRNA. *Mol. Cell. Biol.* **1998**, *18*, 2932–2939. [CrossRef] [PubMed]
205. Maquat, L.E. Evidence that selenium deficiency results in the cytoplasmic decay of GPx1 mRNA dependent on pre-mRNA splicing proteins bound to the mRNA exon-exon junction. *Biofactors* **2001**, *14*, 37–42. [CrossRef] [PubMed]
206. Sachdev, S.W.; Sunde, R.A. Selenium regulation of transcript abundance and translational efficiency of glutathione peroxidase-1 and -4 in rat liver. *Biochem. J.* **2001**, *357*, 851–858.
207. Jiang, X.-Q.; Cao, C.-Y.; Li, Z.-Y.; Li, W.; Zhang, C.; Lin, J.; Li, X.-N.; Li, J.-L. Delineating hierarchy of selenotranscriptome expression and their response to selenium status in chicken central nervous system. *J. Inorg. Biochem.* **2017**, *169*, 13–22. [CrossRef] [PubMed]
208. Jiang, Y.-Y.; Huang, J.-Q.; Lin, G.-C.; Guo, H.-Y.; Ren, F.-Z.; Zhang, H. Characterization and expression of chicken selenoprotein U. *Biol. Trace Elem. Res.* **2015**, *166*, 216–224. [CrossRef] [PubMed]
209. Sunde, R.A.; Sunde, G.R.; Sunde, C.M.; Sunde, M.L.; Evenson, J.K. Cloning, sequencing, and expression of selenoprotein transcripts in the turkey (*Meleagris gallopavo*). *PLoS ONE* **2015**, *10*. [CrossRef] [PubMed]
210. Kumaraswamy, E.; Malykh, A.; Korotkov, K.V.; Kozyavkin, S.; Hu, Y.; Kwon, S.Y.; Moustafa, M.E.; Carlson, B.A.; Berry, M.J.; Lee, B.J. Structure-expression relationships of the 15-kDa selenoprotein gene possible role of the protein in cancer etiology. *J. Biol. Chem.* **2000**, *275*, 35540–35547. [CrossRef] [PubMed]
211. Yoboue, E.D.; Rimessi, A.; Anelli, T.; Pinton, P.; Sitia, R. Regulation of calcium fluxes by GPX8, a type-II transmembrane peroxidase enriched at the mitochondria-associated endoplasmic reticulum membrane. *Antioxid. Redox Signal.* **2017**, *27*, 583–595. [CrossRef] [PubMed]
212. Marino, M.; Stoilova, T.; Giorgi, C.; Bachi, A.; Cattaneo, A.; Auricchio, A.; Pinton, P.; Zito, E. SEPN1, an endoplasmic reticulum-localized selenoprotein linked to skeletal muscle pathology, counteracts hyperoxidation by means of redox-regulating SERCA2 pump activity. *Hum. Mol. Genet.* **2015**, *24*, 1843–1855. [CrossRef] [PubMed]
213. Arbogast, S.; Beuvin, M.; Fraysse, B.; Zhou, H.; Muntoni, F.; Ferreiro, A. Oxidative stress in SEPN1-related myopathy: From pathophysiology to treatment. *Ann. Neurol.* **2009**, *65*, 677–686. [CrossRef] [PubMed]
214. Zalk, R.; Marks, A.R. Ca^{2+} Release Channels Join the 'Resolution Revolution'. *Trends Biochem. Sci.* **2017**, *42*, 543–555. [CrossRef] [PubMed]
215. Program, N.T.; Program, N.T. Report on carcinogens. In *Public Health Service, National Toxicology Program*; U.S. Department of Health and Human Services: Research Triangle Park, NC, USA, 2011.
216. Castets, P.; Bertrand, A.T.; Beuvin, M.; Ferry, A.; Le Grand, F.; Castets, M.; Chazot, G.; Rederstorff, M.; Krol, A.; Lescure, A.; et al. Satellite cell loss and impaired muscle regeneration in selenoprotein n deficiency. *Hum. Mol. Genet.* **2011**, *20*, 694–704. [CrossRef] [PubMed]
217. Zhou, J.; Li, C.; Gu, G.; Wang, Q.; Guo, M. Selenoprotein n was required for the regulation of selenium on the uterine smooth muscle contraction in mice. *Biol. Trace Elem. Res.* **2017**, *183*, 138–146. [CrossRef] [PubMed]
218. Grumolato, L.; Ghzili, H.; Montero-Hadjadje, M.; Gasman, S.; Lesage, J.; Tanguy, Y.; Galas, L.; Ait-Ali, D.; Leprince, J.; Guérineau, N.C. Selenoprotein T is a PACAP-regulated gene involved in intracellular Ca^{2+} mobilization and neuroendocrine secretion. *FASEB J.* **2008**, *22*, 1756–1768. [CrossRef] [PubMed]
219. Boukhzar, L.; Hamieh, A.; Cartier, D.; Tanguy, Y.; Alsharif, I.; Castex, M.; Arabo, A.; El Hajji, S.; Bonnet, J.J.; Errami, M.; et al. Selenoprotein t exerts an essential oxidoreductase activity that protects dopaminergic neurons in mouse models of parkinson's disease. *Antioxid. Redox Signal.* **2016**, *24*, 557–574. [CrossRef] [PubMed]
220. Gladyshev, V.N.; Factor, V.M.; Housseau, F.; Hatfield, D.L. Contrasting patterns of regulation of the antioxidant selenoproteins, thioredoxin reductase, and glutathione peroxidase, in cancer cells. *Biochem. Biophys. Res. Commun.* **1998**, *251*, 488–493. [CrossRef] [PubMed]
221. Korotkov, K.V.; Kumaraswamy, E.; Zhou, Y.; Hatfield, D.L.; Gladyshev, V.N. Association between the 15-kDa selenoprotein and UDP-glucose: Glycoprotein glucosyltransferase in the endoplasmic reticulum of mammalian cells. *J. Biol. Chem.* **2001**, *276*, 15330–15336. [CrossRef] [PubMed]
222. Guariniello, S.; Colonna, G.; Raucci, R.; Costantini, M.; Di Bernardo, G.; Bergantino, F.; Castello, G.; Costantini, S. Structure–function relationship and evolutionary history of the human selenoprotein M (SelM) found over-expressed in hepatocellular carcinoma. *Biochim. Biophys. Acta Proteins Proteom.* **2014**, *1844*, 447–456. [CrossRef] [PubMed]

223. Lee, B.C.; Lee, S.-G.; Choo, M.-K.; Kim, J.H.; Lee, H.M.; Kim, S.; Fomenko, D.E.; Kim, H.-Y.; Park, J.M.; Gladyshev, V.N. Selenoprotein MsrB1 promotes anti-inflammatory cytokine gene expression in macrophages and controls immune response in vivo. *Sci. Rep.* **2017**, *7*. [CrossRef] [PubMed]
224. Kim, H.-Y.; Gladyshev, V.N. Different catalytic mechanisms in mammalian selenocysteine-and cysteine-containing methionine-R-sulfoxide reductases. *PLoS Biol.* **2005**, *3*. [CrossRef] [PubMed]
225. Tarrago, L.; Kaya, A.; Weerapana, E.; Marino, S.M.; Gladyshev, V.N. Methionine sulfoxide reductases preferentially reduce unfolded oxidized proteins and protect cells from oxidative protein unfolding. *J. Biol. Chem.* **2012**, *287*, 24448–24459. [CrossRef] [PubMed]
226. Lee, B.C.; Péterfi, Z.; Hoffmann, F.W.; Moore, R.E.; Kaya, A.; Avanesov, A.; Tarrago, L.; Zhou, Y.; Weerapana, E.; Fomenko, D.E. MsrB1 and MICALs regulate actin assembly and macrophage function via reversible stereoselective methionine oxidation. *Mol. Cell* **2013**, *51*, 397–404. [CrossRef] [PubMed]
227. Mehmeti, I.; Lortz, S.; Avezov, E.; Jörns, A.; Lenzen, S. ER-resident antioxidative GPx7 and GPx8 enzyme isoforms protect insulin-secreting INS-1E β-cells against lipotoxicity by improving the ER antioxidative capacity. *Free Radic. Biol. Med.* **2017**, *112*, 121–130. [CrossRef] [PubMed]
228. Li, M.; Cheng, W.; Nie, T.; Lai, H.; Hu, X.; Luo, J.; Li, F.; Li, H. Selenoprotein K mediates the proliferation, migration, and invasion of human choriocarcinoma cells by negatively regulating human chorionic gonadotropin expression via ERK, p38 MAPK, and Akt signaling pathway. *Biol. Trace Elem. Res.* **2017**. [CrossRef] [PubMed]
229. Rozovsky, S.; Liu, J.; Zhang, Z. The intrinsically disordered membrane enzymes selenoprotein S and selenoprotein K. *FASEB J.* **2017**, *31*. [CrossRef]
230. Gao, Y.; Feng, H.C.; Walder, K.; Bolton, K.; Sunderland, T.; Bishara, N.; Quick, M.; Kantham, L.; Collier, G.R. Regulation of the selenoprotein SelS by glucose deprivation and endoplasmic reticulum stress—SelS is a novel glucose-regulated protein. *FEBS Lett.* **2004**, *563*, 185–190. [CrossRef]
231. Curran, J.E.; Jowett, J.B.; Elliott, K.S.; Gao, Y.; Gluschenko, K.; Wang, J.; Azim, D.M.A.; Cai, G.; Mahaney, M.C.; Comuzzie, A.G. Genetic variation in selenoprotein S influences inflammatory response. *Nat. Genet.* **2005**, *37*, 1234–1241. [CrossRef] [PubMed]
232. Chabory, E.; Damon, C.; Lenoir, A.; Henry-Berger, J.; Vernet, P.; Cadet, R.; Saez, F.; Drevet, J. Mammalian glutathione peroxidases control acquisition and maintenance of spermatozoa integrity. *J. Anim. Sci.* **2010**, *88*, 1321–1331. [CrossRef] [PubMed]
233. Li, M.Z.; Elledge, S.J. Slic: A method for sequence-and ligation-independent cloning. *Methods Mol. Biol.* **2012**, *852*, 51–59. [PubMed]
234. Shema, R.; Kulicke, R.; Cowley, G.S.; Stein, R.; Root, D.E.; Heiman, M. Synthetic lethal screening in the mammalian central nervous system identifies Gpx6 as a modulator of huntington's disease. *Proc. Natl. Acad. Sci. USA* **2015**, *112*, 268–272. [CrossRef] [PubMed]
235. Ursini, F. The world of glutathione peroxidases. *J. Trace Elem. Med. Biol.* **2000**, *14*, 116.
236. Ingold, I.; Berndt, C.; Schmitt, S.; Doll, S.; Poschmann, G.; Buday, K.; Roveri, A.; Peng, X.; Freitas, F.P.; Seibt, T. Selenium utilization by GPX4 is required to prevent hydroperoxide-induced ferroptosis. *Cell* **2017**, *21*, 409–422. [CrossRef] [PubMed]
237. Jiao, Y.; Wang, Y.; Guo, S.; Wang, G. Glutathione peroxidases as oncotargets. *Oncotarget* **2017**, *8*, 80093–80102. [CrossRef] [PubMed]
238. Delaunay-Moisan, A.; Ponsero, A.; Toledano, M.B. Reexamining the function of glutathione in oxidative protein folding and secretion. *Antioxid. Redox Signal.* **2017**, *27*, 1178–1199. [CrossRef] [PubMed]
239. Flohé, L.; Brigelius-Flohé, R. Basics and News on Glutathione Peroxidases. In *Selenium*; Springer Nature: New York, NY, USA, 2016; pp. 211–222.
240. Utomo, A.; Jiang, X.; Furuta, S.; Yun, J.; Levin, D.S.; Wang, Y.-C.J.; Desai, K.V.; Green, J.E.; Chen, P.-L.; Lee, W.-H. Identification of a novel putative non-selenocysteine containing phospholipid hydroperoxide glutathione peroxidase (NPGPx) essential for alleviating oxidative stress generated from polyunsaturated fatty acids in breast cancer cells. *J. Biol. Chem.* **2004**, *279*, 43522–43529. [CrossRef] [PubMed]
241. Toppo, S.; Vanin, S.; Bosello, V.; Tosatto, S.C. Evolutionary and structural insights into the multifaceted glutathione peroxidase (Gpx) superfamily. *Antioxid. Redox Signal.* **2008**, *10*, 1501–1514. [CrossRef] [PubMed]
242. Bianco, A.C.; Larsen, P.R. Selenium, Deiodinases and Endocrine Function. Available online: https://link.springer.com/chapter/10.1007/0-387-33827-6_19 (accessed on 23 March 2018).
243. Köhrle, J.; Gärtner, R. Selenium and thyroid. *Best Pract. Res. Clin. Endocrinol. Metab.* **2009**, *23*, 815–827. [CrossRef] [PubMed]

244. Beckett, G.J.; Arthur, J.R. Selenium and endocrine systems. *J. Endocrinol.* **2005**, *184*, 455–465. [CrossRef] [PubMed]
245. Panee, J.; Stoytcheva, Z.R.; Liu, W.; Berry, M.J. Selenoprotein h is a redox-sensing high mobility group family DNA-binding protein that up-regulates genes involved in glutathione synthesis and phase II detoxification. *J. Biol. Chem.* **2007**, *282*, 23759–23765. [CrossRef] [PubMed]
246. Mendelev, N.; Mehta, S.L.; Witherspoon, S.; He, Q.; Sexton, J.Z.; Li, P.A. Upregulation of human selenoprotein H in murine hippocampal neuronal cells promotes mitochondrial biogenesis and functional performance. *Mitochondrion* **2011**, *11*, 76–82. [CrossRef] [PubMed]
247. Ahmed, M.Y.; Al-Khayat, A.; Al-Murshedi, F.; Al-Futaisi, A.; Chioza, B.A.; Pedro Fernandez-Murray, J.; Self, J.E.; Salter, C.G.; Harlalka, G.V.; Rawlins, L.E. A mutation of EPT1 (SELENOI) underlies a new disorder of kennedy pathway phospholipid biosynthesis. *Brain* **2017**, *140*, 547–554. [PubMed]
248. Nogly, P.; Gushchin, I.; Remeeva, A.; Esteves, A.M.; Borges, N.; Ma, P.; Ishchenko, A.; Grudinin, S.; Round, E.; Moraes, I. X-ray structure of a CDP-alcohol phosphatidyltransferase membrane enzyme and insights into its catalytic mechanism. *Nat. Commun.* **2014**, *5*. [CrossRef] [PubMed]
249. Han, S.-J.; Lee, B.C.; Yim, S.H.; Gladyshev, V.N.; Lee, S.-R. Characterization of mammalian selenoprotein o: A redox-active mitochondrial protein. *PLoS ONE* **2014**, *9*. [CrossRef] [PubMed]
250. Gladyshev, M.I.; Sushchik, N.N.; Gubanenko, G.A.; Demirchieva, S.M.; Kalachova, G.S. Effect of way of cooking on content of essential polyunsaturated fatty acids in muscle tissue of humpback salmon (*Oncorhynchus gorbuscha*). *Food Chem.* **2006**, *96*, 446–451. [CrossRef]
251. Burk, R.F.; Hill, K.E. Selenoprotein P: An extracellular protein with unique physical characteristics and a role in selenium homeostasis. *Annu. Rev. Nutr.* **2005**, *25*, 215–235. [CrossRef] [PubMed]
252. Rayman, M.P. Selenoproteins and human health: Insights from epidemiological data. *BBA-Gen. Subj.* **2009**, *1790*, 1533–1540. [CrossRef] [PubMed]
253. Xia, Y.; Hill, K.E.; Byrne, D.W.; Xu, J.; Burk, R.F. Effectiveness of selenium supplements in a low-selenium area of china. *Am. J. Clin. Nutr.* **2005**, *81*, 829–834. [CrossRef] [PubMed]
254. Yao, H.-D.; Wu, Q.; Zhang, Z.-W.; Li, S.; Wang, X.-L.; Lei, X.-G.; Xu, S.-W. Selenoprotein W serves as an antioxidant in chicken myoblasts. *BBA-Gen. Subj.* **2013**, *1830*, 3112–3120. [CrossRef] [PubMed]
255. Whanger, P. Selenoprotein W: A review. *Cell. Mol. Life Sci.* **2000**, *57*, 1846–1852. [CrossRef] [PubMed]
256. McAllister, K.N.; Bouillaut, L.; Kahn, J.N.; Self, W.T.; Sorg, J.A. Using CRISPR-Cas9-mediated genome editing to generate C. difficile mutants defective in selenoproteins synthesis. *Sci. Rep.* **2017**, *7*. [CrossRef] [PubMed]

9

Cerium Oxide Nanoparticles: A Brief Review of their Synthesis Methods and Biomedical Applications

Atul Dhall [1] and William Self [2,*]

[1] Colleges of Nanoscale Science and Engineering, SUNY Polytechnic Institute, Albany, NY 12203, USA; adhall@sunypoly.edu
[2] Burnett School of Biomedical Sciences, College of Medicine, University of Central Florida, Orlando, FL 32816, USA
* Correspondence: william.self@ucf.edu

Abstract: Cerium oxide nanoparticles (CeNPs) exhibit antioxidant properties both in vitro and in vivo. This is due to the self-regeneration of their surface, which is based on redox-cycling between 3+ and 4+ states for cerium, in response to their immediate environment. Additionally, oxygen vacancies in the lattice structure allow for alternating between CeO_2 and CeO_{2-x} during redox reactions. Research to identify and characterize the biomedical applications of CeNPs has been heavily focused on investigating their use in treating diseases that are characterized by higher levels of reactive oxygen species (ROS). Although the bio-mimetic activities of CeNPs have been extensively studied in vitro, in vivo interactions and associated protein corona formation are not well understood. This review describes: (1) the methods of synthesis for CeNPs, including the recent green synthesis methods that offer enhanced biocompatibility and a need for establishing a reference CeNP material for consistency across studies; (2) their enzyme-mimetic activities, with a focus on their antioxidant activities; and, (3) recent experimental evidence that demonstrates their ROS scavenging abilities and their potential use in personalized medicine.

Keywords: cerium oxide nanoparticles; nanoceria; lanthanide; redox-cycling; antioxidants; oxidative stress; green synthesis; biocompatibility; enzyme mimetics; personalized medicine

---

1. Introduction

Cerium, a rare earth metal, is the first element of the lanthanide series in the periodic table. The 4f orbitals of rare earth metals are adequately shielded by 5p and 4d electrons, leading to interesting catalytic properties [1]. Unlike most rare earth metals, cerium can exist in both 3+ and 4+ states [2]. Thus, cerium oxide exists as both CeO_2 and Ce_2O_3 in the bulk state. At the nanoscale, however, cerium oxide has a mix of cerium in the 3+ and 4+ states on the nanoparticle surface. With a decrease in nanoparticle diameter, the number of 3+ sites on the surface increase and oxygen atoms are lost (oxygen vacancies) [3,4]. This is depicted by an overall structure of CeO_{2-x}.

Cerium oxide nanoparticles (CeNPs, nanoceria) are widely used in chemical mechanical polishing/planarization [5], corrosion protection [6], solar cells [7], fuel oxidation catalysis [8], and automotive exhaust treatment [9]. Pertinent to this review, CeNPs also display many bio-relevant activities-mimicking superoxide dismutase (SOD) [10], catalase [11], peroxidase [12], oxidase [13], and phosphatase [14], and scavenging hydroxyl radicals [15], nitric oxide radicals [16], and peroxynitrite [17].

Reactive Oxygen Species (ROS) are released as by-products in aerobic metabolism and they are routinely linked to oxidative stress (increased levels of intracellular ROS contributing to many diseases). However, ROS primarily act as signaling molecules in physiological processes. For a current and detailed understanding of ROS, readers are referred to an extensive review by Schieber et al. [18] that describes the two faces of ROS—redox signaling and oxidative stress. In this context, antioxidants can be defined as substances that scavenge ROS or inhibit their production. Interest in studying antioxidants grew after a study that described the potential benefits of vitamin E on cardiac health [19]. The activity of metal and metal-based nanoparticle systems and their interactions with ROS depend on their microenvironment. It is well established that metal and metal oxide nanoparticles exhibit antioxidant properties [20]. Since naturally occurring small antioxidant molecules have limited absorption into the body [19], nanoparticles have been investigated as carriers for antioxidant molecules [20]. On the other hand, metal and metal-based nanoparticle systems can also be used for prooxidant treatment strategies [21–24].

The bio-relevant activities of CeNPs earmark them for use in potential pharmacological agents [25], drug delivery [26–28], and bioscaffolding [29,30]. The basis for these activities of CeNPs is the thermodynamic efficiency of redox-cycling between 3+ and 4+ states on their surface [10] and their unique ability to absorb and release oxygen [31]. While it was initially thought that both oxygen vacancies and the redox-cycling between cerium in 3+ and 4+ states are involved in the antioxidant activities of CeNPs [6,10], it is now accepted that redox-cycling is solely responsible for all antioxidant properties [32]. This suggests that the surface ratio of Ce^{3+}/Ce^{4+} plays a key role in all of the bio-relevant activities of CeNPs. It is worth noting that CeNPs can also show prooxidant properties at lower pH values [13] and high doses [33], and they are known to exhibit potential toxicity based on their synthesis method, concentration, and exposure time, as detailed in a review by Yokel et al. [34]. As explained by Xu et al. [35] in their review on CeNPs and their applications, cerium is not found in the human body and there are no known clearance mechanisms for it. This implies that exposure to cerium would lead to systemic toxicity. These reasons necessitate careful optimization of synthesis parameters to generate non-toxic CeNPs that have either prooxidant or antioxidant properties that are based on the treatment strategy being used.

The interactions of a nanoparticle system with its microenvironment need to be considered while designing effective nanocarriers. It is important to note that polymeric nanocarriers and smart polymer systems can be used to encapsulate enzymes for drug delivery applications [36–42] and offer good biocompatibility. Such systems can also offer dual responsive programmable drug release [43]. However, CeNP-based treatment strategies have a unique advantage in that they have a self-regenerative antioxidant capability [44].

In the past decade, there have plenty of studies that demonstrate antibody-directed targeted delivery of antioxidant enzymes, like superoxide dismutase and catalase [45–48]. To achieve similar goals of targeted delivery, there are studies that have demonstrated the use of functionalizing CeNPs with surface groups and stabilizers so that they can be applied for targeted delivery into the body (reviewed by Nelson et al. [44]). Such functionalization though, needs to be fine-tuned to suit the needs of a targeting strategy and ensure that the CeNPs that are involved can self-regenerate their surface. Clearance from the body also needs to be considered while designing effective CeNP-based treatment strategies. Readers are directed to a review by Walkey et al. [49] for detailed information on targeting strategies and the possible routes of clearance.

This review begins with a brief overview of the methods that are routinely used to synthesize CeNPs. Green synthesis methods are highlighted because of their use of biocompatible stabilizers that may provide non-toxic preparation routes. We then briefly describe known enzyme-mimetic and antioxidant activities of CeNPs. Lastly, recent evidence from both in vitro and in vivo studies is presented to provide the reader with an up-to-date account of the potential biomedical applications of CeNPs.

2. Synthesis of Cerium Oxide Nanoparticles

The physicochemical properties of any nanoparticle depend on the method of synthesis. For a bio-relevant nanoparticle, synthesis parameters need to be carefully optimized to select for beneficial physicochemical properties in vivo. Different methods of synthesis result in CeNPs of varying size, morphology, and agglomeration. In general, using a polymer or surfactant during synthesis or a coating post-synthesis results in lowered agglomeration of CeNPs in bio-relevant solutions.

An important consideration while synthesizing nanoparticles for use in vivo is the formation of a protein corona that affects both the uptake and clearance of the nanoparticle. Readers are encouraged to read a review by Lynch et al., on the nanoparticle-protein corona [50]. Common methods used to synthesize CeNPs, including recent green synthesis methods, are listed in Table 1 with a relevant example for each method.

2.1. Traditional Synthesis Methods

Numerous methods for the synthesis of CeNPs have been reported. These include solution precipitation [51], hydrothermal [52], solvothermal [53], ball milling [54], thermal decomposition [55], spray pyrolysis [56], thermal hydrolysis [57], and sol-gel methods [58–60]. While these methods can help to determine the shape and size, Dowding et al. [14] were the first to report fine-tuned control over the surface ratio of Ce^{3+}/Ce^{4+}. As expected, many of the traditional methods suffer from low biocompatibility. In general, biocompatible coatings of nanoparticles provide greater stability, longer retention times, and lower toxicity by decreasing non-specific interactions. CeNPs have been functionalized using a variety of coatings–polyacrylic acid [61], polyethylene glycol (PEG) [62], dextran [63], polyethyleneimine [64], cyclodextrin [27], glucose [26], and folic acid [28]. Additionally, CeNPs can also be doped with chelating MRI contrast agents, such as gadolinium, to improve their safety while also displaying antioxidant properties [65]. For a comprehensive review of traditional synthesis methodologies and the associated physicochemical properties, readers are directed to a review by Das et al. [66].

2.2. Green Synthesis Methods

Recently, bio-directed CeNP synthesis methods that use natural matrices as stabilizing agents have gained importance because they help alleviate concerns of bio-compatibility. Such green chemistry methods provide safer routes for preparing CeNPs [59,60] and they are potentially useful for pharmaceutical applications [67]. In general, these methods provide low-cost and simpler alternatives to traditional synthesis methods. However, conclusions about the biocompatibility of a given green synthesis method should only be made after assessing the protein corona formation for synthesized CeNPs in biological fluid environments. The effect of the surface ratio of Ce^{3+}/Ce^{4+} on the biological properties of CeNPs synthesized via green chemistry methods also needs to be investigated [67].

The main strategies involved in the green synthesis of CeNPs are plant-mediated synthesis, fungus-mediated synthesis, polymer-mediated synthesis, and nutrient-mediated synthesis. Plant-mediated methods (phytosynthesis), where plant extracts act as stabilizing and capping agents, result in relatively large CeNPs [68] that are currently not appropriate for biomedical applications [69]. Fungus-mediated methods (mycosynthesis) resolve this by producing smaller CeNPs [70] that are more stable, have higher water dispersibility, and high fluorescent properties [71]. Natural polymers can also aid in the green synthesis of CeNPs and act as stabilizers [72]. An example is the use of PEG to create dispersible nanopowders in aqueous solutions [73]. Nutrient-mediated synthesis, such as in the use of egg white as a substrate to synthesize CeNPs, are extremely cost-effective [72]. Egg white proteins act as stabilizers that result in controlled isotropic growth of small CeNPs. For further information on the green synthesis methods that are available for CeNPs, readers are directed to a review by Charbgoo et al. [67].

As seen from the table, the sheer breadth of techniques available and the resulting physicochemical properties of synthesized CeNPs warrant the development of a reference CeNP material that has well-characterized properties and can be used to maintain consistency across studies.

Table 1. Common methods used to synthesize cerium oxide nanoparticles.

Method of Preparation		Particle Size (nm)	Morphology	Reference
Traditional approaches	Precipitation	15	Spherical	[51]
	Hydrothermal	5	Octahedral	[52]
	Solvothermal	~8	Polyhedral	[53]
	Spray Pyrolysis	~17	Cubic	[56]
Green approaches	Plant-mediated	36	Spherical	[68]
	Fungus-mediated	5	Spherical	[70]
	Polymer-mediated	~2	Spherical	[73]
	Nutrient-mediated	25	Spherical	[72]

3. Bio-Relevant Activities of Cerium Oxide Nanoparticles

3.1. *Enzyme Mimetic Activities*

3.1.1. Superoxide Dismutase and Catalase Mimetic Activity

Superoxide radicals are one of the most abundant free radicals produced in mammalian cells and that are produced as a result of normal aerobic metabolism. Superoxide radicals are also signaling molecules as well as a key component in the oxidative response to pathogens. An excess of these radicals is normally eradicated by the enzyme superoxide dismutase (SOD) [74]. CeNPs with high 3+/4+ ratios exhibit higher SOD-mimetic activity in comparison to those with lower 3+/4+ ratios [10].

Catalase is responsible for the degradation of H_2O_2, a potentially harmful oxidizing agent [75]. CeNPs with low 3+/4+ ratios exhibit higher catalase-mimetic activity in comparison to those with high 3+/4+ ratios [76]. This is in direct opposition to the trend observed for SOD-mimetic activity. Readers are directed to a review by Celardo et al. [25] for detailed mechanisms of these activities. Since CeNPs have both SOD-mimetic and catalase-mimetic activities, the H^2O^2 that is generated in the SOD-mimetic process can enter the catalase-mimetic process to produce H^2O and O^2. If coordinated, these activities can make CeNPs excellent antioxidants [35].

3.1.2. Phosphatase Mimetic Activity

Phosphatases are enzymes that remove phosphate groups from their substrates by hydrolysis of esters into phosphate ions [77]. CeNPs with low 3+/4+ ratios exhibit phosphatase-mimetic abilities for both artificial phosphate substrates [78] and bio-relevant substrates, like ATP [14,79] while CeNPs with high 3+/4+ ratios do not display phosphatase-mimetic activity [14,79]. This is the same trend as observed for catalase-mimetic activity. However, we recently demonstrated that the phosphatase-mimetic activity has distinct active sites from those for catalase-mimetic activity [79]. Given the abundance phosphate anions in biological solutions, it is also important to consider that interactions of CeNPs with phosphate anions increase the catalase-mimetic activity while decreasing the SOD-mimetic activity [80,81].

3.2. *ROS Scavenging Activities*

3.2.1. Scavenging Hydroxyl Radicals

The hydroxyl radical is one of the most biologically active free radicals [82]. CeNPs have been shown to partly eliminate hydroxyl radicals in a size-dependent manner [83]. One of the earliest studies of this behavior, conducted by Das et al. [15], demonstrated that CeNPs with mixed valence states have a neuroprotective effect on adult rat spinal cord neurons.

3.2.2. Scavenging Nitric Oxide Radicals and Peroxynitrite

The nitric oxide radical is a gaseous free radical with both beneficial and damaging biological effects [84]. Similar to their catalase-mimetic activity, CeNPs with low 3+/4+ ratios exhibit higher scavenging of nitric oxide radicals [16]. Nitric oxide radicals can react with superoxide radicals to make peroxynitrite. CeNPs have also been shown to accelerate the decay of peroxynitrite [17]. Since CeNPs interact with both peroxynitrite and its breakdown products, their scavenging of peroxynitrite is independent of the 3+/4+ ratio.

4. Evidence for Bio-Relevant Activities of Cerium Oxide Nanoparticles

This section provides the reader with recent evidence of CeNPs' antioxidant activities. Each synopsis lists the synthesis method that is used as it is important for researchers to keep these methods in mind before utilizing similar strategies in new experiments. A list of recent literature detailing the biomedical use of CeNPs is shown in Table 2. The sub-sections that follow provide details on each of these studies. Readers are referred to a comprehensive review by Das et al. [66] for similar evidence prior to 2013.

Table 2. Recent literature on the biomedical studies involving cerium oxide nanoparticles (CeNPs).

Type of Testing	Cell Line/Animal Model	Use	Reference
In Vitro	Primary human skin fibroblasts	Alteration of mitochondrial metabolism	[85]
	BV-2 and PC-12	Phenotypic activation of microglia to reshape immune microenvironment	[86]
	A375	Combinational cancer therapy with doxorubicin	[87]
	THP-1	Evaluating uptake and ROS scavenging ability of CeNPs	[88]
	BY-2	Autophagy-mediated antioxidant and geno-protective role of CeNPs	[89]
In Vivo	5XFAD mice	Suppressing neuronal death in Alzheimer's disease	[90]
	Nude Mice	Reduction of tumor growth in ovarian cancer	[91]
	P23H-1 rat	Preventing photoreceptor cell loss in autosomal dominant retinitis pigmentosa	[92]
	Wistar rat	Obesity treatment	[93]
	Sprague Dawley rat	Prophylactic treatment of hepatic ischemia reperfusion injury	[94]

4.1. In Vitro Studies

Pezzini et al. [85] demonstrated the protective effects of CeNPs on primary human skin fibroblasts that were exposed to a pro-oxidative insult. Monodispersed CeNPs with an average diameter of 2 nm were purchased from Alfa Aesar. Fibroblast proliferation was assessed after 24 and 72 h of incubation with CeNPs at concentrations of 0, 100, and 200 μg/mL. It was found that CeNPs were internalized, displayed strong ROS scavenging activity, and did not affect the viability of the fibroblasts. Additionally, CeNPs affected mitochondrial function by leading to an increase in ATP production, but preserved mitochondrial membrane potential. This study serves as a proof-of-principle of the applications of CeNPs for a wide range of conditions that are associated with the accumulation of oxidative stress and alteration of mitochondrial metabolism.

Zeng et al. [86] demonstrated that PEGylated-CeNPs can mitigate pro-inflammatory M1-polarization and advance anti-inflammatory M2-polarization by scavenging ROS triggered by stress stimuli in microglial BV-2 and PC-12 cells. Near-spherical CeNPs were synthesized, as described by Lee et al. [95]. PEGylated-CeNP treated microglia showed neuroprotective effects on the co-cultured neurons after Oxygen and Glucose Deprivation/Reoxygenation stimulus by blocking the pro-inflammatory NF-κB pathway. This study provides a new strategy for reshaping the immune-microenvironment using the phenotypic activation of microglia.

Sack et al. [87] examined the use of redox-active CeNPs in combination with a conventional therapeutic, doxorubicin, for cancer therapy. The CeNPs that were used in this study were synthesized as described by Karakoti et al. [96]. Antitumor activity of doxorubicin is primarily mediated by DNA damage, cell-cycle arrest, and apoptosis. While doxorubicin is effective against cancer cells, it also affects healthy cells [97]. The authors compared the antitumor activity of CeNPs with doxorubicin and demonstrated that CeNPs enhanced the antitumor activity of doxorubicin in human melanoma cells (A375 cells), in context of cytotoxicity, ROS formation, and oxidative damage. While both CeNPs and doxorubicin exerted cytotoxic effects on A375 cells, when used together, the viability of A375 cells decreased further than with each agent alone. Additionally, CeNPs abolished the toxic effects of doxorubicin on human dermal fibroblasts (HDFs). Such approaches involving the supplementation of conventional chemotherapeutics with CeNPs may offer novel strategies in cancer therapy. The same group has also investigated the potential use of CeNPs in brain tumor-related treatment. Sack-Zschauer et al. [98] demonstrated that CeNPs killed malignant glioma cells while protecting healthy cells. CeNPs (water-based suspension of 1.5 mg/mL and 1–10 nm) were purchased from Sciventions and stabilized in sodium polyacrylate (1.27 mg/mL). The authors reported that CeNPs had a cytotoxic effect on anaplastic astrocytoma (grade III glioma) cells while displaying no cytotoxicity towards microvascular endothelial cells.

Patel et al. [88] demonstrated that human monocyte leukemia cells (THP-1 cells) can be used as a model to evaluate the uptake and free radical scavenging ability of CeNPs. CeNPs were synthesized using slight modifications to a basic strategy that was described by Hirst et al. [99]. Internalization of CeNPs was shown to increase in a concentration-dependent manner in THP-1 cells between 10 and 100 µg/mL. Additionally, CeNPs reduced the amount of ROS without exhibiting cytotoxicity. Thus, unlike other oxide nanoparticles, which induce ROS generation in the cytoplasm [100], CeNPs retained their antioxidant activity in the cytoplasm after rapid internalization by THP-1 cells.

Sadhu et al. [89] demonstrated that high CeNP concentrations in tobacco BY-2 cells induce cytotoxicity and impair metabolic activity while low concentrations exhibit antioxidant activity. CeNPs that were used in this study (under 25 nm) were purchased from Sigma-Aldrich Chemical Co., (Bengaluru, India). The authors treated tobacco BY-2 cells with CeNP concentrations of 10, 50, and 250 µg/mL for 24 h. While concentration-dependent accumulation of Ca^{2+} and ROS was observed for all CeNPs sets, significant DNA damage and alterations in antioxidant defense systems were observed for higher CeNP concentrations (50 and 250 µg/mL). Further, CeNPs at 10 µg/mL did not induce genotoxicity and led to reduced DNA breakage in cells tha were exposed to H_2O_2. Their results point to an alternative autophagy-mediated, antioxidant, and geno-protective role of CeNPs.

4.2. In Vivo Studies

Kwon et al. [90] reported the design and synthesis of triphenylphosphonium-conjugated CeNPs that localized to mitochondria and suppressed neuronal death in 5XFAD transgenic mice (Alzheimer's disease model). CeNPs were synthesized using hydrolytic sol-gel reactions. Mitochondrial dysfunction can lead to abnormal levels of ROS and subsequently cause neuronal cell death. Targeting CeNPs to mitochondria is a promising therapeutic approach for neurodegenerative diseases. The authors synthesized small and positively charged triphenylphosphonium-conjugated CeNPs that are capable of localizing to mitochondria in various cell lines and mitigating reactive gliosis while suppressing neuronal death. This can serve as a novel strategy in the development of mitochondrial therapeutics for Alzheimer's disease and other neurodegenerative diseases.

Hijaz et al. [91] demonstrated that CeNPs significantly reduced tumor growth in an ovarian cancer xenograft nude model. A synthesis strategy that is based on methods used by Das et al. [101] and Cimini et al. [102] was used to make CeNPs and folic acid-CeNPs, respectively. A2780 generated mouse xenografts were treated with 0.1 mg/kg CeNPs, 0.1 mg/kg folic acid-CeNPs, and 4 mg/kg cisplatinum by intra-peritoneal injections. Mice that were treated with folic acid-CeNPs had a lower tumor burden when compared to those treated with just CeNPs. Combining folic acid-CeNPs with cisplatinum further decreased the tumor burden. Additionally, folic acid-CeNPs reduced vimentin expression, thus indicating a potential ability to limit ovarian tumor metastasis.

Wong et al. [92] used the P23H-1 rat (autosomal dominant retinitis pigmentosa model) to understand the cellular mechanisms and duration of the CeNPs' catalytic activity in preventing photoreceptor cell loss. CeNPs were prepared using wet chemistry methods, as described by Karakoti et al. [103]. An increase in rod and cone cell function post-injection was observed. Additionally, CeNP treatment led to a reduction in apoptotic cells and lipid peroxidation in the retinas. This study adds to the list of rodent retinal disease models that demonstrate a delay in disease progression with just one application of CeNPs.

Rocca et al. [93] investigated the antioxidant effects of CeNPs as an approach for obesity treatment in Wistar rats. CeNPs interfered with the adipogenic pathway and hindered triglyceride accumulation. CeNPs were purchased from Sigma and it had characteristics that were similar to those used in a study by Ciofani et al. [104]. They were administrated intraperitoneally twice a week for six weeks at a dose of 0.5 mg/kg in 500 μL of sterile water. Transcriptional analysis following in vivo treatment revealed a down-regulation of *Lep*, *Bmp2*, *Twist1*, *Angpt2*, and *Ddit3*, and an up-regulation of *Irs1* and *Klf4* expression. Overall, CeNPs contributed to a reduction in weight gain and lowered the plasma levels of insulin, leptin, glucose, and triglycerides.

Manne et al. [94] investigated the use of CeNPs in the prophylactic treatment of hepatic ischemia reperfusion injury in Sprague Dawley rats. CeNPs were obtained from U.S. Research Nanomaterials and are characterized as in Manne et al. [105]. Partial hepatic ischemia was induced for 1 h in the left lateral and median lobes. This was followed by 6 h of reperfusion. Prophylactic treatment with CeNPs (at 0.5mg/kg) led to a decrease in alanine aminotransaminase, lactate dehydrogenase, hepatocyte necrosis, macrophage derived chemokine, macrophage inflammatory protein-2, keratinocyte chemoattractant (KC)/human growth-regulated oncogene (GRO), myoglobin, and plasminogen activator inhibitor-1.

5. Conclusions and Future Perspectives

Oxidative stress is implicated in the development and progression of many diseases. The broad range of CeNPs' antioxidant activity and their ability to self-regenerate their surface makes them strong candidates for use as in vivo ROS scavengers. However, to be considered as potential therapeutic agents, it is necessary to optimize their synthesis methods, surface chemistry, and concentration to select the beneficial physicochemical properties. For consistency, such endeavors must begin by establishing CeNP reference materials for pertinent disease models. Eventually, all toxicological concerns also need to be addressed.

It is important to note that the physicochemical properties of CeNPs reported in vitro differ from those under physiological conditions. In particular, the natural protein corona associated with CeNPs in vivo is primed to be the focus of studies that describe existing/identify new biomedical applications. Any pharmacokinetic improvement will involve CeNPs with biocompatible coatings and effective targeting strategies.

Green synthesis methods that use biocompatible stabilizers are increasingly gaining relevance in the production of CeNPs and their biomedical applications. Undoubtedly, interdisciplinary studies that are based in material science and tailored towards identifying new biomedical applications of CeNPs will continue to clarify their physicochemical properties and catalytic activities.

Author Contributions: A.D. wrote and structured the manuscript. W.S. critically reviewed and edited the manuscript in addition to handling all corresponding author responsibilities.

Funding: The Self lab is currently participating in an NSF funded REU project, NSF project 1560007.

Conflicts of Interest: The authors declare no conflict of interest.

References

1. Bouzigues, C.; Gacoin, T.; Alexandrou, A. Biological applications of rare-earth based nanoparticles. *ACS Nano* **2011**, *5*, 8488–8505. [CrossRef] [PubMed]
2. Dahle, J.T.; Arai, Y. Environmental geochemistry of cerium: Applications and toxicology of cerium oxide nanoparticles. *Int. J. Environ. Res. Public Health* **2015**, *12*, 1253–1278. [CrossRef] [PubMed]
3. Tsunekawa, S.; Sivamohan, R.; Ito, S.; Kasuya, A.; Fukuda, T. Structural study on monosize CeO_2-x nano-particles. *Nanostruct. Mater.* **1999**, *11*, 141–147. [CrossRef]
4. Tsunekawa, S.; Sivamohan, R.; Ohsuna, T.; Takahashi, H.; Tohji, K. Ultraviolet Absorption Spectra of CeO_2 Nano-Particles. *Mater. Sci. Forum* **1999**, *315–317*, 439–445. [CrossRef]
5. Reed, K.; Cormack, A.; Kulkarni, A.; Mayton, M.; Sayle, D.; Klaessig, F.; Stadler, B. Exploring the properties and applications of nanoceria: Is there still plenty of room at the bottom? *Environ. Sci. Nano* **2014**, *1*, 390–405. [CrossRef]
6. Ivanov, V.K.; Shcherbakov, A.; Usatenko, A. Structure-sensitive properties and biomedical applications of nanodispersed cerium dioxide. *Russ. Chem. Rev.* **2009**, *78*, 855. [CrossRef]
7. Corma, A.; Atienzar, P.; Garcia, H.; Chane-Ching, J.-Y. Hierarchically mesostructured doped CeO_2 with potential for solar-cell use. *Nat. Mater.* **2004**, *3*, 394–397. [CrossRef] [PubMed]
8. Jung, H.; Kittelson, D.B.; Zachariah, M.R. The influence of a cerium additive on ultrafine diesel particle emissions and kinetics of oxidation. *Combus. Flame* **2005**, *142*, 276–288. [CrossRef]
9. Campbell, C.T. Oxygen vacancies and catalysis on ceria surfaces. *Science* **2005**, *309*, 713–714. [CrossRef] [PubMed]
10. Korsvik, C.; Patil, S.; Seal, S.; Self, W.T. Superoxide dismutase mimetic properties exhibited by vacancy engineered ceria nanoparticles. *Chem. Commun.* **2007**, *10*, 1056–1058. [CrossRef] [PubMed]
11. Rzigalinski, B.A.; Meehan, K.; Davis, R.M.; Xu, Y.; Miles, W.C.; Cohen, C.A. Radical nanomedicine. *Nanomedicine* **2006**, *1*, 399–412. [CrossRef] [PubMed]
12. Jiao, X.; Song, H.; Zhao, H.; Bai, W.; Zhang, L.; Lv, Y. Well-redispersed ceria nanoparticles: Promising peroxidase mimetics for H_2O_2 and glucose detection. *Anal. Methods* **2012**, *4*, 3261–3267. [CrossRef]
13. Asati, A.; Santra, S.; Kaittanis, C.; Nath, S.; Perez, J.M. Oxidase-like activity of polymer-coated cerium oxide nanoparticles. *Angew. Chem.* **2009**, *121*, 2344–2348. [CrossRef]
14. Dowding, J.M.; Das, S.; Kumar, A.; Dosani, T.; McCormack, R.; Gupta, A.; Sayle, T.X.T.; Sayle, D.C.; von Kalm, L.; Seal, S.; et al. Cellular interaction and toxicity depend on physicochemical properties and surface modification of redox-active nanomaterials. *ACS Nano* **2013**, *7*, 4855–4868. [CrossRef] [PubMed]
15. Das, M.; Patil, S.; Bhargava, N.; Kang, J.-F.; Riedel, L.M.; Seal, S.; Hickman, J.J. Auto-catalytic ceria nanoparticles offer neuroprotection to adult rat spinal cord neurons. *Biomaterials* **2007**, *28*, 1918–1925. [CrossRef] [PubMed]
16. Dowding, J.M.; Dosani, T.; Kumar, A.; Seal, S.; Self, W.T. Cerium oxide nanoparticles scavenge nitric oxide radical (•No). *Chem. Commun.* **2012**, *48*, 4896–4898. [CrossRef] [PubMed]
17. Dowding, J.M.; Seal, S.; Self, W.T. Cerium oxide nanoparticles accelerate the decay of peroxynitrite ($ONOO^-$). *Drug Deliv. Transl. Res.* **2013**, *3*, 375–379. [CrossRef] [PubMed]
18. Schieber, M.; Chandel, N.S. ROS function in redox signaling and oxidative stress. *Curr. Biol.* **2014**, *24*, R453–R462. [CrossRef] [PubMed]
19. Hutson, S. *Experts Urge a More Measured Look at Antioxidants*; Nature Publishing Group: London, UK, 2008.
20. Sharpe, E.; Andreescu, D.; Andreescu, S. Artificial nanoparticle antioxidants. In *Oxidative Stress: Diagnostics, Prevention, and Therapy*; American Chemical Society: Washington, DC, USA, 2011; pp. 235–253.

21. Yeh, H.P.; Del Valle, A.C.; Syu, M.C.; Qian, Y.; Chang, Y.C.; Huang, Y.F. A new photosensitized oxidation-responsive nanoplatform for controlled drug release and photodynamic cancer therapy. *ACS Appl. Mater. Interfaces* **2018**, *10*, 21160–21172. [CrossRef] [PubMed]
22. Keyvan Rad, J.; Mahdavian, A.R.; Khoei, S.; Shirvalilou, S. Enhanced photogeneration of reactive oxygen species and targeted photothermal therapy of c6 glioma brain cancer cells by folate-conjugated gold-photoactive polymer nanoparticles. *ACS Appl. Mater. Interfaces* **2018**, *10*, 19483–19493. [CrossRef] [PubMed]
23. Neubauer, N.; Palomaeki, J.; Karisola, P.; Alenius, H.; Kasper, G. Size-dependent ROS production by palladium and nickel nanoparticles in cellular and acellular environments—An indication for the catalytic nature of their interactions. *Nanotoxicology* **2015**, *9*, 1059–1066. [CrossRef] [PubMed]
24. Brenneisen, P.; Reichert, A.S. Nanotherapy and reactive oxygen species (ROS) in cancer: A novel perspective. *Antioxidants* **2018**, *7*, 31. [CrossRef] [PubMed]
25. Celardo, I.; Pedersen, J.Z.; Traversa, E.; Ghibelli, L. Pharmacological potential of cerium oxide nanoparticles. *Nanoscale* **2011**, *3*, 1411–1420. [CrossRef] [PubMed]
26. Li, M.; Shi, P.; Xu, C.; Ren, J.; Qu, X. Cerium oxide caged metal chelator: Anti-aggregation and anti-oxidation integrated H_2O_2-responsive controlled drug release for potential alzheimer's disease treatment. *Chem. Sci.* **2013**, *4*, 2536–2542. [CrossRef]
27. Xu, C.; Lin, Y.; Wang, J.; Wu, L.; Wei, W.; Ren, J.; Qu, X. Nanoceria-triggered synergetic drug release based on CeO_2-capped mesoporous silica host-guest interactions and switchable enzymatic activity and cellular effects of CeO_2. *Adv. Healthc. Mater.* **2013**, *2*, 1591–1599. [CrossRef] [PubMed]
28. Vassie, J.A.; Whitelock, J.M.; Lord, M.S. Targeted delivery and redox activity of folic acid-functionalized nanoceria in tumor cells. *Mol. Pharm.* **2018**, *15*, 994–1004. [CrossRef] [PubMed]
29. Karakoti, A.S.; Tsigkou, O.; Yue, S.; Lee, P.D.; Stevens, M.M.; Jones, J.R.; Seal, S. Rare earth oxides as nanoadditives in 3-D nanocomposite scaffolds for bone regeneration. *J. Mater. Chem.* **2010**, *20*, 8912–8919. [CrossRef]
30. Mandoli, C.; Pagliari, F.; Pagliari, S.; Forte, G.; Di Nardo, P.; Licoccia, S.; Traversa, E. Stem cell aligned growth induced by CeO_2 nanoparticles in PLGA scaffolds with improved bioactivity for regenerative medicine. *Adv. Funct. Mater.* **2010**, *20*, 1617–1624. [CrossRef]
31. Deshpande, S.; Patil, S.; Kuchibhatla, S.V.N.T.; Seal, S. Size dependency variation in lattice parameter and valency states in nanocrystalline cerium oxide. *Appl. Phys. Lett.* **2005**, *87*, 133113. [CrossRef]
32. Celardo, I.; De Nicola, M.; Mandoli, C.; Pedersen, J.Z.; Traversa, E.; Ghibelli, L. Ce^{3+} ions determine redox-dependent anti-apoptotic effect of cerium oxide nanoparticles. *ACS Nano* **2011**, *5*, 4537–4549. [CrossRef] [PubMed]
33. Karakoti, A.; Singh, S.; Dowding, J.M.; Seal, S.; Self, W.T. Redox-active radical scavenging nanomaterials. *Chem. Soc. Rev.* **2010**, *39*, 4422–4432. [CrossRef] [PubMed]
34. Yokel, R.A.; Hussain, S.; Garantziotis, S.; Demokritou, P.; Castranova, V.; Cassee, F.R. The yin: An adverse health perspective of nanoceria: Uptake, distribution, accumulation, and mechanisms of its toxicity. *Environ. Sci. Nano* **2014**, *1*, 406–428. [CrossRef] [PubMed]
35. Xu, C.; Qu, X. Cerium oxide nanoparticle: A remarkably versatile rare earth nanomaterial for biological applications. *NPG Asia Mater.* **2014**, *6*, e90. [CrossRef]
36. Dziubla, T.D.; Karim, A.; Muzykantov, V.R. Polymer nanocarriers protecting active enzyme cargo against proteolysis. *J. Control. Release* **2005**, *102*, 427–439. [CrossRef] [PubMed]
37. Dziubla, T.D.; Shuvaev, V.V.; Hong, N.K.; Hawkins, B.J.; Madesh, M.; Takano, H.; Simone, E.; Nakada, M.T.; Fisher, A.; Albelda, S.M.; et al. Endothelial targeting of semi-permeable polymer nanocarriers for enzyme therapies. *Biomaterials* **2008**, *29*, 215–227. [CrossRef] [PubMed]
38. Garnacho, C.; Dhami, R.; Simone, E.; Dziubla, T.; Leferovich, J.; Schuchman, E.H.; Muzykantov, V.; Muro, S. Delivery of acid sphingomyelinase in normal and niemann-pick disease mice using intercellular adhesion molecule-1-targeted polymer nanocarriers. *J. Pharmacol. Exp. Ther.* **2008**, *325*, 400–408. [CrossRef] [PubMed]
39. Hood, E.D.; Chorny, M.; Greineder, C.F.; Alferiev, S.; Levy, R.J.; Muzykantov, V.R. Endothelial targeting of nanocarriers loaded with antioxidant enzymes for protection against vascular oxidative stress and inflammation. *Biomaterials* **2014**, *35*, 3708–3715. [CrossRef] [PubMed]

40. Poole, K.M.; Nelson, C.E.; Joshi, R.V.; Martin, J.R.; Gupta, M.K.; Haws, S.C.; Kavanaugh, T.E.; Skala, M.C.; Duvall, C.L. ROS-responsive microspheres for on demand antioxidant therapy in a model of diabetic peripheral arterial disease. *Biomaterials* **2015**, *41*, 166–175. [CrossRef] [PubMed]
41. Hood, E.; Simone, E.; Wattamwar, P.; Dziubla, T.; Muzykantov, V. Nanocarriers for vascular delivery of antioxidants. *Nanomedicine* **2011**, *6*, 1257–1272. [CrossRef] [PubMed]
42. Gupta, M.K.; Martin, J.R.; Werfel, T.A.; Shen, T.; Page, J.M.; Duvall, C.L. Cell protective, ABC triblock polymer-based thermoresponsive hydrogels with ROS-triggered degradation and drug release. *J. Am. Chem. Soc.* **2014**, *136*, 14896–14902. [CrossRef] [PubMed]
43. Chen, D.; Zhang, G.; Li, R.; Guan, M.; Wang, X.; Zou, T.; Zhang, Y.; Wang, C.; Shu, C.; Hong, H.; et al. Biodegradable, hydrogen peroxide, and glutathione dual responsive nanoparticles for potential programmable paclitaxel release. *J. Am. Chem. Soc.* **2018**, *140*, 7373–7376. [CrossRef] [PubMed]
44. Nelson, B.C.; Johnson, M.E.; Walker, M.L.; Riley, K.R.; Sims, C.M. Antioxidant cerium oxide nanoparticles in biology and medicine. *Antioxidants* **2016**, *5*, 15. [CrossRef] [PubMed]
45. Shuvaev, V.V.; Han, J.; Tliba, S.; Arguiri, E.; Christofidou-Solomidou, M.; Ramirez, S.H.; Dykstra, H.; Persidsky, Y.; Atochin, D.N.; Huang, P.L.; et al. Anti-inflammatory effect of targeted delivery of SOD to endothelium: Mechanism, synergism with no donors and protective effects in vitro and in vivo. *PLoS ONE* **2013**, *8*, e77002. [CrossRef] [PubMed]
46. Shuvaev, V.V.; Han, J.; Yu, K.J.; Huang, S.; Hawkins, B.J.; Madesh, M.; Nakada, M.; Muzykantov, V.R. Pecam-targeted delivery of SOD inhibits endothelial inflammatory response. *FASEB J. Off. Publ. Fed. Am. Soc. Exp. Biol.* **2011**, *25*, 348–357. [CrossRef] [PubMed]
47. Shuvaev, V.V.; Christofidou-Solomidou, M.; Bhora, F.; Laude, K.; Cai, H.; Dikalov, S.; Arguiri, E.; Solomides, C.C.; Albelda, S.M.; Harrison, D.G.; et al. Targeted detoxification of selected reactive oxygen species in the vascular endothelium. *J. Pharmacol. Exp. Ther.* **2009**, *331*, 404–411. [CrossRef] [PubMed]
48. Shuvaev, V.V.; Tliba, S.; Nakada, M.; Albelda, S.M.; Muzykantov, V.R. Platelet-endothelial cell adhesion molecule-1-directed endothelial targeting of superoxide dismutase alleviates oxidative stress caused by either extracellular or intracellular superoxide. *J. Pharmacol. Exp. Ther.* **2007**, *323*, 450–457. [CrossRef] [PubMed]
49. Walkey, C.; Das, S.; Seal, S.; Erlichman, J.; Heckman, K.; Ghibelli, L.; Traversa, E.; McGinnis, J.F.; Self, W.T. Catalytic properties and biomedical applications of cerium oxide nanoparticles. *Environ. Sci. Nano* **2015**, *2*, 33–53. [CrossRef] [PubMed]
50. Lynch, I.; Dawson, K.A. Protein-nanoparticle interactions. *Nano Today* **2008**, *3*, 40–47. [CrossRef]
51. Pelletier, D.A.; Suresh, A.K.; Holton, G.A.; McKeown, C.K.; Wang, W.; Gu, B.; Mortensen, N.P.; Allison, D.P.; Joy, D.C.; Allison, M.R. Effects of engineered cerium oxide nanoparticles on bacterial growth and viability. *Appl. Environ. Microbiol.* **2010**, *76*, 7981–7989. [CrossRef] [PubMed]
52. Rojas, S.; Gispert, J.D.; Abad, S.; Buaki-Sogo, M.; Victor, V.M.; Garcia, H.; Herance, J.R.L. In vivo biodistribution of amino-functionalized ceria nanoparticles in rats using positron emission tomography. *Mol. Pharm.* **2012**, *9*, 3543–3550. [CrossRef] [PubMed]
53. Zhang, H.; He, X.; Zhang, Z.; Zhang, P.; Li, Y.; Ma, Y.; Kuang, Y.; Zhao, Y.; Chai, Z. Nano-CeO_2 exhibits adverse effects at environmental relevant concentrations. *Environ. Sci. Technol.* **2011**, *45*, 3725–3730. [CrossRef] [PubMed]
54. Yadav, T.; Srivastava, O. Synthesis of nanocrystalline cerium oxide by high energy ball milling. *Ceram. Int.* **2012**, *38*, 5783–5789. [CrossRef]
55. Wang, Y.; Mori, T.; Li, J.G.; Ikegami, T. Low-temperature synthesis of praseodymium-doped ceria nanopowders. *J. Am. Ceram. Soc.* **2002**, *85*, 3105–3107. [CrossRef]
56. Demokritou, P.; Gass, S.; Pyrgiotakis, G.; Cohen, J.M.; Goldsmith, W.; McKinney, W.; Frazer, D.; Ma, J.; Schwegler-Berry, D.; Brain, J. An in vivo and in vitro toxicological characterisation of realistic nanoscale CeO_2 inhalation exposures. *Nanotoxicology* **2013**, *7*, 1338–1350. [CrossRef] [PubMed]
57. Hirano, M.; Fukuda, Y.; Iwata, H.; Hotta, Y.; Inagaki, M. Preparation and spherical agglomeration of crystalline cerium (IV) oxide nanoparticles by thermal hydrolysis. *J. Am. Ceram. Soc.* **2000**, *83*, 1287–1289. [CrossRef]
58. He, H.-W.; Wu, X.-Q.; Ren, W.; Shi, P.; Yao, X.; Song, Z.-T. Synthesis of crystalline cerium dioxide hydrosol by a sol–gel method. *Ceram. Int.* **2012**, *38*, S501–S504. [CrossRef]

59. Darroudi, M.; Sarani, M.; Oskuee, R.K.; Zak, A.K.; Hosseini, H.A.; Gholami, L. Green synthesis and evaluation of metabolic activity of starch mediated nanoceria. *Ceram. Int.* **2014**, *40*, 2041–2045. [CrossRef]
60. Darroudi, M.; Sarani, M.; Oskuee, R.K.; Zak, A.K.; Amiri, M.S. Nanoceria: Gum mediated synthesis and in vitro viability assay. *Ceram. Int.* **2014**, *40*, 2863–2868. [CrossRef]
61. Sehgal, A.; Lalatonne, Y.; Berret, J.-F.; Morvan, M. Precipitation-redispersion of cerium oxide nanoparticles with poly (acrylic acid): Toward stable dispersions. *Langmuir* **2005**, *21*, 9359–9364. [CrossRef] [PubMed]
62. Karakoti, A.S.; Singh, S.; Kumar, A.; Malinska, M.; Kuchibhatla, S.V.; Wozniak, K.; Self, W.T.; Seal, S. Pegylated nanoceria as radical scavenger with tunable redox chemistry. *J. Am. Chem. Soc.* **2009**, *131*, 14144–14145. [CrossRef] [PubMed]
63. Perez, J.M.; Asati, A.; Nath, S.; Kaittanis, C. Synthesis of biocompatible dextran-coated nanoceria with pH-dependent antioxidant properties. *Small* **2008**, *4*, 552–556. [CrossRef] [PubMed]
64. Lee, S.S.; Song, W.; Cho, M.; Puppala, H.L.; Nguyen, P.; Zhu, H.; Segatori, L.; Colvin, V.L. Antioxidant properties of cerium oxide nanocrystals as a function of nanocrystal diameter and surface coating. *ACS Nano* **2013**, *7*, 9693–9703. [CrossRef] [PubMed]
65. Eriksson, P.; Tal, A.A.; Skallberg, A.; Brommesson, C.; Hu, Z.; Boyd, R.D.; Olovsson, W.; Fairley, N.; Abrikosov, I.A.; Zhang, X.; et al. Cerium oxide nanoparticles with antioxidant capabilities and gadolinium integration for MRI contrast enhancement. *Sci. Rep.* **2018**, *8*, 6999. [CrossRef] [PubMed]
66. Das, S.; Dowding, J.M.; Klump, K.E.; McGinnis, J.F.; Self, W.; Seal, S. Cerium oxide nanoparticles: Applications and prospects in nanomedicine. *Nanomedicine* **2013**, *8*, 1483–1508. [CrossRef] [PubMed]
67. Charbgoo, F.; Ahmad, M.B.; Darroudi, M. Cerium oxide nanoparticles: Green synthesis and biological applications. *Int. J. Nanomed.* **2017**, *12*, 1401–1413. [CrossRef] [PubMed]
68. Kannan, S.K.; Sundrarajan, M. A green approach for the synthesis of a cerium oxide nanoparticle: Characterization and antibacterial activity. *Int. J. Nanosci.* **2014**, *13*, 1450018. [CrossRef]
69. Jacinthe, G.; Katharina, M.F. Toxicity and protective effects of cerium oxide nanoparticles (nanoceria) depending on their preparation method, particle size, cell type, and exposure route. *Eur. J. Inorg. Chem.* **2015**, *2015*, 4510–4517.
70. Munusamy, S.; Bhakyaraj, K.; Vijayalakshmi, L.; Stephen, A.; Narayanan, V. Synthesis and characterization of cerium oxide nanoparticles using curvularia lunata and their antibacterial properties. *Int. J. Innov. Res. Sci. Eng.* **2014**, *2*, 318–323.
71. Mohanpuria, P.; Rana, N.K.; Yadav, S.K. Biosynthesis of nanoparticles: Technological concepts and future applications. *J. Nanopart. Res.* **2008**, *10*, 507–517. [CrossRef]
72. Kargar, H.; Ghazavi, H.; Darroudi, M. Size-controlled and bio-directed synthesis of ceria nanopowders and their in vitro cytotoxicity effects. *Ceram. Int.* **2015**, *41*, 4123–4128. [CrossRef]
73. Qi, L.; Fresnais, J.; Muller, P.; Theodoly, O.; Berret, J.F.; Chapel, J.P. Interfacial activity of phosphonated-peg functionalized cerium oxide nanoparticles. *Langmuir* **2012**, *28*, 11448–11456. [CrossRef] [PubMed]
74. Heckert, E.; Karakoti, A.; Seal, S.; Self, W.T. The role of cerium redox state in the SOD mimetic activity of nanoceria. *Biomaterials* **2008**, *29*, 2705–2709. [CrossRef] [PubMed]
75. Nicholls, P. Classical catalase: Ancient and modern. *Arch. Biochem. Biophys.* **2012**, *525*, 95–101. [CrossRef] [PubMed]
76. Pirmohamed, T.; Dowding, J.M.; Singh, S.; Wasserman, B.; Heckert, E.; Karakoti, A.S.; King, J.E.; Seal, S.; Self, W.T. Nanoceria exhibit redox state-dependent catalase mimetic activity. *Chem. Commun.* **2010**, *46*, 2736–2738. [CrossRef] [PubMed]
77. Cohen, P. The origins of protein phosphorylation. *Nat. Cell Biol.* **2002**, *4*, E127. [CrossRef] [PubMed]
78. Kuchma, M.H.; Komanski, C.B.; Colon, J.; Teblum, A.; Masunov, A.E.; Alvarado, B.; Babu, S.; Seal, S.; Summy, J.; Baker, C.H. Phosphate ester hydrolysis of biologically relevant molecules by cerium oxide nanoparticles. *Nanomed. Nanotechnol. Biol. Med.* **2010**, *6*, 738–744. [CrossRef] [PubMed]
79. Dhall, A.; Burns, A.; Dowding, J.; Das, S.; Seal, S.; Self, W. Characterizing the phosphatase mimetic activity of cerium oxide nanoparticles and distinguishing its active site from that for catalase mimetic activity using anionic inhibitors. *Environ. Sci. Nano* **2017**, *4*, 1742–1749. [CrossRef]
80. Singh, S.; Dosani, T.; Karakoti, A.S.; Kumar, A.; Seal, S.; Self, W.T. A phosphate-dependent shift in redox state of cerium oxide nanoparticles and its effects on catalytic properties. *Biomaterials* **2011**, *32*, 6745–6753. [CrossRef] [PubMed]

81. Xue, Y.; Zhai, Y.; Zhou, K.; Wang, L.; Tan, H.; Luan, Q.; Yao, X. The vital role of buffer anions in the antioxidant activity of CeO_2 nanoparticles. *Chemistry* **2012**, *18*, 11115–11122. [CrossRef] [PubMed]
82. Lipinski, B. Hydroxyl radical and its scavengers in health and disease. *Oxid. Med. Cell. Longev.* **2011**, *2011*, 809696. [CrossRef] [PubMed]
83. Xue, Y.; Luan, Q.; Yang, D.; Yao, X.; Zhou, K. Direct evidence for hydroxyl radical scavenging activity of cerium oxide nanoparticles. *J. Phys. Chem. C* **2011**, *115*, 4433–4438. [CrossRef]
84. Knott, A.B.; Bossy-Wetzel, E. Nitric oxide in health and disease of the nervous system. *Antioxid. Redox Signal.* **2009**, *11*, 541–553. [CrossRef] [PubMed]
85. Pezzini, I.; Marino, A.; Turco, S.D.; Nesti, C.; Doccini, S.; Cappello, V.; Gemmi, M.; Parlanti, P.; Santorelli, F.M.; Mattoli, V.; et al. Cerium oxide nanoparticles: The regenerative redox machine in bioenergetic imbalance. *Nanomedicine* **2017**, *12*, 403–416. [CrossRef] [PubMed]
86. Zeng, F.; Wu, X.; Li, X.; Ge, X.; Guo, Q.; Lou, X.; Cao, Z.; Hu, B.; Long, N.J.; Mao, Y.; et al. Custom-made ceria nanoparticles show a neuroprotective effect by modulating phenotypic polarization of the microglia. *Angew. Chem. Int. Ed.* **2018**, *57*, 5808–5812.
87. Sack, M.; Alili, L.; Karaman, E.; Das, S.; Gupta, A.; Seal, S.; Brenneisen, P. Combination of conventional chemotherapeutics with redox-active cerium oxide nanoparticles—A novel aspect in cancer therapy. *Mol. Cancer Ther.* **2014**, *13*, 1740–1749. [CrossRef] [PubMed]
88. Patel, P.; Kansara, K.; Singh, R.; Shukla, R.K.; Singh, S.; Dhawan, A.; Kumar, A. Cellular internalization and antioxidant activity of cerium oxide nanoparticles in human monocytic leukemia cells. *Int. J. Nanomed.* **2018**, *13*, 39–41. [CrossRef] [PubMed]
89. Sadhu, A.; Ghosh, I.; Moriyasu, Y.; Mukherjee, A.; Bandyopadhyay, M. Role of cerium oxide nanoparticle-induced autophagy as a safeguard to exogenous H_2O_2-mediated DNA damage in tobacco by-2 cells. *Mutagenesis* **2018**, *33*, 161–177. [CrossRef] [PubMed]
90. Kwon, H.J.; Cha, M.Y.; Kim, D.; Kim, D.K.; Soh, M.; Shin, K.; Hyeon, T.; Mook-Jung, I. Mitochondria-targeting ceria nanoparticles as antioxidants for Alzheimer's disease. *ACS Nano* **2016**, *10*, 2860–2870. [CrossRef] [PubMed]
91. Hijaz, M.; Das, S.; Mert, I.; Gupta, A.; Al-Wahab, Z.; Tebbe, C.; Dar, S.; Chhina, J.; Giri, S.; Munkarah, A.; et al. Folic acid tagged nanoceria as a novel therapeutic agent in ovarian cancer. *BMC Cancer* **2016**, *16*, 220. [CrossRef] [PubMed]
92. Wong, L.L.; Pye, Q.N.; Chen, L.; Seal, S.; McGinnis, J.F. Defining the catalytic activity of nanoceria in the p23h-1 rat, a photoreceptor degeneration model. *PLoS ONE* **2015**, *10*, e0121977. [CrossRef] [PubMed]
93. Rocca, A.; Moscato, S.; Ronca, F.; Nitti, S.; Mattoli, V.; Giorgi, M.; Ciofani, G. Pilot in vivo investigation of cerium oxide nanoparticles as a novel anti-obesity pharmaceutical formulation. *Nanomed. Nanotechnol. Biol. Med.* **2015**, *11*, 1725–1734.
94. Manne, N.; Arvapalli, R.; Graffeo, V.A.; Bandarupalli, V.V.K.; Shokuhfar, T.; Patel, S.; Rice, K.M.; Ginjupalli, G.K.; Blough, E.R. Prophylactic treatment with cerium oxide nanoparticles attenuate hepatic ischemia reperfusion injury in sprague dawley rats. *Cell. Physiol. Biochem. Int. J. Exp. Cell. Physiol. Biochem. Pharmacol.* **2017**, *42*, 1837–1846. [CrossRef] [PubMed]
95. Lee, S.S.; Zhu, H.; Contreras, E.Q.; Prakash, A.; Puppala, H.L.; Colvin, V.L. High temperature decomposition of cerium precursors to form ceria nanocrystal libraries for biological applications. *Chem. Mater.* **2012**, *24*, 424–432. [CrossRef]
96. Karakoti, A.; Kuchibhatla, S.V.; Babu, K.S.; Seal, S. Direct synthesis of nanoceria in aqueous polyhydroxyl solutions. *J. Phys. Chem. C* **2007**, *111*, 17232–17240. [CrossRef]
97. Minotti, G.; Menna, P.; Salvatorelli, E.; Cairo, G.; Gianni, L. Anthracyclines: Molecular advances and pharmacologic developments in antitumor activity and cardiotoxicity. *Pharmacol. Rev.* **2004**, *56*, 185–229. [CrossRef] [PubMed]
98. Sack-Zschauer, M.; Bader, S.; Brenneisen, P. Cerium oxide nanoparticles as novel tool in glioma treatment: An in vitro study. *J. Nanomed. Nanotechnol.* **2017**, *8*, 474.
99. Hirst, S.M.; Karakoti, A.S.; Tyler, R.D.; Sriranganathan, N.; Seal, S.; Reilly, C.M. Anti-inflammatory properties of cerium oxide nanoparticles. *Small* **2009**, *5*, 2848–2856. [PubMed]
100. Kansara, K.; Patel, P.; Shah, D.; Shukla, R.K.; Singh, S.; Kumar, A.; Dhawan, A. Tio_2 nanoparticles induce DNA double strand breaks and cell cycle arrest in human alveolar cells. *Environ. Mol. Mutagen.* **2015**, *56*, 204–217. [CrossRef] [PubMed]

101. Das, S.; Singh, S.; Dowding, J.M.; Oommen, S.; Kumar, A.; Sayle, T.X.; Saraf, S.; Patra, C.R.; Vlahakis, N.E.; Sayle, D.C.; et al. The induction of angiogenesis by cerium oxide nanoparticles through the modulation of oxygen in intracellular environments. *Biomaterials* **2012**, *33*, 7746–7755. [CrossRef] [PubMed]
102. Cimini, A.; D'Angelo, B.; Das, S.; Gentile, R.; Benedetti, E.; Singh, V.; Monaco, A.M.; Santucci, S.; Seal, S. Antibody-conjugated PEGylated cerium oxide nanoparticles for specific targeting of Aβ aggregates modulate neuronal survival pathways. *Acta Biomater.* **2012**, *8*, 2056–2067. [CrossRef] [PubMed]
103. Karakoti, A.; Monteiro-Riviere, N.; Aggarwal, R.; Davis, J.; Narayan, R.J.; Self, W.; McGinnis, J.; Seal, S. Nanoceria as antioxidant: Synthesis and biomedical applications. *JOM* **2008**, *60*, 33–37. [CrossRef] [PubMed]
104. Ciofani, G.; Genchi, G.G.; Liakos, I.; Cappello, V.; Gemmi, M.; Athanassiou, A.; Mazzolai, B.; Mattoli, V. Effects of cerium oxide nanoparticles on PC12 neuronal-like cells: Proliferation, differentiation, and dopamine secretion. *Pharm. Res.* **2013**, *30*, 2133–2145. [CrossRef] [PubMed]
105. Manne, N.D.; Arvapalli, R.; Nepal, N.; Thulluri, S.; Selvaraj, V.; Shokuhfar, T.; He, K.; Rice, K.M.; Asano, S.; Maheshwari, M.; et al. Therapeutic potential of cerium oxide nanoparticles for the treatment of peritonitis induced by polymicrobial insult in sprague-dawley rats. *Crit. Care Med.* **2015**, *43*, e477–e489. [CrossRef] [PubMed]

10

Selenium-Rich Ricegrass Juice Improves Antioxidant Properties and Nitric Oxide Inhibition in Macrophage Cells

Rattanamanee Chomchan [1], Panupong Puttarak [2], Adelheid Brantner [3] and Sunisa Siripongvutikorn [4,*]

1 Interdisciplinary Graduate School of Nutraceutical and Functional Food, Prince of Songkla University, Hat-Yai, Songkla 90112, Thailand; pui_galz@hotmail.com
2 Department of Pharmaceutical Sciences, Prince of Songkla University, Hat-Yai, Songkla 90112, Thailand; panupong.p@psu.ac.th
3 Department of Pharmacognosy, Institute of Pharmaceutical Sciences, University of Graz, Graz 8010, Austria; adelheid.brantner@uni-graz.at
4 Department of Food Technology, Faculty of Agro-Industry, Prince of Songkla University, Hat-Yai, Songkla 90112, Thailand
* Correspondence: sunisa.s@psu.ac.th

Abstract: Ricegrass juice (*Oryza sativa* L.) was introduced as a functional food as the consumption of sprouts or seedlings has been claimed to provide high nutritive value. Selenium (Se) is a trace mineral that plays a key role in the human antioxidation scheme. Supplementation of Se into plants is one strategy to enhance plant bioactivities, and the consumption of Se plant foods may confer superior health benefits. In this study, ricegrass juice extract was analyzed for its major phenolic components. The effect of ricegrass juice extracts bio-fortified with 0, 10 and 40 mg Se/L named as RG0, RG10, and RG40, respectively, were investigated for a percentage of cell viability, changes of endogenous antioxidant enzymes, lipid peroxidation, and nitric oxide inhibition in RAW264.7 macrophage cells. Flavone glycosides, namely chrysoeriol arabinosyl arabinoside derivatives, were found to be the foremost bioactive components in ricegrass juice extract indicated by UHPLC-MS. The results of cell culture assessment revealed that RG40 showed an ability to promote macrophage cell proliferation at low concentration. Ricegrass juice extract in all treatments possessed the ability to reduce malondialdehyde content, which may be regarded as the bioactivity of phenolic compounds. Moreover, Se also played a role in this effect since RG40 showed the greatest ability via increasing the level of GPx enzyme. It was also discovered that phenolic compounds in the extracts played a role in inhibiting nitric oxide in LPS-induced RAW264.7 cells. Furthermore, RG40 expressed significantly higher NO inhibition properties at IC_{50} 118.76 µg/mL compared to RG0 and RG10, at 147.02 and 147.73 µg/mL, respectively. Se bio-fortified ricegrass juice could be considered as a new potent functional food that can lower the risk of oxidative stress and chronic inflammation diseases.

Keywords: selenium; ricegrass juice; antioxidant enzymes; lipid peroxidation; nitric oxide inhibition

---

1. Introduction

At present, new directions in human consumption consider daily nutrition to include essential nutrients and energy and bioactive compounds that demonstrate the additional benefits to human health [1]. Since plants at the beginning of their growing stage have been reported to contain large amounts of quality phytonutrients such as amino acids, trace elements, vitamins, and various phytochemicals to protect them from danger and prepare for expansion, sprouts or young plant of cereals, grains, or legumes are currently of interest as a new kind of vegetable [2]. Consequently, the consumption of sprouts in the usual diet may deliver many bioactive components and improve well-being. Wheatgrass juice, the eminent sprout juice squeezed from young leaves of wheat, has long been used as a health-promoting drink and has been the subject of health-supportive pharmacological studies. Ricegrass is a brand-new sprout which was recently introduced to substitute the use of wheatgrass, especially in high rice production areas as an economy ingredient. The use of ricegrass also arouses the utilization of low-cost variety rice seeds since it was proven to contain higher levels of polyphenol and possess comparable antioxidant activities to wheatgrass juice [3,4]. Additionally, many varieties of young ricegrass in Thailand had been earlier reported to inhibit lipid peroxidation and provide DNA protective properties against exposure to Fenton reaction due to numerous secondary metabolite components such as anthocyanin and phenolics [5].

Currently, a study on how to produce or improve the functional foods or ingredients quality is of interest since there are many methods available to boost the benefits of ingredients [6]. Minerals are the basic elements required for every unit of living cells. The procedure of mineral supplementation into plants is one of the outstanding methods to provide additional competence to ingredients [7]. It is an inexpensive technique which can provide mineral supplementation as well as possibly improve the biological properties of plants from the combined effects of phytochemical compounds and an increased content of minerals. Selenium (Se) is an essential trace mineral required by humans. It has a major function in the antioxidant system, and it is claimed to have outstanding efficiency among antioxidant minerals involved in many endogenously antioxidant enzymes [8]. Moreover, it has various roles in improving wellness as well as preventing disorder conditions or diseases, including boosting immunity, helping defense against cancer, anti-diabetic, regulation of thyroid function, anti-inflammation, and anti-aging [9]. Se has been supplemented with plentiful plants worldwide to improve plant nutritional values and exert advantageous effects on plant bioactivities [10]. Therefore, the supplementation of Se into ricegrass may possibly be a key to improving the typical ricegrass to be a novel functional food.

Humans currently face many harmful radicals stimulating in everyday life. Diet, stress and pollution are major factors that lead to oxidative stress and cause various health complications. To fight these damages, antioxidant protection is needed to prevent ROS related diseases [11]. Also, in response to injury or invaders, the immune system reacts by generating inflammation. Inflammatory cytokines like nitric oxide (NO) are released for host defense response. Under normal conditions, it plays a part in the regulation of vasodilatation and neurological issues. On the other hand, overproduction of NO induces tissue damage and associated with chronic inflammation [12]. As many of the synthetic antioxidants and anti-inflammation have been widely used, risk of toxicity should be of concern. Accordingly, growing attention has been paid to the development of efficient compounds from natural resources that can naturally modulate the antioxidant protection and inflammation responses. The objective of this study is to identify the type of phenolic compounds present and the Se content of ricegrass juice extract in relation to the supplementation of sodium selenite into ricegrass. The effect of ricegrass juice (RG0) and the Se bio-fortified ricegrass juice (RG10, RG40) was then investigated for a percentage of cell viability, antioxidant enzymes activity, lipid peroxidation, and the inhibition of nitric oxide in RAW264.7 murine macrophage cells.

2. Materials and Methods

2.1. Reagents

Reduced glutathione (GSH), 5,50-dithiobis-(2-nitrobenzoic acid) (DTNB), riboflavin, L-methionine, nitroblue tetrazolium chloride (NBT), bovine serum albumin (BSA), Coomassie brilliant blue G-250 dye, malondialdehyde (MDA), 2-thiobarbituric acid (TBA), formic acid, HPLC grade acetonitrile (ACN), HPLC grade methanol, lipopolysaccharide (LPS) from *E. coli*, L-nitro-arginine

(LNA), and 3-(4,5-dimethylthiazol-2-yl)-2,5-diphenyltetrazolium bromide (MTT) were acquired from Sigma Aldrich Co. (St. Louis, MO, USA). Hydrogen peroxide (H_2O_2) and trichloroacetic acid (TCA) were purchased from Thermo Fisher Scientific Co. (San Jose, CA, USA). Reagents and media for cell line included trypan blue dye, trypsin-EDTA, fetal bovine serum (FBS), penicillin, streptomycin, and Roswell Park Memorial Institute (RPMI) 1640 medium were purchased from Gibco BRL, Life Technologies Inc. (Rockville, MD, USA) and Griess reagent was from Merck (Darmstadt, Germany).

2.2. Plantation and Plant Extract Preparation

Rice grains (*Oryza sativa* L. cv. Chainat 1), provided by the Phatthalung Rice Research Center, Thailand, were soaked in water for 24 h, drained and washed with distilled water. Soaked rice seeds were planted in trays and left in darkness for 48 h to allow the germination. Se solution was prepared by divided into 3 groups of supplementation containing (1) control (without Se) (2) 10 mg Se/L and (3) 40 mg Se/L using sodium selenite as Se source. Se solution was applied into germinated rice seeds at a ratio 1:1 *v/w*. Ricegrass was cultivated hydroponically without any supporting materials under natural light with a day/night average temperature of 33/25 °C, relative humidity 63% ± 5.0%, and photoperiod 12/12 (day/night). Leaves of rice plants or ricegrass at day 8 were harvested and extracted with water at a ratio of 1:2 (*w/v*) using a juicer (DA-900, Hurom Co., Ltd., Gimhae-si, Gyeongsangnam-do, South Korea). The samples were filtered and centrifuged at 10,000× *g* for 10 min. The supernatant was subjected to freeze-drying and the obtained plant powder extracts were stored at 4 °C in dark bottle.

2.3. Selenium Content Determination

Total Se content of plant extracts was determined using an inductively coupled plasma optical electron spectrophotometer (ICP-OES). Approximate 0.1 g of extracts were digested with 3 mL of concentrated HNO_3 and 1 mL of 30% H_2O_2 in a digestive stove heated at 180 °C for 1.5 h. The digested product was reconstituted to 10 mL with Milli-Q water and an auto-sampler for total Se content [13].

2.4. Total Polyphenol Content

The total extractable phenolic content of ricegrass juice extracts was measured using a method modified from Singleton and Rossi [14]. Briefly, 20 µL of the extract was added to 96-well microplate. Then, 100 µL of Folin reagent (10% *v/v*) and 80 µL of Na_2CO_3 (7.5% *w/v*) were added and mixed thoroughly. After incubation for 30 min in the dark at ambient temperature, the absorbance was measured at 765 nm using a microplate reader and expressed as mg pyrogallol equivalent (PYE)/g extract.

2.5. Phenolic Profiles Identification Using UHPLC-DAD-ESI-MS

Main polyphenol compounds in ricegrass juice extracts were investigated using a Thermo Scientific (Dionex Softron GmbH., Germering, Germany) Ultimate 3000 Ultra High-Performance Liquid Chromatography (UHPLC) system equipped with Diode Array Absorbance Detector, Electron Spray Ionization, and LTQ XL mass detector (DAD-ESI-MS) The extracts of 10 mg/mL were dissolved in HPLC water and filtered with a sterile syringe filter of 0.45 µm. Separation was carried out using a Purosper STAR (250 mm × 4.6 mm) with LiChrocart, RP-18 column end-capped with 5 µm diameter particles (Merck, Darmstadt, Germany) as the stationary phase. The mobile phase consisted of H_2O containing 0.5% formic acid (solvent A) and acetonitrile (solvent B), using the following gradient of solvent B: 0.00–10.00 min, 0–10.0%; 10.00–15.00 min, 10.0%; 15.00–20.00 min, 10.0–15.0%; 20.00–30.00 min, 15.0–25.0%; 30.00–35.00 min, 25.0%; 35.00–45.00 min; 25.0–100% followed by washing with 100% methanol and re-equilibration. The flow rate was 0.8 mL/min, and the column temperature was 40 °C with the injection volume of 20 µL. The MS parameters were as follows for both the negative and positive mode: heater temperature: 250 °C; capillary temperature: 330 °C; sheath gas flow: 50 arbitrary units; auxiliary gas flow: 10 arbitrary units. The mass data for the molecular ions were processed with Thermo XcaliburTM software version 2.2.44 (Thermo Scientific., Hemel Hempstead, UK).

2.6. Cell Culture Model

RAW264.7, mouse murine macrophage cells were purchased from the American Type Culture Collection (Manassas, VA, USA). Roswell Park Memorial Institute (RPMI) 1640 medium supplemented with 1.5% sodium bicarbonate, 10% fetal bovine serum (FBS), and 1% penicillin-streptomycin was used for the maintenance of cells at 37 °C, 5% CO_2, in a fully humidified incubator. Phosphate buffer saline (PBS) at pH 7.2 was used to wash the cells and throughout the experiment.

2.7. Cell Viability Assay

The MTT assay was used to determine the percentage of cell viability. Cells grown at 80–90% confluence were harvested with 0.25% trypsin—EDTA and suspended in a fresh medium. Cell counts were determined using a standard haemocytometer based trypan blue cell counting technique [15]. RAW264.7 cells at the density of 1×10^6 cells/mL were seeded in 96-well tissue culture plates and allow to adhere for 2 h. After washing the cells with PBS (pH 7.2), they were allowed to react with the medium mixed with various concentrations of the extracts (0.25–5 mg/mL) followed by 24 h incubation. 24 h incubation time was examined to be the stage that cells remain in the vigorous stage, then suitable to determine the effect on viability. Cell viability was checked after 24 h by removing 100 μL of supernatant and 10 μL of MTT solution was added. After 2 h, the MTT solution was removed, and 100 μL of 0.04 N·HCl in isopropanol was added to dissolve the formazan crystals. Absorbances were recorded at 570 nm using a microplate reader. The percentage of cell viability was calculated by the following Equation (1):

$$\% \text{ Cell viability} = [\text{Absorbance of sample}/\text{Absorbance of control}] \times 100 \quad (1)$$

2.8. Preparation of Endogenous Cellular Extracts

RAW264.7 cells at the density of 1×10^6 cells/mL were seeded in 60 mm tissue culture plates and incubated for 2 h to allow the cells to adhere to the tissue culture plates. Cells were washed with 2 mL of PBS (pH 7.2) before being treated with 6 mL of the extracts at the concentration of 250 and 1000 μg/mL for 24 h. The endogenous cellular fluid was extracted according to a method modified from Du, et al. [16]. Supernatants were removed; cells were washed with PBS and harvested with 0.5 mL of 0.25% trypsin-EDTA. Then, 1 mL of the culture medium was added to stop the reaction, followed by centrifugation at $1000\times g$ for 10 min. Cell pellets were washed with PBS until clean and re-suspended in 1 mL of cold PBS. Cells were lysed using a probe-type sonicator (Vibra-Cell, Sonics and Materials Inc., Newtown, CT, USA) by pulsing at 15 s on and 10 s off for 5 cycles on ice. The cell extracts were centrifuged at $10{,}000\times g$ (4 °C) to discard the cell debris, while supernatants were used for the determination of antioxidant enzymes activity and lipid peroxidation assay.

2.9. Determination of Endogenous Antioxidant Enzyme Activity

Total superoxide dismutase (SOD) assay was performed using a mixture of 20 μM riboflavin (0.3 mL), 130 mM methionine (0.3 mL), and 100 μM di-sodium ethylenediaminetetraacetic acid ($EDTA\text{-}Na^2$) (0.3 mL), 50 mM potassium phosphate buffer at pH 7.8 (1.5 mL), deionized water (0.25 mL), 750 μmol/L NBT (0.3 mL), and followed by 0.05 mL of the endogenous cellular extracts. The mixture was placed under light at a photon flux density of 78 μmol photons s^{-1} m^{-2} for 20 min. The absorbance was measured under UV light at 560 nm [17]. The level of glutathione peroxidase (GPx) activity which was the main selenoenzyme involved in antioxidant protection system was measured [18]. The mixture of 0.2 mL endogenous cellular extracts, 0.4 mL of 0.1 mM reduced L-glutathione (GSH) and 0.2 mL of 0.067 M $KNaHPO_4$ was pre-heated at 25 °C for 5 min. Afterward, 0.2 mL of 1.3 mM of H_2O_2 was added to initiate the reaction and left for 10 min. 1 mL of 1% of trichloroacetic acid was added to terminate the reaction followed by incubation on an ice bath for 30 min. The mixture was centrifuged at 1000× g for 10 min and the supernatant (0.48 mL) was then mixed with 0.32 M of Na_2HPO_4 (2.2 mL) and 1 mM of DTNB (0.32 mL) in the cuvette. The absorbance at 412 nm was measured under UV light after 5 min (E = 39.4 $mM^{-1}cm^{-1}$). Catalase (CAT) assay was investigated from the mixture of 0.3% H_2O_2 in 50 mM potassium phosphate buffer pH 7.0 (1.9 mL) with the endogenous cellular extracts (0.1 mL) in the cuvette. Activity of CAT was measured from absorbance change in 60 s at 240 nm (E = 39.4 $mM^{-1}cm^{-1}$) [19]. All enzyme activities were calculated according to protein content expressed from the calibration curve of BSA as a standard and expressed as a percentage of the control. The assay of Bradford [20] was used to determined protein content. Reagent was made by dissolving 100 mg of Coomassie brilliant blue G-250 dye in 50 mL of 95% ethanol. The solution was mixed with 100 mL of 85% phosphoric acid and made up to 1 L with distilled water. The reagent was filtered, and 5 mL was added to 0.1 mL of endogenous cellular extract. Absorbance at 595 nm was measured.

2.10. Determination of Lipid Peroxidation

Lipid peroxidation assay was measured using thiobarbituric acid reactive substances assay (TBARS) [21]. 1 mL of endogenous cellular extracts was mixed with 4 mL of 20% TCA containing 0.8% of TBA (*w/v*). The mixtures were heated at 95 °C for 60 min, then cooled on ice and centrifuged at 3000× g for 10 min. The absorbance was measured at 532 nm. The amount of red complexes was compared to an external standard of MDA. The amount of TBARS was expressed as nmol MDA/mg protein.

2.11. Nitric Oxide Synthesis Inhibition Determination

Nitric oxide (NO) synthesis inhibition determination was measured as the screening method for anti-inflammatory properties of ricegrass juice extracts. Briefly, RAW 264.7 cells at the density of 1×10^6 cells/mL were seeded into 96-well plates and allowed to adhere for 2 h. Cells were induced to produce NO by treating them with 100 µL of 100 µg/mL lipopolysaccharide (LPS) from *E. coli* as a foreign matter. 100 µL of extracts at various concentrations from 0.1–1 mg/mL were further added and incubated for 24 h. L-nitro arginine was used as a positive control. Sodium selenite and Se-methionine (Se-Met) from Se-yeast were also used as the sample control. The percentage of NO synthesis inhibition was determined by measuring the accumulation of nitrite in the culture supernatant using the Griess reagent. The supernatant (100 µL) was transferred to 96-well tissue culture plates and then added with 100 µL of Griess reagent. The mixtures were measured using a microplate reader at 570 nm. The percentage of NO synthesis inhibition (%) was calculated from Equation (2). The rest of cells in 96-well plates were rechecked for the number of cell viability with MTT assay to confirm the effectiveness of the extract on the inhibition of NO synthesis.

$$\%\ \text{Inhibition of NO synthesis} = \frac{[(\text{Control} - \text{Blank of control}) - (\text{Sample} - \text{Blank of sample})]}{(\text{Control} - \text{Blank of control})} \times 100 \quad (2)$$

2.12. Statistical Analysis

All data were expressed as means (n = 3) ± standard deviation (S.D.). Comparison between groups was carried out by one-way analysis of variance using SPSS (SPSS Inc., Chicago, IL, USA). Duncan's test was used to determine significant differences ($p < 0.05$).

3. Results and Discussion

3.1. Changes in Se Content and Total Polyphenol Content

Rice is a plant in the Poaceae family and has been classified as a moderate selenium (Se) accumulating plant. This study aimed to bio-fortify Se in young rice plants, which can exert extra biological properties in combination with polyphenols compounds in ricegrass. According to the preliminary results, however, ricegrass was revealed to have the limitation of not accumulating Se compounds more than 40 mg Se/L, since higher levels of Se concentration led to toxicity, which resulted in significant growth limitation. The addition of Se at 10 and 40 mg Se/L revealed no significant changes in the physiology and yield of ricegrass collected on the day of harvesting [22]. In the present experiment, Se compounds were found to be accumulated in ricegrass in a dose-dependent manner. The supplementation of sodium selenite compounds in the plantation at 10 and 40 mg Se/L resulted in higher levels of Se accumulation than when feeding with water alone. After the aqueous extraction of ricegrass, the highest level of Se compounds that would be achieved in ricegrass juice extract was at the level of 59.76 ± 1.52 µg/g extract at treatment 40 mg Se/L supplementation (Figure 1).

In previous research work, the technique of Se supplementation into plants had been proposed as an alternative path to trigger some of the phytochemical constituents in numerous plants [10]. For example, an enhancement of naringin chalcone and kaempferol level in tomato fruits [23], and a promotion of catechin accumulation in Assam tea has been observed [24]. However, the supplementation of Se compounds into ricegrass during plantation in this study showed a minor modification in the total polyphenol content (TPC) of its aqueous extract. The addition of 10 mg Se/m^3 led to slightly higher accumulative in TPC level. This may result from a stimulating effect of Se compounds on phenylalanine ammonia lyase (PAL) which is the main enzyme responsible for the synthesis of phenol secondary metabolites in the phenylpropanoids pathway [22,25]. However, plants return to their homeostasis when higher levels were supplemented (treatment 40 mg Se/m^3).

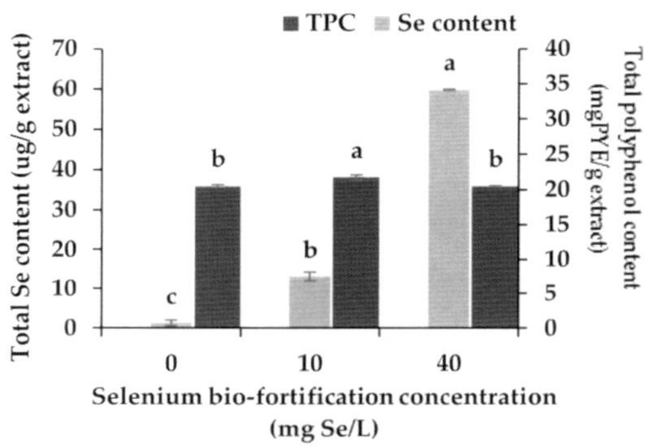

Figure 1. Total selenium (Se) content (µg/g extract) (left axis) and total polyphenol content (right axis) of ricegrass juice extract after being bio-fortified with various concentrations of sodium selenite (0, 10 and 40 mg Se/L) during plantation. Each treatment was tested in triplicate. Data are means ± standard deviation (SD). Different letters indicated significant differences ($p < 0.05$) in Duncan's significant differences test. PYE: pyrogallol equivalent.

3.2. Phenolic Profiles Identification Using UHPLC-DAD-ESI-MS

In this study, the supplementation of Se compounds into ricegrass appeared to have minimal effects on both the number of phenolic compounds as reported by TPC level and the quality of phenolic compounds. The types of phenolic compounds detected in ricegrass juice extract (RG0) and Se-ricegrass juice extract (RG10, RG40) investigated using HPLC were similar (data not shown). Therefore, ricegrass juice extract (control) was chosen as a representative to identify the main type of phenolic compounds which can be a major substance exhibited the bioactivities using the reversed-phase UHPLC-DAD-ESI-MS, since there was only limited data on the specific types of phenolic compounds found in the aqueous extract of young ricegrass or rice seedlings. The compounds in the present extract were identified based on the UV spectra and a mass ion of each peak was compared to the existing literature.

Figure 2 presents the reversed-phase UHPLC-DAD chromatogram of ricegrass juice extract cultivar Chainat 1 obtained using the suitable gradient elution program. In total, 11 compounds were tentatively identified through the ESI-MS in negative mode considering the UV and MS spectral data. Data concerning the identification of the peaks are shown in Table 1, where the retention time, molecular weight and electrospray ionization mass spectrometry of all the compounds detected are also reported. Peak 1 was observed to represent a base molecular anion at m/z 191, thus it was identified as quinic acid. Peaks 3 and 4 were identified as phenolic glycosides according to the m/z of base ions at 315 and 385 resembling the spectrum of protocatechuic glucoside and 1-*o*-sinapoyl-β-D-glucose, respectively. The ion found at the retention time 23.87 min (peak 5), with the m/z of 367, presented a fragment at m/z 193 which resembles the m/z of the ferulic acid fragment. Thus, this compound was consistent with 3-*o*-feruloyl-quinic acid. The large group of secondary metabolite compounds in the leaves of *Oryza sativa* have been reported earlier to be flavone glycosides [26]. The spectra of peaks 6–9 showed a similar base peak of 563 which resembles the spectrum of chrysoeriol arabinosyl arabinoside derivatives. This compound has been formerly found in the literature investigating the compounds in rice leaves using MS/MS with the same m/z recorded [27]. Peak 7 was recognized as the main compound in ricegrass juice extract. The ESI-MS on negative ion of this peak is presented in Figure 3. Peaks 2, 10 and 11 were the group of compounds which also tentatively identified as flavone glycosides referred to the literature. The m/z of 325, 445, 491 were detected and they were identified as tricin, swertisin, and tricin-7-*o*-β-D-glucopyranoside, respectively, which are the compounds existing in the leaves of rice and wheat [27–29].

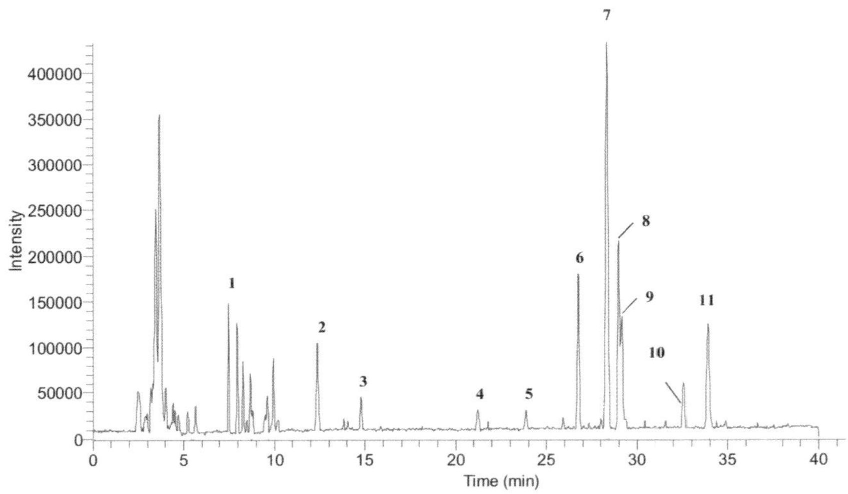

Figure 2. Reversed-phase Ultra High-Performance Liquid Chromatography with diode array detection (UHPLC-DAD) chromatogram of Thai ricegrass juice extract (*Oryza sativa*., Chainat1) with identified peak (1–11).

Table 1. Tentative identification of phenolic compounds in ricegrass juice extract analyzed by Ultra High-Performance Liquid Chromatography with electrospray ionization-mass spectrometry (UHPLC-ESI-MS).

Peak No. [a]	RT (min)	Tentative Compounds	MW	[M − H] − (*m/z*)	Fragment Ion	Ref.
1	7.95	Quinic acid	192	191	111, 192, 613	[30]
2	12.38	Tricin	330	329	175, 461	[27,28]
3	14.79	Protocatechuic glucoside	316	315	175, 445, 575	[31,32]
4	21.20	1-*o*-Sinapoyl-β-D-glucose	386	385	175, 469, 599	[27]
5	23.87	3-*o*-Feruloylquinic acid	368	367	193, 435, 497	[27,33]
6	26.75	Chrysoeriol arabinosyl arabinoside derivatives	564	563	175, 305, 693	[26,27]
7	28.31	Chrysoeriol arabinosyl arabinoside derivatives	564	563	565, 693	[26,27]
8	29.00	Chrysoeriol arabinosyl arabinoside derivatives	564	563	693	[26,27]
9	29.14	Chrysoeriol arabinosyl arabinoside derivatives	564	563	693	[26,27]
10	32.56	Swertisin	446	445	175, 305	[27]
11	33.90	Tricin-7-*o*-β-D-glucopyranoside	492	491	769, 983	[27]

[a] Peak numbers and retention times refer to Figure 1. RT: retention time. MW: Molecular weight.

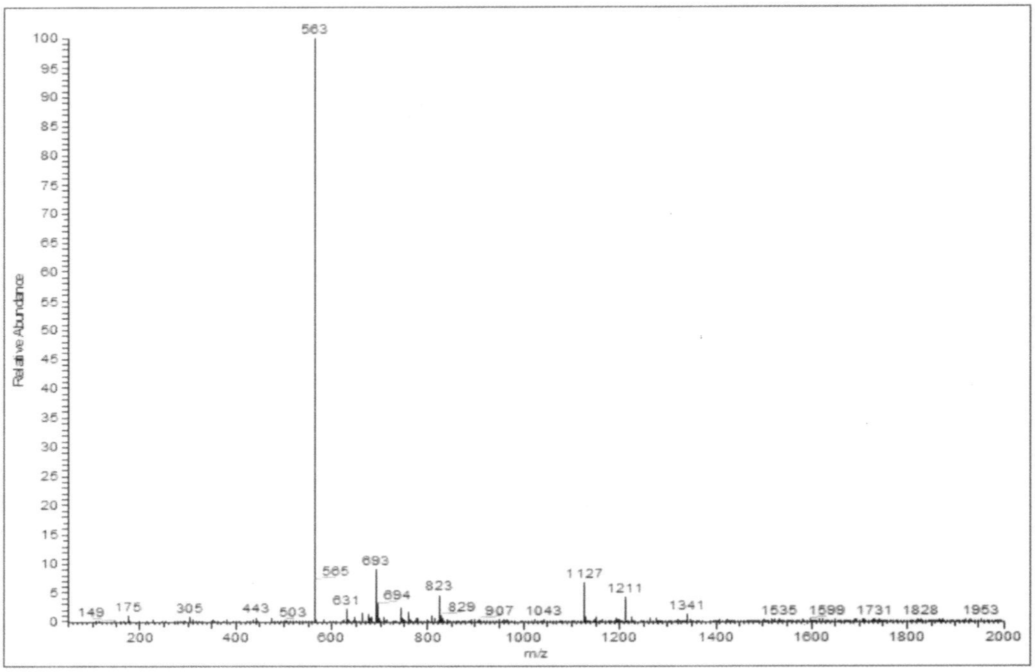

Figure 3. Electro-spray ionization mass spectrum on negative ion of peak 7 (RT 28.71) in ricegrass juice extract.

3.3. Cell Viability and Cell Proliferation

The safety aspect was stated as it is necessary for introducing each functional food product into the market. Reliable evidence is needed to make a claim on the cytotoxicity of the extract on mammalian cells. The cytotoxicity of the extracts on RAW264.7, a murine macrophage cell, was chosen since it can represent the influence of compounds specifically on an essential immune system, which is the first defense step in the human body. Macrophages are phagocytic cells which play a crucial role in the clearance of microorganisms, pathogens, and harmful disturbances. Thus, it is also important for the function of antigen presentation, cytokine production and anti-tumor activity [34]. The experiment measured the number of viable cells and cell proliferation after incubating the healthy macrophage cells with the extracts for 24 h.

Figure 4 reveals the number of cell viability and cell proliferation of RAW264.7 cells after incubating with various concentrations of three extracts (RG0, RG10, RG40), ranging from 250–5000 μg/mL compared to the control. The macrophage cell number slightly decreased through an increased concentration of extracts because an excessive concentration of phenolic compounds, as well as Se compounds in the extract, can act as pro-oxidant molecules which cause damage to cells and lead to cell death. However, the results still confirmed that all of the extracts had no or low toxicity to the RAW264.7 macrophage cells. According to the system of drug screening for neglected diseases, the 50% cytotoxicity concentration (CC_{50}) of any substance which was higher than 90 μg/mL was classified as no toxicity [35], thus the extracts were confidently claimed as safe when displaying CC_{50} over 5000 μg/mL. Furthermore, it was found that RG40 greatly promoted the proliferation of RAW264.7 cells ($p < 0.05$) compared to the control especially at low concentration, while RG0 and RG10 did not. All the extracts caused a reduction in the number of the viable cells while the concentration has been increased. The effect of ricegrass juice extract on cell viability in this study can be stated mainly from phenolics and Se. Other literature that checked the effect of Se on mouse monocyte-macrophage cell line (TIB69) also claimed that supplementation of Se influences cell proliferation [36]. Both phenolic and Se compounds have been claimed individually for the positive effects over the cell viability at low amount by being involved as a source of nutrition and possibly playing a role in antioxidant protection in the metabolism of the cells, however, the higher level of both Se and phenolic compounds can cause the oxidative damage to cells and result in cell death. It could be assumed that RG40 at low concentration (250 μg/mL) is the most suitable condition for RAW264.7 cells to grow while RG10 at about 1000 or 2000 μg/mL, though provide similar level of Se compounds to RG40 at 250 μg/mL, it provides higher level of phenolic compounds and may indicate in the reduction in cell viability. Moreover, the bio-fortification of Se into ricegrass may propose changes in various components not only phenolic compounds and selenium content. The LCMS analysis may only visible some compounds contained in the extracts which do not differ from each other. The other compounds may play some role in the cell proliferation as well as cell reduction.

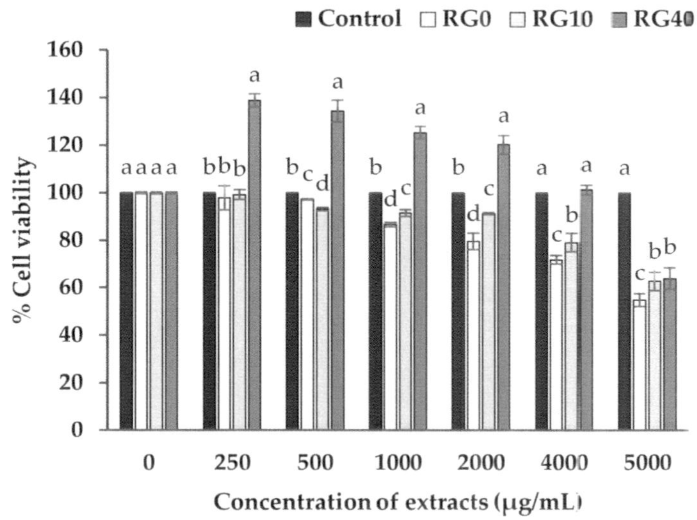

Figure 4. Cell viability and cell proliferation of RAW264.7 murine macrophage cells after incubating with various concentrations of extracts from 250–5000 μg/mL for 24 h: RG0; ricegrass juice extract (control), RG10; ricegrass juice fortified with 10 mg Se/m^3 extract, RG40; ricegrass juice fortified with 40 mg Se/m^3 extract. Data are means ± standard deviation (SD). Different letters indicated significant differences ($p < 0.05$) in Duncan's significant differences test.

3.4. Lipid Peroxidation and Antioxidant Enzymes Activity

Oxygen is the primary agent used for the respiration and the metabolism of living organisms. ROS are a natural byproduct of the normal metabolism of oxygen. Generally, it has had an important role in cellular signaling and defense against pathogens [37]. However, during times of environmental stress, ROS levels can increase dramatically, and the elevated amounts include superoxide anion ($O_2\bullet^-$), hydroperoxyl (perhydroxyl) radical ($HO_2\bullet$), hydroxyl radical ($\bullet OH$), and nitric oxide (NO), resulting in significant damage to cell structures. Living organisms contain lipid as the main structure of cellular membranes [38]. Thus, lipid peroxidation can be stated as a crucial step in the pathogenesis of several disease states in humans such as atherosclerosis, Alzheimer's disease, and cancer. Therefore, the extent of lipid peroxidation byproducts produced like malondialdehyde (MDA) can reflect the extent of oxidative damage to cells [39].

The level of MDA detected from the cellular extracts of RAW264.7 cells after treatment with the extracts, therefore, revealed the effect of ricegrass juice extract and Se-enriched ricegrass juice extract on the role of oxidative stress protection (Figure 5). Outcomes indicated that ricegrass juice extracts of all treatments can significantly reduce the level detected of MDA from RAW264.7 cellular compared to the normal cells. The role of phenolic compounds in the extracts was considered as having the major effects. Phenolic compounds possess a mechanism to lower the MDA level through the ability as an electron donor, which can stabilize the hydroxyl radicals and lipid peroxyl radicals, thereby lowering the extent of oxidative damage to the lipid cell membrane. In addition, an increased level of

Se content in the RG10 and RG40 showed more reduction in MDA content compared to the RG0 at dose 1000 μg/mL.

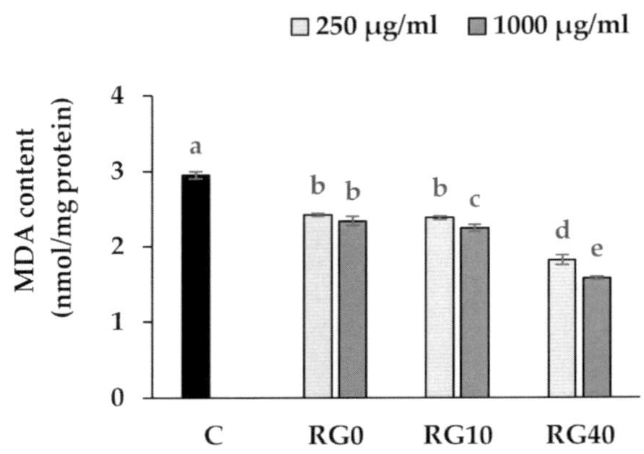

Figure 5. Level of malondialdehyde (MDA) in RAW264.7 cell line treated with selenium biofortified ricegrass juice extract (RG0, RG10, RG40) at level 250 and 1000 μg/mL compared to control. RG0; ricegrass juice extract (control), RG10; ricegrass juice fortified with 10 mg Se/m^3 extract, RG40; ricegrass juice fortified with 40 mg Se/m^3 extract. Data are means ± standard deviation (SD). Different letters indicated significant differences ($p < 0.05$) in Duncan's significant differences test.

In order to clarify the conceivable mechanism of the extracts in lowering the level of lipid peroxidation, their ability to regulate three main endogenous antioxidant enzymes including SOD, CAT, and GPx was also studied. SOD is the defense enzyme that deals with superoxide radicals (O_2•) which are the first radicals generated from oxygen metabolism and convert them to hydrogen peroxide (H_2O_2) which CAT and GPx are occupied and further transformation to harmless water (H_2O) which terminates the damaging chain reaction [40].

All the extracts at low concentration seemed to have no effect on the level of total SOD. Yet, at a higher concentration, the was a slight increase total SOD. No effect was detected from the different concentration of Se in the extracts (Figure 6a). The addition of extracts to RAW264.7 cells in all treatments was able to promote the activity of GPx which are classified as the seleno-enzymes. It appeared that the RG40 at 1000 μg/mL can increase the highest proportion of GPX activity, up to 73% above the control (Figure 6b). Since Se is the main cofactor of this enzyme, extracts that contain a high level of Se can then logically promote a greater level of GPx activity. In the CAT assay, low level of the extracts at RG10 and RG40 treatment showed an increasing CAT activity above the level of normal cells (C), while the level of CAT in RG0 showed no change. However, a higher level of the extracts at 1000 μg/mL suppressed CAT activity (Figure 6c). This phenomenon can be explained by the fact that GPx and CAT had grossing similar roles in converting H_2O_2 to H_2O. While GPx was high enough to reduce the level of the substrate, the CAT was probably sparing in the cells to remain in homeostasis. According to the results, ricegrass juice extracts revealed the supportive activity on all three antioxidant enzymes above the regular one. Animal studies on the effect of dietary supplementation of phenolic compounds on antioxidant enzymes levels in rat suggested that phenolic compounds selectively induced the mRNA expression through the upregulation of gene transcription and Nrf2 transcription factor [41]. Moreover, it was noticed that the tested extracts provided larger effects on CAT and GPx enzymes compared to total SOD. The reduction in MDA content from the cellular extracts of cells treated with the test samples especially in RG40 treatment, thus indicating that the proposed role of these two enzymes is via both Se element and phenolics functions.

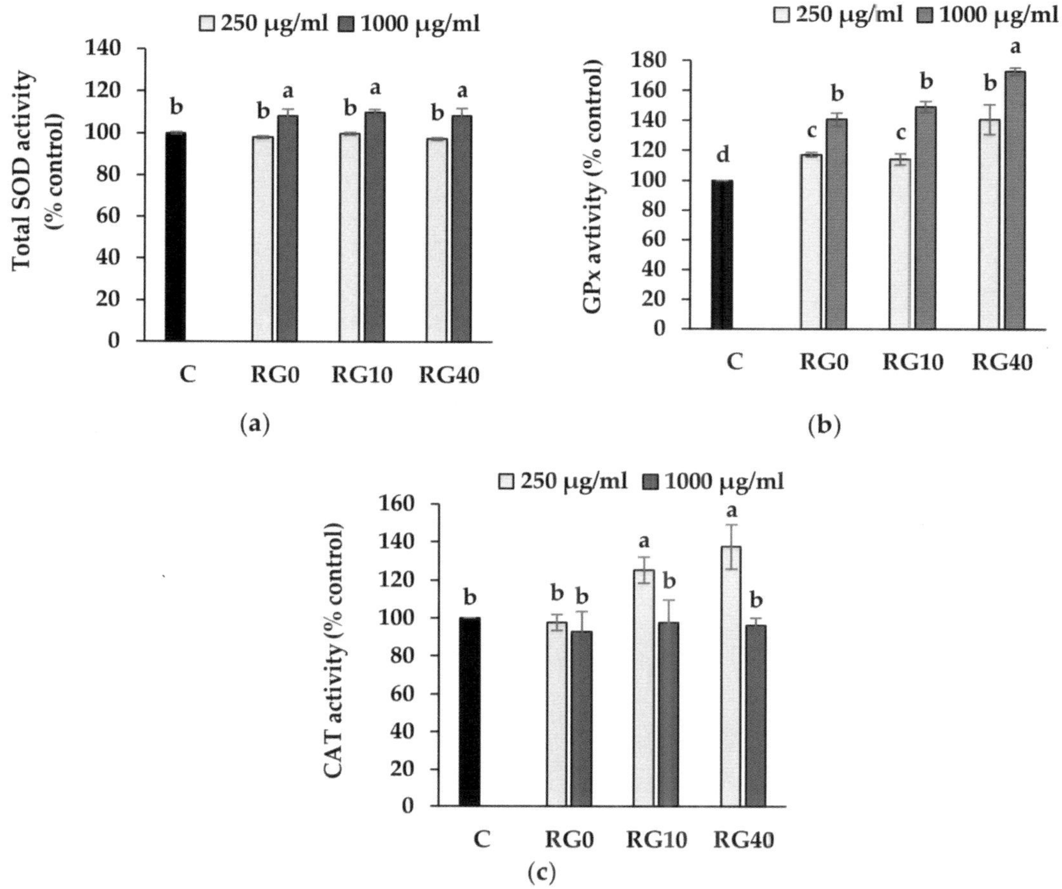

Figure 6. Level of SOD (**a**), GPx (**b**), and CAT (**c**) in RAW264.7 cell line treated with RG0, RG10, and RG40 compare to control. RG0; ricegrass juice extract (control), RG10; ricegrass juice fortified with 10 mg Se/L extract, RG40; ricegrass juice fortified with 40 mg Se/L extract. Data are means ± standard deviation (SD). Different letters indicated significant differences ($p < 0.05$) in Duncan's significant differences test.

3.5. Nitric Oxide Inhibition Properties

Nitric oxide (NO) is a major mediator produced by macrophages during inflammation responses. It is produced by the enzyme inducible nitric oxide synthase (iNOS) from the substrate, arginine [42]. NO is vital for many physiological functions such as being a neurotransmitter and affecting blood flow and synaptic plasticity. On the other hand, an excess amount of NO can destroy and induce dysfunction in the macrophages themselves as well as in surrounding normal cells [43]. Therefore, the study on plant foods that can modulate the level of NO produced by its homeostasis is an important issue because they are safer, have limited side effects, and are relatively low cost compared with medication. In this study, LPS from *E. coli* as a foreign matter was applied to RAW264.7 cells to initiate the production of NO. Then, RG0, RG10, and RG40 were co-treated to analyze their NO production inhibitory effects. The concentration of ricegrass juice extracts which did not affect the percentage of cell viability to be lower than 80% was 2000 µg/mL. Thus, this range was the maximum concentration used for the determination of nitric oxide inhibition properties to verify that NO was truly produced. The level of LPS which did not affect cell viability and could stimulate the highest level of NO was scanned and the level of LPS at 0.5 µg/mL was chosen. The percentage of NO production inhibition was measured using the Griess assay and it was shown as the percentage of negative control (Figure 7). The co-incubation experiment of LPS and the extracts at various concentration showed a dose-dependent inhibition of NO production. Results revealed that NO from

LPS-induced RAW264.7 was significantly inhibited by ricegrass juice extracts. The Se biofortified one, RG40, showed the greatest ability to inhibit NO compared to other treatments. The IC_{50} of RG0, RG10, and RG40 were 147.02, 147.73, and 118.76 μg/mL, respectively. Although the IC_{50} values were still higher compared to the positive control, L-nitro-arginine (LNA), which is known as the enzyme iNOS inhibitor (IC_{50} = 30.05 μg/mL). Therefore, ricegrass juice in all treatments was still on a considerable amount that can be classified as functional food.

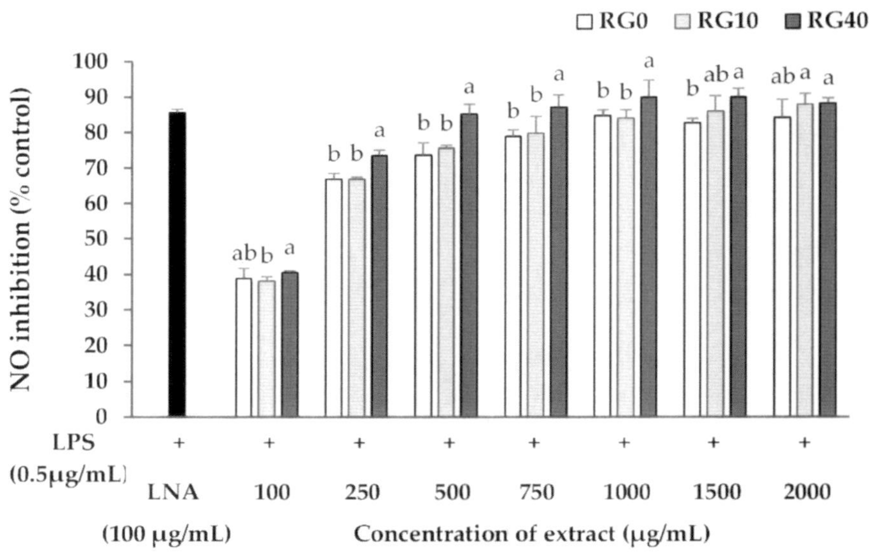

Figure 7. The effect of extracts on the inhibition of nitric oxide (NO) in RAW264.7 murine macrophage cells after co-incubation of LPS from *E. coli* (0.5 μg/mL) with various concentrations of extracts from 100–1000 μg/mL for 24 h using LNA as a positive control (100 μg/mL): RG0; ricegrass juice extract (control), RG10; ricegrass juice fortified with 10 mg Se/L extract, RG40; ricegrass juice fortified with 40 mg Se/L extract. Data are means ± standard deviation (SD). Different letters indicate significant differences ($p < 0.05$) in Duncan's significant differences test.

The NO inhibition of ricegrass juice extract can be initially attributed to the role of phenolic compounds. A correlation between high intake of phenolic compound rich food and the ability to downregulate the inflammatory responses in vitro and in vivo has been previously reported [44,45]. It has been hypothesized that phenolic compounds exert anti-inflammatory activity by inhibiting the synthesis of pro-inflammatory mediators, modification of eicosanoid synthesis, inhibition of activated immune cells, or inhibition of iNOS and cyclooxygenase-2 via inhibitory effects on nuclear factor NF-κβ [46]. Main components of phenolic compounds found in ricegrass juice extract were in the group of flavone glycosides. The previous study has reported on the effect of flavonoid compounds like apigenin and quercetin on NO; the results indicated that the inhibition of NO was due to the reduction of iNOS expression [47]. Moreover, flavone compounds may possess scavenging ability since NO is one of the reactive oxygen species (ROS) that is a by-product formed during the mitochondrial respiratory process [41]. Phenolic compounds can effectively scavenge the radicals as well as NO radical through the antioxidation process by stabilizing the radicals through the active site of -OH group and the planar ring. Thus, a reduction in the NO level in cell surrounding was found.

Another segment that influences the reduction of NO production may relate to the activity of Se. Since RG40 exerted approximately an extra 5% on NO inhibition activity compared to RG0 and RG10, the effect of Se itself on NO inhibition was then studied to confirm the additional benefit (Figure 8). The experiment was designed to use two forms of Se compounds including sodium selenite as inorganic Se supplement and seleno-methionine (Se-Met) from Se yeast as organic Se supplement. Se in both forms exerted NO inhibition properties at a low dose, which less than 0.15 μg/mL, while a higher dose of the pure compounds was toxic to the cells. Furthermore, Se-Met exerted higher ability than sodium selenite to reduce the level of NO. The underlying mechanisms of Se to inhibit the production of NO might be that Se as an essential part of the enzyme glutathione peroxidase (GPx), Se-GPx active site may exert its chemo-preventive effect by inhibiting the expression of iNOS and subsequently inhibiting NO production [48]. Moreover, the organic form of Se provided higher ability could be due to the bioavailability of the organic Se in which the element was already bound to amino acid and could be utilized straightforwardly as a part of the enzyme while inorganic form like selenite needs to initially be transformed to the organic form before being utilized, so an extra stage is required [49]. Since the majority of Se in the ricegrass juice extract was supposed to be an organic form, the RG40 treatment that contained five times of Se content than the control may provide more advantages from the higher level of organic Se. These outcomes provided evidence for the beneficial effects of dietary Se supplementation in the prevention and or treatment of oxidative-stress-mediated inflammatory diseases.

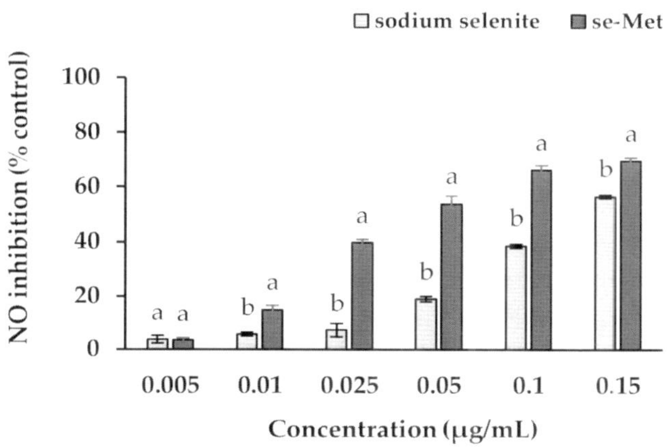

Figure 8. The effect of extracts on the inhibition of nitric oxide (NO) in RAW264.7 murine macrophage cells after co-incubation of LPS from *E. coli* (0.5 μg/mL) with sodium selenite, seleno-methionine (se-Met) from Se-yeast for 24 h. Data are means ± standard deviation (SD). Different letters indicate significant differences ($p < 0.05$) in Duncan's significant differences test.

The experiment was designed to test the effect of the ricegrass juice extract on antioxidant activities in the non-stimulating model because it represented the normal condition of healthy people because we would like to examine whether the consumption of ricegrass juice can promote the antioxidant defense system in a normal human body, since the oxidative damage naturally occurred all the time even in the normal condition. However, the inflammation is the more complex process which did not occur naturally. Thus, the induction of nitric oxide production using foreign matter (LPS) is required to examine this property. However, future work could also further examine the effect of the extracts on stimulating condition like H_2O_2 oxidative stress or Cd stress induction.

4. Conclusions

Se-rich ricegrass juice extract can be classified as safe since it had no toxicity on RAW264.7 murine macrophage cells. Additionally, RG40 promoted proliferation of the cells. Flavone glycosides were identified as the main phenolic compounds in ricegrass juice extracts and possessed biological properties on the reduction of oxidative stress and NO inhibition. This finding was the first work to report the ability of ricegrass juice to play a part in the treatment of anti-inflammation. Moreover, Se supplemented treatment (RG40) reduced the greatest level of MDA content and inhibited NO production in which the mechanism was related to an increase in CAT and GPx activities. Therefore, Se-rich ricegrass juice can be considered for production as a value-added functional drink from rice that can lower risk of oxidative stress and chronic inflammatory disease and promote human well-being.

Acknowledgments: This work was carried out with the financial support of Thailand's Education Hub for Southern Region of ASEAN Countries Scholarship, Graduate School Dissertation Funding for Thesis, the Overseas Thesis Research Scholarship and Revenue Budget Fund (AGR600544S) from Prince of Songkla University, Thailand. The authors would like to thank Alan F. Geater and Maria Mullet for English copy editing.

Author Contributions: Rattanamanee Chomchan, Sunisa Siripongvutikorn, and Panupong Puttrak conceived and designed the experiments; Adelheid Brantner encouraged the analysis of extracts on LC-MS; Rattanamanee Chomchan performed the experiments, analyzed the data, and wrote the paper, which was reviewed, edited, and approved by all the authors.

Conflicts of Interest: The authors declare no conflict of interest.

References

1. Fardet, A.; Rock, E. Toward a new philosophy of preventive nutrition: From a reductionist to a holistic paradigm to improve nutritional recommendations. *Adv. Nutr.* **2014**, *5*, 430–446. [CrossRef] [PubMed]
2. Wigmore, A. *The Sprouting Book*; Penguin Putnam Inc.: East Rutherford, NJ, USA, 1986.
3. Chomchan, R.; Siripongvutikorn, S.; Puttarak, P.; Rattanapon, R. Investigation of phytochemical constituents, phenolic profiles and antioxidant activities of ricegrass juice compared to wheatgrass juice. *Funct. Food. Health Dis.* **2016**, *6*, 822–835.
4. Rattanapon, R.; Siripongvutikorn, S.; Usawakesmanee, W.; Thongraung, C. Improvement nutritional value and bioactivity of ricegrass as affected of priming induced by fish protein hydrolysate. *Funct. Foods Health Dis.* **2016**, *6*, 219–233.
5. Khanthapoka, P.; Muangpromb, A.; Sukronga, S. Antioxidant activity and DNA protective properties of rice grass juices. *Sci. Asia* **2015**, *41*, 119–129. [CrossRef]
6. Baenas, N.; García-Viguera, C.; Moreno, D. Elicitation: A tool for enriching the bioactive composition of foods. *Molecules* **2014**, *19*, 13541–13563. [CrossRef] [PubMed]
7. White, P.J.; Broadley, M.R. Biofortifying crops with essential mineral elements. *Trends Plant Sci.* **2005**, *10*, 586–593. [CrossRef] [PubMed]
8. McDowell, L.R.; Wilkinson, N.; Madison, R.; Felix, T. *Vitamins and Minerals Functioning as Antioxidants with Supplementation Considerations*; Florida Ruminant Nutrition Symposium, Best Western Gateway Grand: Gainesville, FL, USA, 2007; pp. 30–31.
9. Rayman, M.P. The importance of selenium to human health. *Lancet* **2000**, *356*, 233–241. [CrossRef]
10. Chomchan, R.; Siripongvutikorn, S.; Puttarak, P. Selenium bio-fortification: An alternative to improve phytochemicals and bioactivities of plant foods. *Funct. Foods Health Dis.* **2017**, *7*, 263–279.
11. Devasagayam, T.P.A.; Tilak, J.C.; Boloor, K.K.; Sane, K.S.; Ghaskadbi, S.S.; Lele, R.D. Free radicals, and antioxidants in human health: current status and future prospects. *J. Assoc. Physicians India* **2004**, *52*, 794–804. [PubMed]
12. McGeer, P.L.; McGeer, E.G. Inflammation and the degenerative diseases of aging. *Ann. N. Y. Acad. Sci.* **2004**, *1035*, 104–116. [CrossRef] [PubMed]
13. Wang, Y.D.; Wang, X.; Wong, Y.S. Generation of selenium-enriched rice with enhanced grain yield, selenium content, and bioavailability through fertilisation with selenite. *Food Chem.* **2013**, *141*, 2385–2393. [CrossRef] [PubMed]
14. Singleton, V.L.; Rossi, J.A. Colorimetry of total phenolics with phosphomolybdic-phosphotungstic acid reagents. *Am. J. Enol. Vitic.* **1965**, *16*, 144–158.
15. Louis, K.S.; Siegel, A.C. Cell viability analysis using trypan blue: Manual and automated methods. *Mamm. Cell Viability Methods Protoc.* **2011**, *740*, 7–12.
16. Du, Y.; Esfandi, R.; Willmore, W.G.; Tsopmo, A. Antioxidant activity of oat proteins derived peptides in stressed hepatic HepG2 cells. *Antioxid* **2016**, *5*, 39. [CrossRef] [PubMed]
17. Giannopolitis, C.N.; Ries, S.K. Superoxide dismutases. *Plant Physiol.* **1977**, *59*, 315–318. [CrossRef] [PubMed]
18. Flohé, L.; Günzler, W.A. Assays of glutathione peroxidase. *Methods Enzymol.* **1984**, *105*, 114–120. [PubMed]
19. Brennan, T.; Frenkel, C. Involvement of hydrogen peroxide in the regulation of senescence in pear. *Plant Physiol.* **1977**, *59*, 411–416. [CrossRef] [PubMed]
20. Bradford, M.M. A rapid and sensitive method for the quantitation of microgram quantities of protein utilizing the principle of protein-dye binding. *Anal. Biochem.* **1976**, *72*, 248–254. [CrossRef]

21. Chen, L.; Yang, X.; Jiao, H.; Zhao, B. Tea catechins protect against lead-induced cytotoxicity, lipid peroxidation and membrane fluidity in HepG2 cells. *Toxicol. Sci.* **2002**, *69*, 149–156. [CrossRef] [PubMed]
22. Chomchan, R.; Siripongvutikorn, S.; Puttarak, P.; Rattanapon, R. Influence of selenium bio-fortification on nutritional compositions, bioactive compounds content and anti-oxidative properties of young ricegrass (*Oryza sativa* L.). *Funct. Foods Health Dis.* **2017**, *7*, 195–209.
23. Schiavon, M.; dall'Acqua, S.; Mietto, A.; Pilon-Smits, E.A.; Sambo, P.; Masi, A.; Malagoli, M. Selenium fertilization alters the chemical composition and antioxidant constituents of tomato (*Solanum lycopersicon* L.). *J. Agric. Food Chem.* **2013**, *61*, 10542–10554. [CrossRef] [PubMed]
24. Sae-Lee, N.; Kerdchoechuen, O.; Laohakunjit, N. Chemical qualities and phenolic compounds of Assam tea after soil drench application of selenium and aluminium. *Plant Soil* **2012**, *356*, 381–393. [CrossRef]
25. Hahlbrock, K.; Scheel, D. Physiology and molecular biology of phenylpropanoid metabolism. *Annu. Rev. Plant Biol.* **1989**, *40*, 347–369. [CrossRef]
26. Besson, E.; Dellamonica, G.; Chopin, J.; Markham, K.R.; Kim, M.; Koh, H.-S.; Fukami, H. C-glycosylflavones from *Oryza sativa*. *Phytochemistry* **1985**, *24*, 1061–1064. [CrossRef]
27. Yang, Z.; Nakabayashi, R.; Okazaki, Y.; Mori, T.; Takamatsu, S.; Kitanaka, S.; Kikuchi, J.; Saito, K. Toward better annotation in plant metabolomics: Isolation and structure elucidation of 36 specialized metabolites from *Oryza sativa* (rice) by using MS/MS and NMR analyses. *Metabolomics* **2014**, *10*, 543–555. [CrossRef] [PubMed]
28. Kim, J.H.; Cheon, Y.M.; Kim, B.-G.; Ahn, J.-H. Analysis of flavonoids and characterization of the OsFNS gene involved in flavone biosynthesis in rice. *J. Plant Biol.* **2008**, *51*, 97. [CrossRef]
29. Moheb, A.; Agharbaoui, Z.; Kanapathy, F.; Ibrahim, R.K.; Roy, R.; Sarhan, F. Tricin biosynthesis during growth of wheat under different abiotic stresses. *Plant Sci.* **2013**, *201*, 115–120. [CrossRef] [PubMed]
30. Zhao, X.-Q.; Wang, W.-S.; Zhang, F.; Zhang, T.; Zhao, W.; Fu, B.-Y.; Li, Z.-K. Temporal profiling of primary metabolites under chilling stress and its association with seedling chilling tolerance of rice (*Oryza sativa* L.). *Rice* **2013**, *6*, 23. [CrossRef] [PubMed]
31. Fang, N.; Yu, S.; Prior, R.L. LC/MS/MS characterization of phenolic constituents in dried plums. *J. Agric. Food Chem.* **2002**, *50*, 3579–3585. [CrossRef] [PubMed]
32. Sulaiman, C.; Gopalakrishnan, V.; Balachandran, I. Reverse phase liquid chromatography coupled with quadra pole-time of flight mass spectrometry for the characterization of phenolics from *Acacia catechu* (L.f.) willd. *Int. J. Phytomed.* **2012**, *4*, 403–408.
33. Markham, K.R.; Tanner, G.J.; Caasi-Lit, M.; Whitecross, M.I.; Nayudu, M.; Mitchell, K.A. Possible protective role for 3′,4′-dihydroxyflavones induced by enhanced UV-B in a UV-tolerant rice cultivar. *Phytochemistry* **1998**, *49*, 1913–1919. [CrossRef]
34. Cekici, A.; Kantarci, A.; Hasturk, H.; Van Dyke, T.E. Inflammatory and immune pathways in the pathogenesis of periodontal disease. *Periodontology 2000* **2014**, *64*, 57–80. [CrossRef] [PubMed]
35. Ioset, J.-R.; Brun, R.; Wenzler, T.; Kaiser, M.; Yardley, V. Drug Screening for Kinetoplastids Diseases—A Training Manual for Screening in Neglected Diseases. Available online: https://www.dndi.org/wp-content/uploads/2009/04/kinetoplastid_drug_screening_manual_final.pdf (accessed on 20 February 2018).
36. Genuardi, J.; Eskew, M.; Zeligs, B.; Bellanti, J. The effects of vitamin E and selenium on the nitric oxide production of macrophages. *Pediatr. Res.* **1999**, *45*, 771. [CrossRef]
37. Halliwell, B. Reactive oxygen species in living systems: Source, biochemistry, and role in human disease. *Am. J. Med.* **1991**, *91*, S14–S22. [CrossRef]
38. Ray Halder, S.; Bhattacharyya, M. Oxidative stress: Lipid peroxidation products as predictors in disease progression. *J. Exp. Integr. Med.* **2014**, *4*, 151–164. [CrossRef]
39. Ayala, A.; Muñoz, M.F.; Argüelles, S. Lipid peroxidation: Production, metabolism, and signaling mechanisms of malondialdehyde and 4-hydroxy-2-nonenal. *Oxid. Med. Cell. Longev.* **2014**, *2014*, 1–31. [CrossRef] [PubMed]
40. Mates, J. Effects of antioxidant enzymes in the molecular control of reactive oxygen species toxicology. *Toxicology* **2000**, *153*, 83–104. [CrossRef]
41. Yeh, C.T.; Yen, G.C. Induction of hepatic antioxidant enzymes by phenolic acids in rats is accompanied by increased levels of multidrug resistance-associated protein 3 mRNA expression. *J. Nutr.* **2006**, *136*, 11–15. [CrossRef] [PubMed]

42. Sharma, J.; Al-Omran, A.; Parvathy, S. Role of nitric oxide in inflammatory diseases. *Inflammopharmacology* **2007**, *15*, 252–259. [CrossRef] [PubMed]
43. Kim, Y.J.; Park, W. Anti-inflammatory effect of quercetin on raw 264.7 mouse macrophages induced with polyinosinic-polycytidylic acid. *Molecules* **2016**, *21*, 450. [CrossRef] [PubMed]
44. Panico, A.; Cardile, V.; Avondo, S.; Garufi, F.; Gentile, B.; Puglia, C.; Bonina, F.; Santagati, N.; Ronsisvalle, G. The in vitro effect of a lyophilized extract of wine obtained from Jacquez grapes on human chondrocytes. *Phytomed* **2006**, *13*, 522–526. [CrossRef] [PubMed]
45. Terra, X.; Montagut, G.; Bustos, M.; Llopiz, N.; Ardèvol, A.; Bladé, C.; Fernández-Larrea, J.; Pujadas, G.; Salvadó, J.; Arola, L. Grape-seed procyanidins prevent low-grade inflammation by modulating cytokine expression in rats fed a high-fat diet. *J. Nutr. Biochem.* **2009**, *20*, 210–218. [CrossRef] [PubMed]
46. Chuang, C.C.; McIntosh, M.K. Potential mechanisms by which polyphenol-rich grapes prevent obesity-mediated inflammation and metabolic diseases. *Annu. Rev. Nutr.* **2011**, *31*, 155–176. [CrossRef] [PubMed]
47. Chen, Y.C.; Shen, S.C.; Lee, W.R.; Hou, W.C.; Yang, L.L.; Lee, T.J. Inhibition of nitric oxide synthase inhibitors and lipopolysaccharide-induced inducible nos and cyclooxygenase-2 gene expressions by rutin, quercetin, and quercetin pentaacetate in RAW264.7 macrophages. *J. Cell. Biochem.* **2001**, *82*, 537–548. [CrossRef] [PubMed]
48. Prabhu, K.S.; Zamamiri-Davis, F.; Stewart, J.B.; Thompson, J.T.; Sordillo, L.M.; Reddy, C.C. Selenium deficiency increases the expression of inducible nitric oxide synthase in RAW264.7 macrophages: Role of nuclear factor-κb in up-regulation. *Biochem. J.* **2002**, *366*, 203–209. [CrossRef] [PubMed]
49. Verma, A.K.; Kumar, A.; Rahal, A.; Kumar, V.; Roy, D. Inorganic versus organic selenium supplementation: A review. *Pak. J. Biol. Sci.* **2012**, *15*, 418–425.

Effect of the Extraction Process on the Biological Activity of Lyophilized Apricot Extracts Recovered from Apricot Pomace

Dina Cheaib [1], Nada El Darra [2,*], Hiba N. Rajha [3], Iman El-Ghazzawi [2], Richard G. Maroun [3] and Nicolas Louka [3]

1 Faculty of Sciences, Beirut Arab University, P.O. Box 115020, Riad El Solh, Beirut 1107 2809, Lebanon; dac273@student.bau.edu.lb
2 Faculty of Health Sciences, Beirut Arab University, Tarik El Jedidah—Beirut, P.O. Box 115020, Riad El Solh, Beirut 1107 2809, Lebanon; i.ghazzawi@bau.edu.lb
3 Unité de Recherche Technologies et Valorisation Agro-alimentaire, Centre d'Analyses et de Recherche, Faculté des Sciences, Université Saint-Joseph de Beyrouth, B.P. 11-514 Riad El Solh, Beirut 1107 2050, Lebanon; hiba.rajha@usj.edu.lb (H.N.R.); richard.maroun@usj.edu.lb (R.G.M.); nicolas.louka@usj.edu.lb (N.L.)
* Correspondence: n.aldarra@bau.edu.lb

Abstract: The preservation of polyphenols in fruits by lyophilization has gained great interest in the recent decades. The present study aims to assess the impact of the pre-treatment extraction methods heat-assisted extraction (HAE) and infrared (IR) on lyophilized apricot pomace extracts. Then to test the conservation of polyphenols quantities as well as their bioactivities (antiradical and antibacterial) in lyophilized extract. An aqueous extract was obtained through either heat-assisted extraction or infrared pre-treatments then lyophilized to obtain a dried form. Results showed that the content of polyphenols, the antiradical and antibacterial activities in lyophilized extracts exhibited a slighter decrease in infrared sample compared to the heat-assisted extraction ones. The High-performance liquid chromatography (HPLC) analysis showed that lyophilized extracts IR and HAE preserved the same phenolic molecules (rutin, catechin and epicatechin) detected in liquid extracts (IR and HAE) with a smaller yield. Lyophilization can be used as a widely process in the food industry to conserve many bioactive molecules.

Keywords: lyophilization; apricot pomace; heat-assisted extraction; infrared; polyphenols

1. Introduction

In the last decade, phenolic compounds have gained a considerable interest due to their different biological properties [1]. They are closely linked with the nutritional and sensory quality of fruits and vegetables [2,3]. The phenolic composition and the biological properties of fruits can be affected by different factors such as variety, climate, harvest time, storage as well as post-harvest processes like drying, cutting, storage, packaging, fermentation, and cooking processing [4,5]. In order to preserve the nutritional components of fruits (such as vitamins and carotenoids), it is generally recommended to dry product by lyophilization or (freeze-drying). The latter is known to be an effective method used to preserve a wide variety of materials (such as proteins, microbes, tissues and plasma), produce commercial products (pharmaceutical, natural additives, and preservatives for food industries) and to extend the shelf-life of foods by preventing the microbial growth, inhibiting enzymatic degradation, and retarding lipid oxidation [6–9]. On the other hand, during the lyophilization process, there might be a chance of decrease in the antioxidant property caused by the degradation of certain bioactive compounds (such as phenolic compounds, ascorbic acid) [10,11]. In order to protect polyphenols from freeze-drying, a maltodextrin precoating process may be applied before the drying process [12]. Many studies compared the nutritional composition of fresh and freeze-dried fruits and vegetables. A loss of certain vitamins (vitamins A and C) was noted, as well as a decrease in the nutritional value in some vegetables due to the freeze-drying process [9,10,13]. Moreover, a decrease in total phenolic content in freeze-dried mango fruits compared to fresh ones (from 14 to 17 mg gallic acid equivalent (GAE)/100 g dry sample) was showed by Rahman et al. (2015) [14]. However, the comparison between liquid and lyophilized extract compositions obtained by different extraction techniques have not been well explored. The infrared-assisted extraction (IRAE) technique (with wavelength range between 1.72 and 16.66 μm) is conducted with an infrared lamp. IRAE is used as a heat source due to its highest efficiency when its wavelength matches the absorption properties of the material it is warming [15,16]. Compared to other conventional techniques (heat assisted extraction and microwave assisted extraction), infrared is easy to use and could enhance the extraction yield of many bioactive molecules from medicinal plants [17].

Due to the diverse application fields of phenolic compounds, their extraction and isolation from fruits byproducts have been widely studied. However, the impact of extraction methods (as a pre-treatment) on the lyophilization process has not been yet documented.

The present work aims first to study the impact of the extraction methods; heat-assisted extraction (HAE) and infrared (IR) on lyophilized apricot pomace extracts and second, to test the conservation of polyphenols quantities as well as their bioactivities (antiradical and antibacterial) in lyophilized extract (powder-dried form).

2. Materials and Methods

2.1. Raw Materials

Apricot pomace was obtained from Conserves Modernes Chtaura (Chtaura, Lebanon); this industry is specialized in the production of fruit purees and jams. The pomace is made of pressed skins and pulp residues (of fresh apricots).

2.2. Extraction Experiments

The extraction conditions were conducted at different durations in order to reach the same energy consumption of 2290.90 kJ/kg for the infrared and the heat-assisted extraction methods.

2.2.1. Infrared-Assisted Extraction

The infrared-assisted extraction apparatus was designed at Faculté des Sciences, Université Saint Joseph de Beyrouth (Beirut, Lebanon). It consists of a ceramic infrared transmitter with a power between 63 and 170 W to conduct the heating process connected to a proportional–integral–derivative (PID) control and temperature adjustment system. The temperature and the voltage can be regulated manually or automatically. This apparatus utilize infrared energy from the ceramic to heat the solvent sample mixture placed in a round bottom flask and set at a variable distance away from the ceramic transmitter. An amount of 10 g of apricot pomace was mixed with 100 mL of preheated water (75 °C) in the round-bottom flask and placed on the top of the ceramic transmitter. The temperature was fixed at 75 °C for 60 min (according to a preliminary study). The infrared (IR) energy W_{IR} (kJ/kg) was calculated:

$$W_{IR} = \frac{P_{IR} \times t_{IR}}{m} \tag{1}$$

where P_{IR} is the generator power (70 W), t_{IR} is the total extraction duration (s), and m is the product mass (g). Note that m = 110 g (100 g water + 10 g dry matter) and W_{IR} is the energy consumed (2290.90 kJ/kg).

2.2.2. Heat-Assisted Extraction

The heat-assisted extraction was conducted using a water bath with a power of 660 W. The glass flask containing 10 g of apricot pomace mixed in 100 mL of preheated water at 75 °C, and then covered by aluminum foil in order to avoid polyphenol degradation. The temperature of the water bath was fixed at 75 °C.

The time required for the heat-assisted extraction t_{HAE} (s) to reach the same energy of infrared technique was calculated as follows:

$$t_{HAE} = \frac{W_{HAE} \times m}{P_{HAE}} \quad (2)$$

where W_{HAE} is the energy consumed (2290.90 kJ/kg), P_{HAE} is the generator power (660 W), m is the product mass (g) and t_{HAE} is the total extraction duration (s) (which is 6 min).

The extracts were then filtered using glass wool before analysis.

2.3. Lyophilization

Liquid samples were placed in petri dishes (7 mm), then frozen at −20 °C and finally lyophilized at −55 °C under vacuum (Ilshin Lab. Co., Ltd., Yangju-si, Korea) for 48 h.

2.4. Analysis

2.4.1. Dry Matter Content

The analysis of the dry matter content of the raw material was carried out by weighing an specific amount of sample and drying it for 24 h using a ventilated oven at 105 °C [18].

2.4.2. Quantification of Total Polyphenol Content by Folin-Ciocalteu Method

In accordance with the Folin Ciocalteu (FC) method, 0.2 mL of the extract, 0.1 mL of commercial FC reagent and 0.8 mL of sodium carbonate solution (75 mg/L) were mixed and kept for 10 min at 60 °C [19]. The absorbance of the extracts was then read at 750 nm by a spectrophotometer UV-VIS (Gold S54T UV-VIS, Shanghai, China). The absorbance values were compared to a standard curve of prepared gallic acid solutions and expressed as milligram of gallic acid equivalents (GAE) per gram (g) of dry matter (mg GAE/g DM).

2.4.3. Determination of the Antiradical Activity

The free radical scavenging activity was determined by the capacity of the phenolic molecules in the samples to reduce DPPH (2,2-diphenyl-picrylhydrazyl), a stable free radical. In brief, 4 mL of 1 mM DPPH was mixed with 0.2 mL of the extract. The absorbance at 517 nm of the extracts was measured after 30 min at room temperature using methanol as a blank. The decrease in the absorbance allowed the calculation of the inhibition percentage. Two models were represented; the percentage of inhibition at the initial concentration of the extracts and the inhibition percentage at a fixed concentration of polyphenols (2.7 mg GAE/g DM) in order to determine the influence of their diversity [20].

2.4.4. HPLC-DAD Analysis

Polyphenol analyses of the liquid extracts and lyophilized dried from prepared from apricot pomace were performed by High-Performance Liquid Chromatography (HPLC). Prior to analytical chromatography.

The samples were purified by filtration through 0.2 μm syringe filters to remove interferences of sugars and organic acids from the crude samples. An equipment consisting of liquid-chromatography-Agilent 1100 Series system (Teknokroma Professional Friendly Lichrospher 100 RP18 5 μM, 25 × 0.46, Serial number NF-21378, Barcelona, Spain), equipped with an autosampler, a Zorbax column oven (Barcelona, Spain), coupled to a diode array detector. The separation of polyphenols was performed through a C18 Column (25 × 0.46 mm). The standards used for identification and quantification purchased from Sigma (Aldrich) were: trans-cinnamic acid, caffeic acid, epicatechin, hydroxybenzoic acid, chlorogenic acid, catechin, rutin, gallic acid, kaempferol, catechin gallate and myrecetin (purity $\geq$ 98%). The mobile phase consisted of acidified nanopure water at pH 2.3 with HCl (A) and acetonitrile (B) HPLC grade. The elution was done under isocratic conditions from 0 to 5 min with (85%) A and (15%) B. Gradient profile was from 5 to 30 min, beginning with (85%) A and (15%) B and ending with (0%) A and (100%) B. It was followed by isocratic conditions from 30 to 35 min with (0%) A and (100%) B. The injection volume was 10 μL and the flow rate was 1 mL/min. Based on the retention time and the spectra of the original standard each peak was identified. Quantification was accomplished using the phenolic standards solutions [21].

2.4.5. Determination of the Antibacterial Activity

Bacterial Strains, Culture Media and Growth Conditions

For the antibacterial activity; eight clinical bacterial strains were studied: two strains of *Staphylococcus aureus*, amongst which, one is *Methicillin-Resistant Staphylococcus Aureus* (MRSA 3); one strain of *Coagulase-negative Staphylococci* (1530), one strain of *Staphylococcus epidermidis* (2080), two strains of *Klebsiella*, amongst which, one is Metallo-beta-lactamase producer and two strains of *Escherichia coli* amongst which, one is extended spectrum beta lactamase (ESBL 2238).

Preparation of the Bacterial Inocula for Minimum Inhibitory Concentration (MIC)

All strains were subcultured using freshly-prepared blood agar. Part of five colonies of each strain were inoculated in 3 mL of cation adjusted Mueller Hinton broth. After reaching a turbidity of 0.5 McFarland, a dilution of 1/100 was made into tubes of adjusted Mueller Hinton broth.

Phenolic Extracts Preparation for MIC Assessment

Five serial dilutions of each extracts (infrared and solid-liquid) were conducted (starting from 1.6 to 26 μg/mL). Before the analysis, all stocks were sterilized using 0.4 μm disposable syringe filters. After the addition of equal volumes (100 μL) of each concentration of the four extracts to the bacterial strains (100 μL) in a 96 well (U shape) microtiter plates, the final concentrations of the different phenolic extracts were reduced to: 13.5 μg/mL up to 0.8 μg/mL. Two plates were utilized in this experiment. Finally, the plates of each of the phenolic extracts were read for the MIC that inhibits the bacterial growth after an overnight incubation at 37 °C.

2.4.6. Statistical Analysis

Each experiment was conducted in duplicates and analysis repeated twice. Means and standard deviations of data were calculated. The error bars in all figures correspond to the standard errors. Variance analyses (ANOVA) and Least Significant Difference test (LSD) were conducted to evaluate the significant differences between the results. STATGRAPHICS® Centurion XV (StatPoint Technologies, Inc., Warrenton, VA, USA) was used to perform statistical analysis.

3. Results and Discussion

3.1. Total Polyphenols Content

Figure 1 represents the total phenolic content of apricot pomace extracts liquid and lyophilized (HAE and IR). IR lyophilized gave higher phenolic content compared to HAE lyophilized. On the other hand HAE lyophilized showed a decrease of 32% (ranging from 4 to 2.7 mg GAE/g DM) of phenolic content compared to HAE liquid extract while IR lyophilized showed a slight decrease 16% (ranging from 10.8 to 9 mg GAE/g DM) of the total phenolic content compared to IR liquid extract. Many studies showed a reduction in polyphenolic yield from lyophilized fruits and vegetables compared to fresh ones. Georgé et al. (2010) found that the total polyphenol content of yellow tomatoes, decreased by 30% in lyophilized tomato compared to fresh ones [22]. Moreover the level of phenolic compounds in some tropical fruits (watermelon, papaya, mango and melon) decreased by 48.23%, 39.73%, 23.19% and 10.41% respectively after freeze drying process [10].

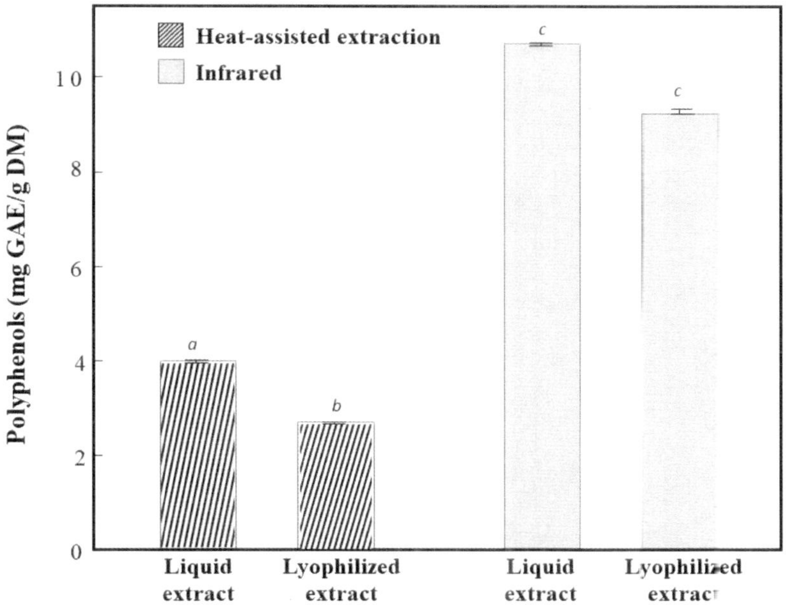

Figure 1. Polyphenol content of heat-assisted extraction and infrared apricot pomace extracts (liquid and lyophilized). Different superscript letters indicate significant statistical difference ($p < 0.05$).

This decrease in the polyphenols content in lyophilized fruits and vegetables products could be due to the rupture of the cell wall caused by ice crystals formation and the subsequent release of hydrolytic and oxidative enzymes (which are not fully deactivated) which cause a degradation in phenolic compounds [22–24]. However, in our study a liquid extract was subjected to lyophilization and, thus, no cells were found in the lyophilized sample. This decrease in polyphenolic yield in lyophilized extract could be attributed to the changes in the structure of the extracted molecules (phenolic compounds) which was reported by Deladino et al. (2013) who showed a reduction in polyphenol content by 20% in lyophilized extract compared to liquid one from Yerba mate (*Ilex paraguariensis*) [25]. Although freeze-drying appears to be an effective method of preservation, its effect on polyphenolic molecules is variable depending on the method of extraction, type of solvent used and sample matrix [26]. Regarding the extraction technique, the slight decrease of phenolic content in IR lyophilized compared to the HAE one could be explained by the mode of action of the extraction method which affects the cellular structure differently. IR radiation directly heats the sample matrix which could extract more bioactive compounds, while in conventional techniques more time is required to heat the vessel before the energy of heating is transferred to the sample mixture [15]. Moreover, the efficiency of the IR recovery can be attributed to the matching between the infrared wavelength and the absorption characteristics of the solvent [17].

3.2. Biological Activities

3.2.1. Antiradical Activity (AA)

Figure 2a represents the antiradical activity (AA) of apricot pomace liquid extracts and lyophilized (HAE and IR) at their initial concentration. HAE lyophilized showed a decrease of 46% of AA compared to HAE liquid extract, while IR lyophilized showed a 10% decrease compared to IR liquid extract. These findings could be correlated to the higher decrease in polyphenols content in HAE lyophilized compared to IR lyophilized (Figure 1). On the other hand, at the same polyphenol concentration (Figure 2b), IR lyophilized exhibited a better AA than HAE lyophilized sample. These results could be attributed to the different polyphenol composition, responsible for the enhancement of the radical scavenging activity in each method of extraction [27]. To confirm this hypothesis, HPLC analysis was conducted in our study to identify the phenolic compounds responsible for the antiradical activity. The antiradical activity results showed that lyophilized sample exhibited an AA, which was more conserved in the infrared sample than in the heat-assisted extraction extract.

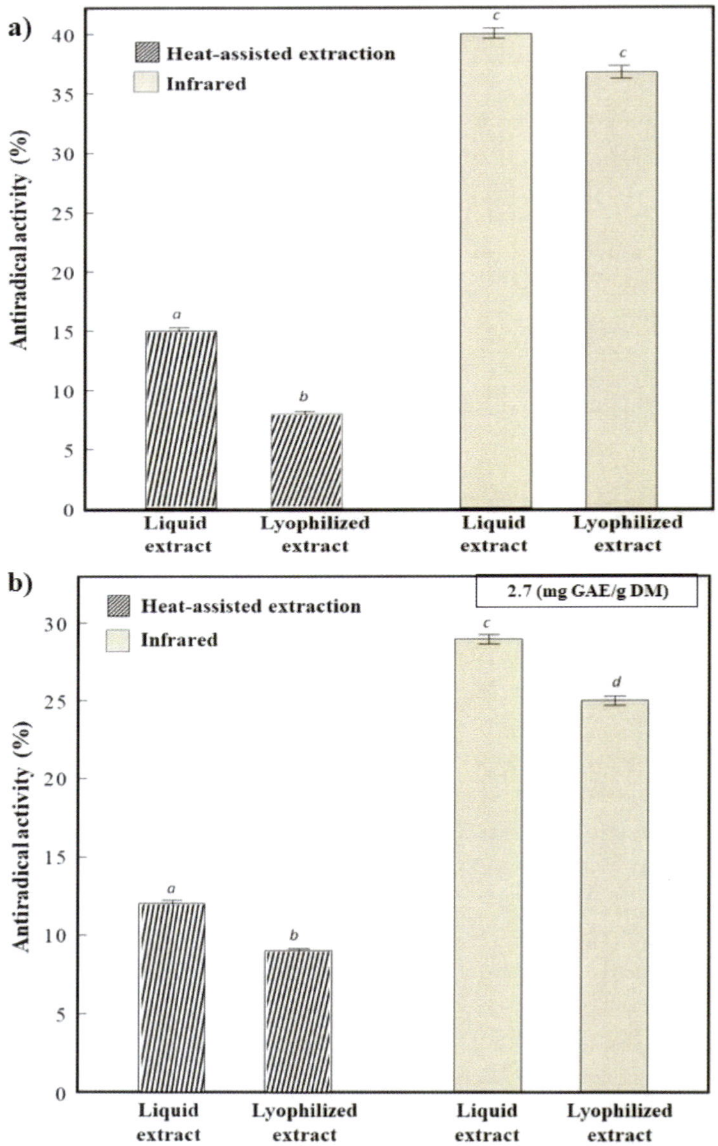

Figure 2. Antiradical activity of heat-assisted extraction and infrared apricot pomace extracts (liquid and lyophilized). (**a**) at their initial concentration and (**b**) at 2.7 mg GAE/g DM of polyphenols. Different superscript letters indicate significant statistical difference ($p < 0.05$).

3.2.2. Antibacterial Activity of the Apricot Pomace Liquid and Lyophilized Extracts

The antibacterial activity of apricot pomace liquid and lyophilized extracts treated by HAE and IR technique were tested against different Gram-positive strains and Gram-negative bacterial strains

(Table 1) using MIC for the different concentrations 13.5 μg/mL, 6.75 μg/mL, 3.3 μg/mL, 1.6 μg/mL, and 0.8 μg/mL. HAE and IR lyophilized samples showed antibacterial activity. IR liquid extract exhibited the lowest inhibitory concentration denoting the highest inhibitory bacterial activity against all Gram-positive strains and one Gram-negative strain. IR lyophilized showed antibacterial activity against the same bacterial strains tested for IR liquid but the minimum inhibitory concentration (MIC) was higher for the IR lyophilized. On the other hand, HAE (liquid and lyophilized extracts) showed the highest MIC exhibiting, the lowest inhibition against only two Gram-positive in comparison with IR liquid and lyophilized extracts respectively. The antibacterial results are in concordance with the radical scavenging activity, where the IR liquid extract gave the highest activity followed by IR lyophilized and HAE liquid extract. The HAE lyophilized gave the lowest antibacterial activity. Table showed that the effect of polyphenols was only against one Gram-negative bacterial strain compared to Gram-positive ones. Those results can be explained by the fact that phenolic molecules have higher activity against gram-positive bacteria in comparison to gram-negative ones. The latter have an outer membrane in their cell wall which plays a role of a barrier and thus decreasing the uptake. Moreover, the reduction of the activity of polyphenols in some bacteria could be also due to other mechanism of resistance such as the mutation in porin protein or the efflux phenomena [28,29]. Our findings showed that lyophilized samples preserved their antibacterial activity with increased inhibition concentrations compared to (IR and HAE) liquid extracts.

Table 1. Minimum inhibitory concentration (μg/mL) of different Gram-positive and Gram-negative bacteria from heat-assisted extraction (HAE) and infrared (IR) apricot pomace extracts (liquid and lyophilized).

	Minimum Inhibitory Concentration (μg/mL)			
	Heat-Assisted Extraction		Infrared	
Bacterica/POMs	Liquid Extract	Lyophilized Extract	Liquid Extract	Lyophilized Extract
Methicillin Resistant Staphylococcus aureus (MRSA3) (gram+)	-	-	6.75	13.5
Staphylococcus aureus 1966 (gram+)	6.75	13.5	3.3	6.75
Coagulase-negative Staphylococci 1530 (gram+)	-	-	3.3	6.75
Staphylococcus epidermidis 2080 (gram+)	6.75	13.5	3.3	6.75
Klebsiella 118 metallo beta lactamase + (gram−)	-	-	-	-
Klebsiella (gram−)	-	-	-	-
E. coli ESBL 2238 (gram−)	-	-	-	-
Escherichia coli (1250) (gram−)	-	-	6.75	13.5

- indicates absence of antibacterial activity.

3.3. *Quantification of Polyphenol Extracts by High-Performance Liquid Chromatography*

The composition of polyphenol in apricot pomace extracts and lyophilized (IR and HAE) was shown in Figure 3a. The chromatographic profile of the several phenolic compounds from different extracts was shown in Figure 3b. The main polyphenols were rutin, catechin and epicatechin which was consistent with the results of Veberic and Stampar (2005) on the polyphenol composition in apricot varieties [30]. Rutin was found in all samples. However, catechin and epicatechin were only detected in infrared liquid and lyophilized extracts suggesting the selectivity of IR towards those compounds. IR liquid and lyophilized extracts showed the highest extraction yield for all the detected polyphenol compounds compared to HAE extract and HAE lyophilized respectively.

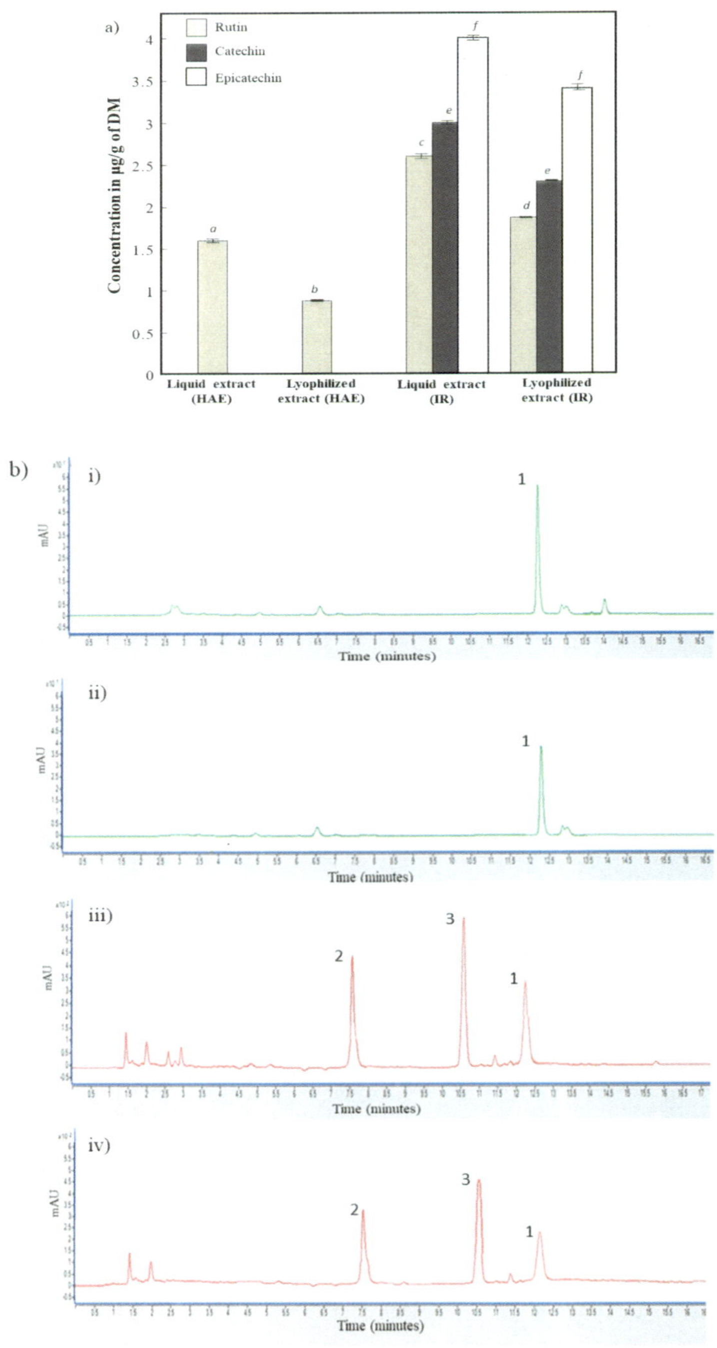

Figure 3. (**a**) Polyphenols composition of heat-assisted extraction and infrared apricot pomace extracts (liquid and lyophilized). Different superscript letters indicate significant statistical difference ($p < 0.05$). **(b)** Chromatographic profile of the several phenolic compounds 1: Rutin, 2: catechin and 3: epicatechin of: i: liquid HAE, ii: lyophilized HAE, iii: liquid IR and iv: lyophilized IR.

Figure 3 showed that lyophilized samples (IR and HAE) preserved the same phenolic molecules detected in liquid extracts (IR and HAE) with a smaller yield. Rutin in HAE lyophilized decreased by 45% compared to IR lyophilized which showed a reduction of 34%. Our results are in accordance with those of Lorena Deladino et al. (2013) who found that the amounts of rutin in the lyophilized sample was lower (by 28%) than in the liquid extract from Yerba mate [25]. Concerning catechin and epicatechin, their concentrations decreased by 26% and 22% in IR lyophilized, respectively.

Those results showed that lyophilization process depends not only on the technique of extraction (pretreatment) but also on the structure of the extracted molecules [22]. The Freeze-drying process can alter some phenolic compounds (rutin) more than others (catechin and epicatechin) as shown in Figure 3.

4. Conclusions

In conclusion, the content of polyphenols and the antiradical and antibacterial activities in the lyophilized samples showed a slighter decrease in infrared samples than in heat-assisted extraction ones. After lyophilization process, the same phenolic compounds were identified in lyophilized extracts, which could explain the preservation of their biological activities especially in infrared samples. The latter seems to better preserve the structure of the extracted molecules in comparison to heat assisted extraction method which showed more decrease in polyphenol yield. This difference in polyphenolic content could be due to mode of action of each technique; the heat-assisted extraction method seems to fragilize more the extracted molecules which become more vulnerable to lyophilization treatment. Since the freeze-drying process is a widely used technique to stabilize plant material over a long duration, it could be of interest to determine the factors or mechanisms that could affect the phenolic content and biological activities during this process.

Author Contributions: Dina Cheaib, the main author, is a PhD student at the Faculty of Sciences, Beirut Arab University. Dina Cheaib proposed the idea, performed the experiments as well as analyzed the data and wrote the manuscript. Nada El Darra is the co-supervisor, who assisted Dina Cheaib in the design of the experimental setup, and contributed to the writing and correction of the manuscript. Hiba N. Rajha assisted Dina Cheaib in the implementation of some experiments and contributed to the correction of the manuscript. Iman El-Ghazzawi assisted Dina Cheaib in the implementation of the antibacterial experiment. Nicolas Louka is the main supervisor, who assisted in the development of the proposal and, the design of the experiments, and contributed to writing and correction of the manuscript. Richard G. Maroun initiated the work and contributed to the project design.

Conflicts of Interest: The authors declare no conflict of interest. We hereby certify that the work we are submitting is original and that all authors have contributed significantly and are in agreement with the manuscript.

References

1. Balasundram, N.; Sundram, K.; Samman, S. Phenolic compounds in plants and agri-industrial by-products: Antioxidant activity, occurrence, and potential uses. *Food Chem.* **2006**, *99*, 191–203. [CrossRef]
2. Rinaldo, D.; Mbéguié-A-Mbéguié, D.; Fils-Lycaon, B. Advances on polyphenols and their metabolism in sub-tropical and tropical fruits. *Trends Food Sci. Technol.* **2010**, *21*, 599–606. [CrossRef]
3. Ames, B.N.; Shigenaga, M.K.; Hagen, T.M. Oxidants, antioxidants, and the degenerative diseases of aging. *Proc. Natl. Acad. Sci. USA* **1993**, *90*, 7915–7922. [CrossRef] [PubMed]
4. Patthamakanokporn, O.; Puwastien, P.; Nitithamyong, A.; Sirichakwal, P.P. Changes of antioxidant activity and total phenolic compounds during storage of selected fruits. *J. Food Compos. Anal.* **2008**, *21*, 241–248. [CrossRef]
5. Rodrigues, A.S.; Pérez-Gregorio, M.R.; García-Falcón, M.S.; Simal-Gándara, J. Effect of curing and cooking on flavonols and anthocyanins in traditional varieties of onion bulbs. *Food Res. Int.* **2009**, *42*, 1331–1336. [CrossRef]
6. Franks, F. Freeze-drying of bioproducts: Putting principles into practice. *Eur. J. Pharm. Biopharm.* **1998**, *45*, 221–229. [CrossRef]
7. Abdelwahed, W.; Degobert, G.; Stainmesse, S.; Fessi, H. Freeze-drying of nanoparticles: Formulation, process and storage considerations. *Adv. Drug Deliv. Rev.* **2006**, *58*, 1688–1713. [CrossRef] [PubMed]
8. Pérez-Gregorio, M.R.; Regueiro, J.; González-Barreiro, C.; Rial-Otero, R.; Simal-Gándara, J. Changes in antioxidant flavonoids during freeze-drying of red onions and subsequent storage. *Food Control* **2011**, *22*, 1108–1113. [CrossRef]
9. Chang, C.H.; Lin, H.Y.; Chang, C.Y.; Liu, Y.C. Comparisons on the antioxidant properties of fresh, freeze-dried and hot-air-dried tomatoes. *J. Food Eng.* **2006**, *77*, 478–485. [CrossRef]
10. Shofian, N.M.; Hamid, A.A.; Osman, A.; Saari, N.; Anwar, F.; Pak Dek, M.S.; Hairuddin, M.R. Effect of freeze-drying on the antioxidant compounds and antioxidant activity of selected tropical fruits. *Int. J. Mol. Sci.* **2011**, *12*, 4678–4692. [CrossRef] [PubMed]

11. Marques, L.G.; Silveira, A.M.; Freire, J.T. Freeze-drying characteristics of tropical fruits. *Dry. Technol.* **2006**, *24*, 457–463. [CrossRef]
12. Cai, Y.Z.; Corke, H. Production and Properties of Spray-dried Amaranthus Betacyanin Pigments. *J. Food Sci.* **2000**, *65*, 1248–1252. [CrossRef]
13. Murcia, M.A.; López-Ayerra, B.; Martinez-Tomé, M.; Vera, A.M.; García-Carmona, F. Evolution of ascorbic acid and peroxidase during industrial processing of broccoli. *J. Sci. Food Agric.* **2000**, *80*, 1882–1886. [CrossRef]
14. Rahman, M.M.; Das, R.; Hoque, M.M.; Zzaman, W. Effect of freeze drying on antioxidant activity and phenolic contents of mango (Mangifera indica). *Int. Food Res. J.* **2015**, *22*, 613–617.
15. Cai, Y.; Yu, Y.; Duan, G.; Li, Y. Study on infrared-assisted extraction coupled with high performance liquid chromatography (HPLC) for determination of catechin, epicatechin, and procyanidin B2 in grape seeds. *Food Chem.* **2011**, *127*, 1872–1877. [CrossRef]
16. Qu, Y.; Li, C.; Zhang, C.; Zeng, R.; Fu, C. Optimization of infrared-assisted extraction of *Bletilla striata* polysaccharides based on response surface methodology and their antioxidant activities. *Carbohydr. Polym.* **2016**, *148*, 345–353. [CrossRef] [PubMed]
17. Chen, Y.; Duan, G.; Xie, M.; Chen, B.; Li, Y. Infrared-assisted extraction coupled with high-performance liquid chromatography for simultaneous determination of eight active compounds in *Radix Salviae miltiorrhizae*. *J. Sep. Sci.* **2010**, *33*, 2888–2897. [CrossRef] [PubMed]
18. Madrau, M.A.; Piscopo, A.; Sanguinetti, A.M.; Del Caro, A.; Poiana, M.; Romeo, F.V.; Piga, A. Effect of drying temperature on polyphenolic content and antioxidant activity of apricots. *Eur. Food Res. Technol.* **2009**, *228*, 441–448. [CrossRef]
19. Slinkard, K.; Singleton, V. Total phenol analysis: Automation and comparison with manual methods. *Am. J. Enol. Vitic.* **1977**, *28*, 49–55.
20. Zhang, D.; Hamauzu, Y. Phenolic compounds, ascorbic acid, carotenoids and antioxidant properties of green, red and yellow bell peppers. *J. Food Agric. Environ.* **2003**, *1*, 22–27.
21. Vizzotto, M.; Cisneros-zevallos, L.; Byrne, D.H. Large Variation Found in the Phytochemical and Antioxidant Activity of Peach and Plum Germplasm. *J. Am. Soc. Hortic. Sci.* **2007**, *132*, 334–340.
22. Georgé, S.; Tourniaire, F.; Gautier, H.; Goupy, P.; Rock, E.; Caris-Veyrat, C. Changes in the contents of carotenoids, phenolic compounds and vitamin C during technical processing and lyophilisation of red and yellow tomatoes. *Food Chem.* **2011**, *124*, 1603–1611. [CrossRef]
23. Liliana, S.-C.; Diana, P.V.-M.; Alfredo, A.A. Structural, physical, functional and nutraceutical changes of freeze-dried fruit. *Afr. J. Biotechnol.* **2015**, *14*, 442–450. [CrossRef]
24. Alfaro, S.; Mutis, A.; Quiroz, A.; Seguel, I.; Scheuermann, E. Effects of Drying Techniques on Murtilla Fruit Polyphenols and Antioxidant Activity. *J. Food Res.* **2014**, *3*, 73. [CrossRef]
25. Deladino, L.; Teixeira, A.S.; Reta, M.; García, A.D.M.; Navarro, A.S.; Martino, M.N. Major phenolics in yerba mate extracts (*Ilex paraguariensis*) and their contribution to the total antioxidant capacity. *Food Nutr. Sci.* **2013**, *4*, 154–162. [CrossRef]
26. Abascal, K.; Ganora, L.; Yarnell, E. The effect of freeze-drying and its implications for botanical medicine: A review. *Phytother. Res.* **2005**, *19*, 655–660. [CrossRef] [PubMed]
27. Hasmida, M.N.; Nur Syukriah, A.R.; Liza, M.S.; Mohd Azizi, C.Y. Effect of different extraction techniques on total phenolic content and antioxidant activity of quercus infectoria galls. *Int. Food Res. J.* **2014**, *21*, 1039–1043.
28. Delcour, A.H. Outer Membrane Permeability and Antibiotic Resistance. *Biochim. Biophys. Acta* **2009**, *1794*, 808–816. [CrossRef] [PubMed]
29. Russell, A.D. Similarities and differences in the responses of microorganisms to biocides 1. *J. Antimicrob. Chemother.* **2003**, *52*, 750–763. [CrossRef] [PubMed]
30. Veberic, R.; Stampar, F. Selected polyphenols in fruits of different cultivars of genus Prunus. *Phyton—Ann. Rei Bot.* **2005**, *45*, 375–383.

12

Inhibitory Effects of Auraptene and Naringin on Astroglial Activation, Tau Hyperphosphorylation, and Suppression of Neurogenesis in the Hippocampus of Streptozotocin-Induced Hyperglycemic Mice

Satoshi Okuyama *, Tatsumi Nakashima, Kumi Nakamura, Wakana Shinoka, Maho Kotani, Atsushi Sawamoto, Mitsunari Nakajima and Yoshiko Furukawa

Department of Pharmaceutical Pharmacology, College of Pharmaceutical Sciences, Matsuyama University, 4-2 Bunkyo-cho, Matsuyama, Ehime 790-8578, Japan; mu.yakuri.009@gmail.com (T.N.); mu.yakuri.008@gmail.com (K.N.); mu.yakuri.010@gmail.com (W.S.); mu.yakuri.011@gmail.com (M.K.); asawamot@g.matsuyama-u.ac.jp (A.S.); mnakajim@g.matsuyama-u.ac.jp (M.N.); furukawa@g.matsuyama-u.ac.jp (Y.F.)
* Correspondence: sokuyama@g.matsuyama-u.ac.jp

Abstract: Auraptene, a citrus-related compound, exerts anti-inflammatory effects in peripheral tissues, and we demonstrated these effects in the brains of a lipopolysaccharide-injected systemic inflammation animal model and a brain ischemic mouse model. Naringin, another citrus-related compound, has been shown to exert antioxidant effects in several animal models. Hyperglycemia induces oxidative stress and inflammation and causes extensive damage in the brain; therefore, we herein evaluated the anti-inflammatory and other effects of auraptene and naringin in streptozotocin-induced hyperglycemic mice. Both compounds inhibited astroglial activation and the hyperphosphorylation of tau at 231 of threonine in neurons, and also recovered the suppression of neurogenesis in the dentate gyrus of the hippocampus in hyperglycemic mice. These results suggested that auraptene and naringin have potential effects as neuroprotective agents in the brain.

Keywords: auraptene; naringin; hyperglycemia; neurogenesis; tau phosphorylation; anti-inflammation; anti-oxidation

---

1. Introduction

Recent research shows that hyperglycemia induces inflammation, reactive oxygen species production and neuronal dysfunction in the central nervous system, and those are linked to a number of disorders [1]. Diabetes was recently identified as a risk factor for Alzheimer's disease (AD) [2–4]. The AD brain is frequently associated with severe inflammation, oxidative stress, neuronal dysfunction, amyloid-beta accumulation, tau hyperphosphorylation, and memory impairment [5]. A well-established hyperglycemia diabetes model is induced by streptozotocin (STZ), a glucosamine-nitrosourea compound. STZ induces insulin-secreting pancreatic beta cell death through DNA methylation [6], resulting in chronic hyperglycemia and hypoinsulinemia. Severe oxidative stress, inflammation, tau hyperphosphorylation, and neuronal dysfunction have been observed in the brain of the STZ-induced hyperglycemia model [7,8].

We previously demonstrated that auraptene (AUR), a coumarin compound from citrus fruit, exerted anti-inflammatory and neuroprotective effects in the brain of a lipopolysaccharide (LPS)-injected inflammation model [9]. In this experiment, an intranigral injection of LPS induced microglial activation and dopaminergic neuronal death; on the other hand, an AUR treatment suppressed microglial activation and neuronal cell death. Furthermore, AUR exerted suppressive effects on astrocyte activation and neuronal cell death in the hippocampus of a transient global cerebral ischemic mouse model [10]. Naringin (NGI) is also a biologically active flavonoid substance from citrus that has been shown to exert antioxidant, anti-inflammatory, and neuroprotective effects in the brains of several brain disorder models [11–14]. Therefore, the aim of the present study was to investigate whether both AUR and NGI show anti-inflammatory and anti-tau hyperphosphorylation effects in the STZ-induced hyperglycemia mouse brain.

2. Materials and Methods

2.1. Experiment Schedule

C57BL/6 mice (nine-week-old, male) were purchased from Japan SLC, Inc. (Hamamatsu, Japan). All animal experiments were performed with the approved protocol by the Animal Care and Use Committee of Matsuyama University (#9-002; 2 September, 2009). Mice were housed in a room maintained at a constant temperature of 23 ± 1 °C with 12-h light/dark cycle (lights on 8:00–20:00). Mice were given food and water ad libitum for the duration of the study [15].

Randomly, mice were divided into the following four groups ($n = 9$ each). Intraperitoneally with vehicle (saline) treatment and the oral administration of vehicle (5% dimethyl sulfoxide/H_2O) were the control (CON) group. Intraperitoneal STZ treatment and the oral administration of the vehicle group were the STZ. STZ treatment and the oral administration of AUR (50 mg/kg; Ushio ChemiX Corp, Omaezaki, Japan) group, named AUR, and STZ treatment and the oral administration of NGI (100 mg/kg; LKT Laboratories, Inc., St. Paul, MN, USA) group, named NGI. Saline or 165 mg/kg of STZ (Wako, Osaka, Japan) was administered intraperitoneally depending on the groups on day 1. On day 8, test sample-administered groups were started to receive each sample orally once a day for 14 days. On day 22, mice were transcardially perfused with ice-cold phosphate-buffered saline (PBS) after the measurement of blood glucose, and the brains were removed.

2.2. Blood Glucose Measurement

To measure fasting glucose concentration on day 22, stock diets were removed from 8:00, and blood glucose was measured at 16:00. A Blood Glucose Monitoring System (Glucose Pilot; Iwai Chemicals Company, Tokyo, Japan) was used to measure blood glucose concentrations with a blood drop from the tail.

2.3. Immunohistochemistry and Immunofluorescence

Sagittal frozen brain sections were prepared at a thickness of 30 μm using a cryostat (CM3050S; Leica Microsystems, Heidelberger, Germany). Immunohistochemistry and immunofluorescence was performed as described in our previous study [15] with the specific primary antibodies (Table 1). Immunopositive signals in the micrographic images were quantified using ImageJ software (National Institute of Health, Bethesda, MD, USA) as described previously [15]. The positive signal densities were quantified using the "measure" tool in ImageJ software.

2.4. Western Blotting Analysis

Equal amounts of protein (25 μg) of hippocampal tissues were separated on 10% sodium dodecyl sulfate-polyacrylamide gels and electroblotted onto an Immun-Blot® PVDF Membrane (Bio-Rad, Hercules, CA, USA) as described in our previous study [16]. Western blotting analysis was performed with the specific primary antibodies (Table 1), and immunoreactive bands were visualized by Amersham ECL Prime Western Blotting Detection Reagent (GE Healthcare Life Sciences, Little Chalfont, UK). The band intensity was captured and measured using a LAS-3000 imaging system (Fujifilm, Tokyo, Japan).

2.5. Statistical Analysis

Data were analyzed by an unpaired *t*-test between two groups (CON vs STZ) and a one-factor ANOVA followed by Dunnett's multiple comparison test among three groups (STZ vs AUR or NGI) (Prism 6; GraphPad Software, La Jolla, CA, USA).

Table 1. Summary of primary antibodies used for immunohistochemiatry, immunofluorescence and western blotting analysis.

Antibody	Epitope Protein/Amino Acids	Host	Dilution	Resource
Iba1	ionized calcium-binding adaptor molecule 1	rabbit	1:1000	Wako, Osaka, Japan
GFAP	glial fibrillary acidic protein	mouse	1:200	Sigma-Aldrich, St. Louis, MO, USA
p-Thr231	phosphorylated-tau Threonine 231	rabbit	1:1000	AnaSpec, Fremont, CA, USA
p-Ser396	phosphorylated-tau Serine 396	rabbit	1:1000	AnaSpec
NeuN	neuronal nuclei	mouse	1:200	Millipore, Temecula, CA, USA
DCX	doublecortin	goat	1:50	Santa Cruz Biotechnology, Santa Cruz, CA, USA
PPARγ	peroxisome proliferator-activated receptor-gamma	rabbit	1:1000	Abcam, Cambridge, UK
Actin	actin	rabbit	1:1000	Sigma-Aldrich

3. Results

3.1. Suppressive Effects of AUR and NGI on Astrocyte Activation

Blood glucose concentrations were significantly elevated in the STZ group (Figure 1; *** $p < 0.001$); however, no significant changes were observed in the AUR and NGI groups.

Hyperglycemia induces inflammation and oxidative stress in the brain [7,8], and excess glial cell activation is known to be responsible for oxidative stress and inflammatory reactions in the brain [17]. Micoglia (Iba1-positive cells) activation were not confirmed in all groups (Figure 2a,b); however, the number of reactive astrocytes that is immunostained with the GFAP antibody significantly increased in the stratum lacunosum-moleculare in the hippocampus of the STZ group (Figure 3a,b; ** $p < 0.01$). In contrast, the GFAP-positive signals were significantly suppressed in the AUR and NGI groups (Figure 3a,b; ## $p < 0.01$, ### $p < 0.001$).

PPARγ regulates the cell signaling of the inflammation process and exerts anti-inflammatory effects [18], and the expression of PPARγ in the hippocampus was significantly suppressed in the STZ group (Figure 4; * $p < 0.05$); however, no significant changes were observed in the AUR and NGI groups.

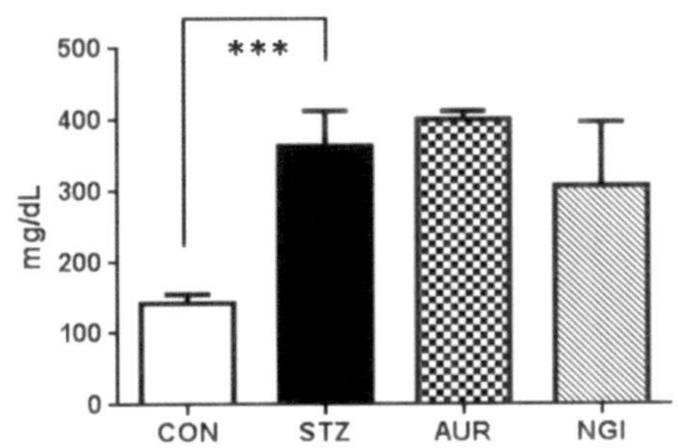

Figure 1. Blood glucose concentrations on Day 22. Values are means ± SEM. The symbol shows a significant difference between CON (control) and STZ (streptozotocin) (*** $p < 0.001$). AUR: auraptene; NGI: naringin.

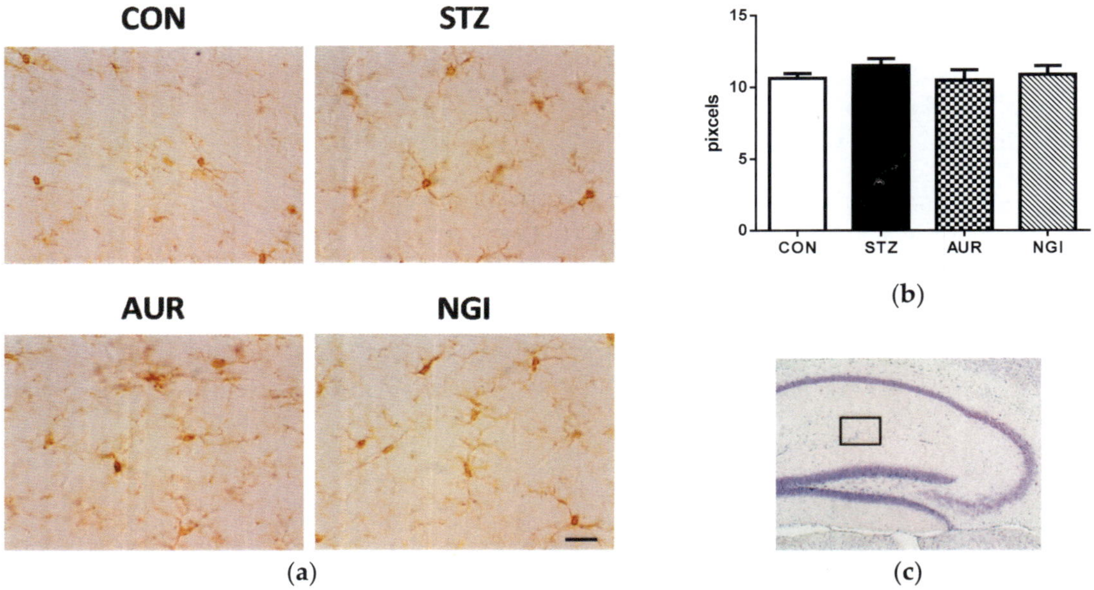

Figure 2. Effects of auraptene and naringin on Iba1 immunoreactivity in the hippocampus. (**a**) Sagittal sections were stained with an anti-Iba1 antibody. The scale bar shows 50 μm. (**b**) Quantitative analysis data of Iba1-positive signals using ImageJ software. (**c**) The location of the captured images. Values are means ± SEM.

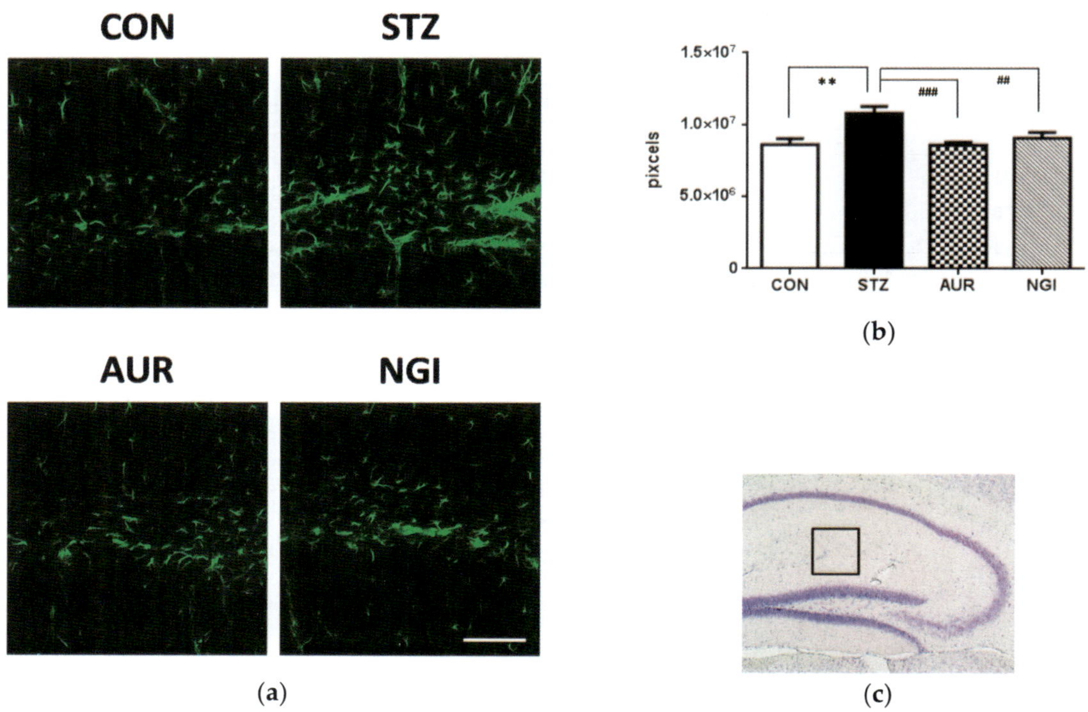

Figure 3. Effects of auraptene and naringin on GFAP immunoreactivity in the hippocampus. (**a**) Sagittal sections were stained with an anti-GFAP antibody. The scale bar shows 100 μm. (**b**) Quantitative analysis data of GFAP-positive signals using ImageJ software. (**c**) The location of the captured images. Values are means ± SEM. Symbols show significant differences between the following conditions: CON vs STZ (** $p < 0.01$), and STZ vs AUR or NGI (## $p < 0.01$, ### $p < 0.001$).

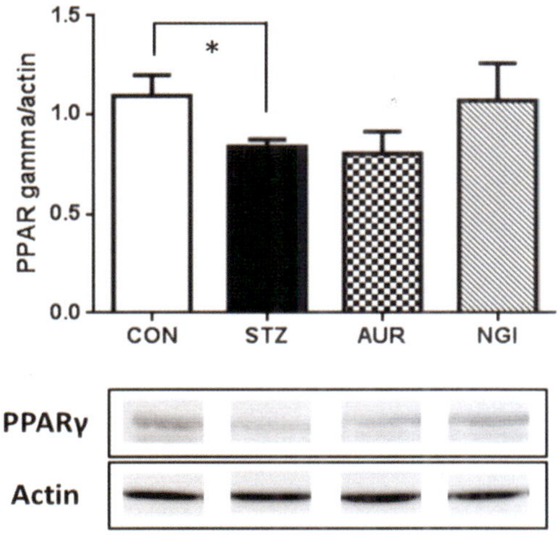

Figure 4. Effects of auraptene and naringin on the expression of PPARγ in the hippocampus. Values are means ± SEM. The symbol shows a significant difference between CON and STZ (* $p < 0.05$).

3.2. *Effects of AUR and NGI on Tau Hyperphosphorylation*

Tau, a microtubule-associated cytoskeletal protein, in the neuron has been understanding to relate to the molecular mechanisms for neurofibrillary tangle (NFT) formation through its multiple phosphorylative and conformational changes. It was previously shown that inflammation and oxidative stress induce tau hyperphosphorylation [19,20], and this was confirmed in STZ-injected mice brain [21]. We evaluated tau phosphorylation levels at 231 of threonine (p-Thr231) and 396 of serine (p-Ser396) in the hippocampus (Figures 5 and 6). Strong positive signals for p-Thr231 were confirmed in the CA3 region pyramidal cell layer and in the stratum lacunosum-moleculare in the hippocampus. The integrated densities of the immune-positive signals were evaluated, and that was significantly higher in the STZ group (Figure 5a,b; ** $p < 0.01$); however, significant suppressive effects on its phosphorylation was observed in the AUR and NGI treated groups (Figure 5a,b; # $p < 0.05$). Similar to p-Thr231, the levels of p-Ser396 in the hippocampus were significantly higher in the STZ group than in the CON group (Figure 6a,b; * $p < 0.05$). The signals were confirmed in hippocampal mossy fibers and the stratum lacunosum-moleculare. On the other hand, the AUR and NGI treatments exerted a tendency of suppressive effects (Figure 6a,b; $p = 0.056$ and $p = 0.087$, respectively).

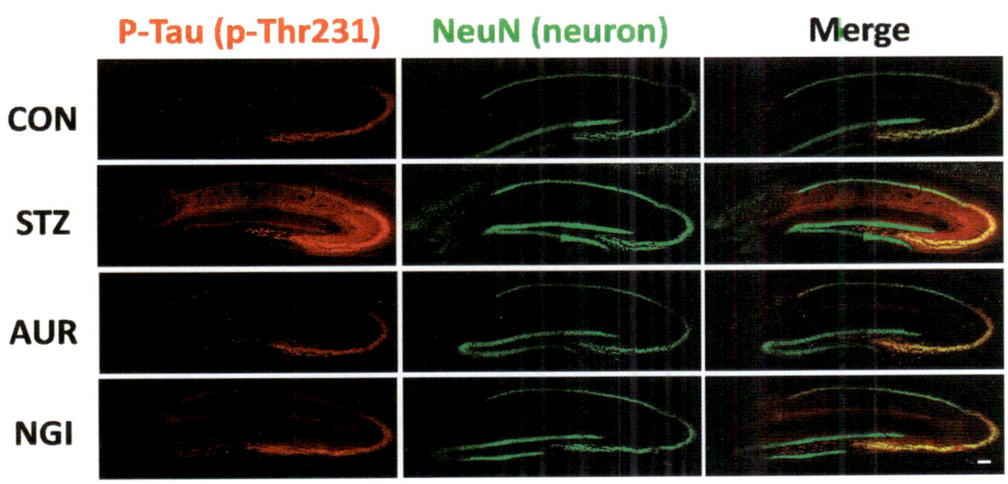

(a)

Figure 5. *Cont.*

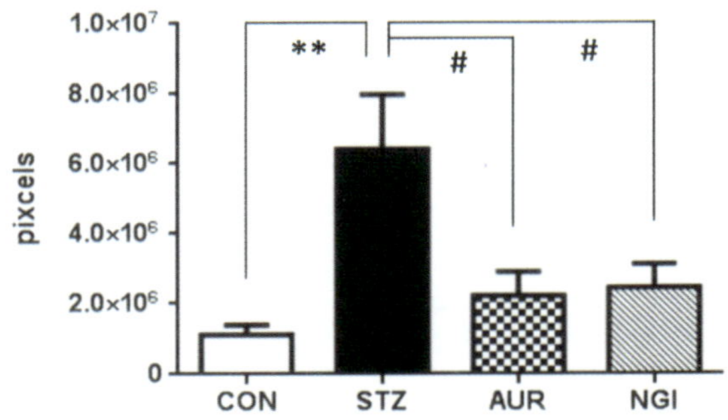

(b)

Figure 5. Effects of auraptene and naringin on the expression of phosphorylated Tau at 231 of threonine in the hippocampus. (**a**) Sagittal sections were stained with the anti-pThr231 (red) and NeuN (green) antibodies. The scale bar shows 100 μm. (**b**) Quantitative analysis data of pThr231-positive signals using ImageJ software. Values are means ± SEM. Symbols show significant differences between the following conditions: CON vs STZ (** $p < 0.01$), and STZ vs AUR or NGI (# $p < 0.05$).

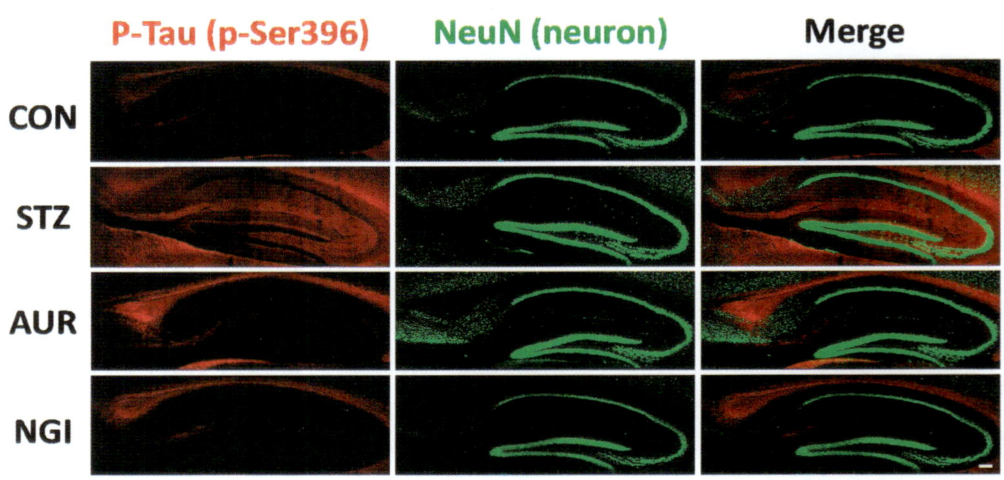

(a)

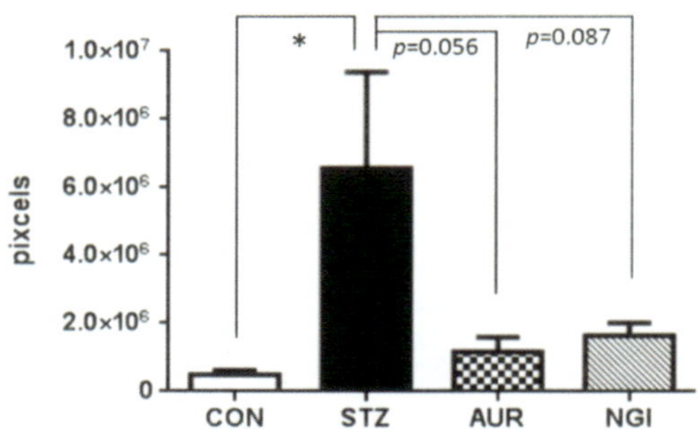

(b)

Figure 6. Effects of auraptene and naringin on the expression of phosphorylated Tau at 396 of serine in the hippocampus. (**a**) Sagittal sections were stained with the anti-pSer396 (red) and NeuN (green) antibodies. The scale bar shows 100 μm. (**b**) Quantitative analysis data of pSer396-positive signals using ImageJ software. Values are means ± SEM. Symbols show significant differences between CON vs STZ (* $p < 0.05$).

3.3. Enhancement of Neurogenesis by AUR and NGI in the Hippocampus

The subgranular zone (SGZ) of the dentate gyrus (DG) is one of the areas in which neurogenesis occurs in the hippocampus [22], and adult neurogenesis is known to play an important role in learning and memory. A previous report showed that suppression of the neurogenesis in the DG was confirmed, following a STZ administration [23]. Figure 6 shows the immunoreactivity of DCX, a marker for immature neurons, in the SGZ. DCX-positive cells were suppressibility observed in the STZ group, but markedly higher number in the AUR and NGI groups (Figure 7a). We manually counted the DCX-positive neurons, with checking the soma and nucleus, in the SGZ under the fluorescence microscopy and evaluated the number of DCX-positive newborn neurons in the SGZ. The numbers of the STZ group showed significantly suppressed expression (Figure 7b; *** $p < 0.001$); in contrast, the AUR and NGI groups ameliorated this suppression (Figure 7b; # $p < 0.05$, ## $p < 0.01$).

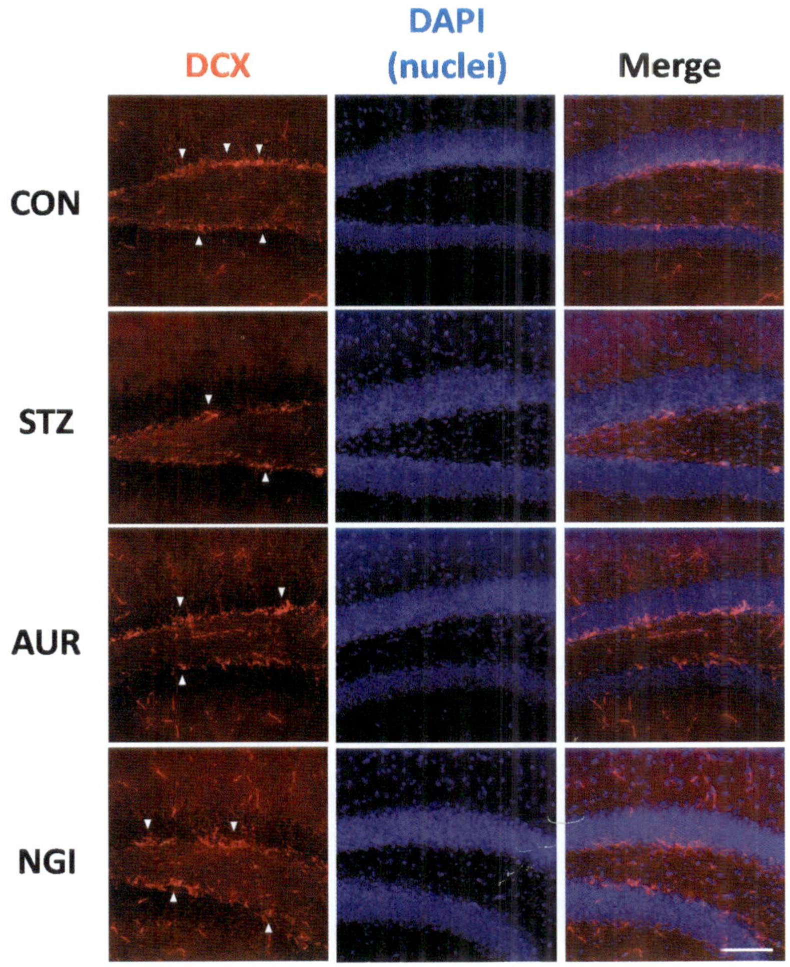

(a)

Figure 7. *Cont.*

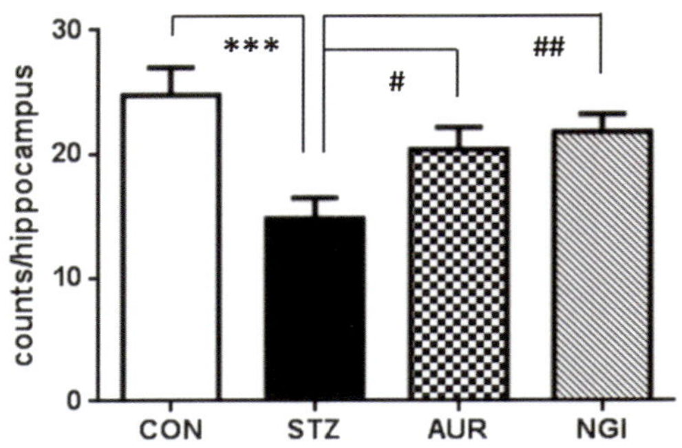

(b)

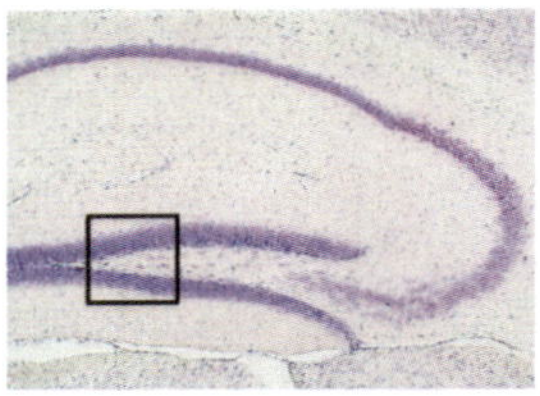

(c)

Figure 7. Effects of auraptene and naringin on doublecortin immunoreactivity in the hippocampus. (**a**) Sagittal sections were stained with the anti-DCX antibody (red) and DAPI (blue). The white arrowheads indicate typical DCX-positive cells in the DG (dentate gyrus). The scale bar shows 100 μm. (**b**) Counting data of DCX-positive signals in the dentate gyrus. (**c**) The location of the captured images is shown with a square in the figure. Values are means ± SEM. Symbols show significant differences between the following conditions: CON vs STZ (*** $p < 0.001$), and STZ vs AUR or NGI (# $p < 0.05$, ## $p < 0.01$).

4. Discussion

Hyperglycemia induces inflammation and oxidative stress in the central nervous system [24], and diabetes is currently regarded as one of the risk factors for dementia, such as AD and vascular dementia [2–4]. The AD brain is frequently associated with severe inflammation, oxidative stress, neuronal dysfunction, amyloid-beta accumulation, tau hyperphosphorylation, and memory impairment [5]. Several studies indicate inflammation and oxidative stress increased tau hyperphosphorylation of neurons in the brain [19,20]; therefore, our primary focus was to clarify the anti-inflammatory and tau hyperphosphorylation suppression effects of AUR and NGI in a hyperglycemia model.

STZ-treated mice showed significantly elevated blood glucose concentrations, whereas suppressive effects were not observed in the NGI and AUR groups (Figure 1). Previous studies reported that the administration of 100 mg/kg of NGI suppressed blood glucose concentrations in STZ-treated rats, or 0.2% of AUR administration resulted in suppressive effects on high-fat diet-induced obese mice, respectively [25,26]. These findings suggested that NGI and AUR have the potential to reduce blood glucose concentrations in several diabetic models. However, treatments with NGI and AUR did not reduce blood glucose concentrations in our experiment.

In hyperglycemia models, astrocyte activation is related to immune response in the brain [27,28]. Treatments with AUR and NGI suppressed astrocyte activation in this experiment (Figure 3), and we previously demonstrated that the activation of astrocytes was inhibited by the AUR treatment in a transient global cerebral ischemic mouse model [10]. Strong microglial activation, also an immune response cell in the brain, was not observed in the STZ group (Figure 2) in this experiment, whereas astrocytes were detected. Microglia is activated earlier than astrocytes in a manner that is dependent on disease conditions [29]; therefore, we considered strong microglial activation to only occur in the early phase of the STZ treatment. In fact, we previously demonstrated that microglial activation was confirmed one week after the administration of STZ [30]; however, the time point of sacrifice in this experiment was two weeks after the STZ treatment. PPARγ is an important target in diabetes therapy, and regulates the cell signaling of the inflammation process [18]. AUR and NGI did not significantly affect the protein expression of PPARγ in the hippocampus in this experiment (Figure 4); on the other hand, a previous study reported that NGI ameliorated cognitive deficits via oxidative stress and proinflammatory factor suppression, and activated the protein expression of PPAR in the hippocampus of an STZ-injected rat model [25]. AUR also activates PPARγ in adipocytes [31]. Collectively, these findings in our experiment indicated that AUR and NGI exerted anti-inflammatory effects by suppressing the activation of astrocytes in the hippocampus, though we still have to do further experiments to see the detail mechanism.

Increases in inflammation and oxidative stress induce the hyperphosphorylated tau protein in neurons and this is enhanced in the hyperglycemic brain [19,20]. The microtubule function of neurons is maintained by the phosphorylation of the tau protein, and the regulation of kinases (including CDK-5 and GSK-3β) and phosphatases (such as PP2A) are very important; however, the hyperphosphorylation of tau induces microtubule dysfunction, leading to the formation of NFT, which is often observed in the AD brain [32]. In tau protein, several strong phosphorylation sites have been identified, such as Thr231 and Ser396, in hyperglycemic animal brains [21,33], and oxidative stress and inflammation may induce a kinase and phosphatase imbalance [34]. We focused on phosphorylation sites in Thr231 and Ser396 in the present study, and AUR and NGI treatment exerted suppressive effects on tau phosphorylation in the hippocampus in STZ-treated mice (Figures 5 and 6). Neurogenesis in the SGZ of the DG in the hippocampus is of particular importance for hippocampal-dependent memory function [35,36]. It is suppressed by a number of conditions, including depression, AD, and aging; in addition, hyperglycemia has also been shown to suppress neurogenesis [37,38]. Staining for neurogenesis with DCX, the AUR and NGI treatments enhanced its expression (Figure 7). Inhibitory effects of AUR and NGI on tau hyperphosphorylation and suppression of neurogenesis were our new findings.

5. Conclusions

When AUR and NGI were administered to STZ-injected hyperglycemia mice, they (1) suppressed astroglial activation; (2) diminished tau phosphorylation; and (3) stimulated neurogenesis in the SGZ of the DG in the hippocampus. These results suggest that AUR and NGI, citrus-related compounds, exert anti-inflammatory and antioxidative effect against hyperglycemia-induced changes in the brain, and have potential as novel neuroprotective agents obtained from food materials.

Author Contributions: S.O. designed and performed the research, and wrote the manuscript; T.N., K.N., W.S., M.K., and A.S. performed the research; M.N. and Y.F. supervised this research project.

Funding: This work was funded by The Tojuro Iijima Foundation for Food Science and Technology, year of 2015 and 2017, and JSPS KAKENHI Grant Number JP26750058.

Acknowledgments: The authors wish to thank Ushio ChemiX Corporation for kindly supplying AUR.

Conflicts of Interest: The authors declare no conflict of interest.

References

1. Dinel, A.L.; André, C.; Aubert, A.; Ferreira, G.; Layé, S.; Castanon, N. Cognitive and emotional alterations are related to hippocampal inflammation in a mouse model of metabolic syndrome. *PLoS ONE* **2011**, *6*, e24325. [CrossRef] [PubMed]
2. Kim, B.; Backus, C.; Oh, S.; Feldman, E.L. Hyperglycemia-induced tau cleavage in vitro and in vivo: A possible link between diabetes and Alzheimer's disease. *J. Alzheimer's Dis.* **2013**, *34*, 727–739. [CrossRef] [PubMed]
3. Kimura, N. Diabetes Mellitus Induces Alzheimer's Disease Pathology: Histopathological Evidence from Animal Models. *Int. J. Mol. Sci.* **2016**, *17*, 503. [CrossRef] [PubMed]
4. Bosco, D.; Fava, A.; Plastino, M.; Montalcini, T.; Pujia, A. Possible implications of insulin resistance and glucose metabolism in Alzheimer's disease pathogenesis. *J. Cell Mol. Med.* **2011**, *15*, 1807–1821. [CrossRef] [PubMed]
5. McKee, A.C.; Carreras, I.; Hossain, L.; Ryu, H.; Klein, W.L.; Oddo, S.; LaFerla, F.M.; Jenkins, B.G.; Kowall, N.W.; Dedeoglu, A. Ibuprofen reduces Abeta, hyperphosphorylated tau and memory deficits in Alzheimer mice. *Brain Res.* **2008**, *1207*, 225–236. [CrossRef] [PubMed]
6. Ho, N.; Balu, D.T.; Hilario, M.R.; Blendy, J.A.; Lucki, I. Depressive phenotypes evoked by experimental diabetes are reversed by insulin. *Physiol. Behav.* **2012**, *105*, 702–708. [CrossRef] [PubMed]

7. Cai, Z.; Yan, Y.; Wang, Y. Minocycline alleviates beta-amyloid protein and tau pathology via restraining neuroinflammation induced by diabetic metabolic disorder. *Clin. Interv. Aging* **2013**, *8*, 1089–1095. [CrossRef] [PubMed]
8. Sharma, R.; Buras, E.; Terashima, T.; Serrano, F.; Massaad, C.A.; Hu, L.; Bitner, B.; Inoue, T.; Chan, L.; Pautler, R.G. Hyperglycemia induces oxidative stress and impairs axonal transport rates in mice. *PLoS ONE* **2010**, *5*, e13463. [CrossRef] [PubMed]
9. Okuyama, S.; Semba, T.; Toyoda, N.; Epifano, F.; Genovese, S.; Fiorito, S.; Taddeo, V.A.; Sawamoto, A.; Nakajima, M.; Furukawa, Y. Auraptene and Other Prenyloxyphenylpropanoids Suppress Microglial Activation and Dopaminergic Neuronal Cell Death in a Lipopolysaccharide-Induced Model of Parkinson's Disease. *Int. J. Mol. Sci.* **2016**, *17*, 1716. [CrossRef] [PubMed]
10. Okuyama, S.; Morita, M.; Kaji, M.; Amakura, Y.; Yoshimura, M.; Shimamoto, K.; Ookido, Y.; Nakajima, M.; Furukawa, Y. Auraptene Acts as an Anti-Inflammatory Agent in the Mouse Brain. *Molecules* **2015**, *20*, 20230–20239. [CrossRef] [PubMed]
11. Gaur, V.; Aggarwal, A.; Kumar, A. Protective effect of naringin against ischemic reperfusion cerebral injury: Possible neurobehavioral, biochemical and cellular alterations in rat brain. *Eur. J. Pharmacol.* **2009**, *616*, 147–154. [CrossRef] [PubMed]
12. Leem, E.; Nam, J.H.; Jeon, M.T.; Shin, W.H.; Won, S.Y.; Park, S.J.; Choi, M.S.; Jin, B.K.; Jung, U.J.; Kim, S.R. Naringin protects the nigrostriatal dopaminergic projection through induction of GDNF in a neurotoxin model of Parkinson's disease. *J. Nutr. Biochem.* **2014**, *25*, 801–806. [CrossRef] [PubMed]
13. Golechha, M.; Chaudhry, U.; Bhatia, J.; Saluja, D.; Arya, D.S. Naringin protects against kainic acid-induced status epilepticus in rats: Evidence for an antioxidant, anti-inflammatory and neuroprotective intervention. *Biol. Pharm. Bull.* **2011**, *34*, 360–365. [CrossRef] [PubMed]
14. Okuyama, S.; Yamamoto, K.; Mori, H.; Sawamoto, A.; Amakura, Y.; Yoshimura, M.; Tamanaha, A.; Ohkubo, Y.; Sugawara, K.; Sudo, M.; et al. Neuroprotective effect of *Citrus kawachiensis* (*Kawachi Bankan*) peels, a rich source of naringin, against global cerebral ischemia/reperfusion injury in mice. *Biosci. Biotechnol. Biochem.* **2018**, *82*, 1216–1224. [CrossRef] [PubMed]
15. Okuyama, S.; Morita, M.; Miyoshi, K.; Nishigawa, Y.; Kaji, M.; Sawamoto, A.; Terugo, T.; Toyoda, N.; Makihata, N.; Amakura, Y.; et al. 3,5,6,7,8,3′,4′-Heptamethoxyflavone, a citrus flavonoid, on protection against memory impairment and neuronal cell death in a global cerebral ischemia mouse model. *Neurochem. Int.* **2014**, *70*, 30–38. [CrossRef] [PubMed]
16. Okuyama, S.; Shimada, N.; Kaji, M.; Morita, M.; Miyoshi, K.; Minami, S.; Amakura, Y.; Yoshimura, M.; Yoshida, T.; Watanabe, S.; et al. Heptamethoxyflavone, a citrus flavonoid, enhances brain-derived neurotrophic factor production and neurogenesis in the hippocampus following cerebral global ischemia in mice. *Neurosci. Lett.* **2012**, *528*, 190–195. [CrossRef] [PubMed]
17. Wilms, H.; Sievers, J.; Rickert, U.; Rostami-Yazdi, M.; Mrowietz, U.; Lucius, R. Dimethylfumarate inhibits microglial and astrocytic inflammation by suppressing the synthesis of nitric oxide, IL-1beta, TNF-alpha and IL-6 in an in vitro model of brain inflammation. *J. Neuroinflamm.* **2010**, *7*, 30. [CrossRef] [PubMed]
18. Collino, M.; Aragno, M.; Mastrocola, R.; Gallicchio, M.; Rosa, A.C.; Dianzani, C.; Danni, O.; Thiemermann, C.; Fantozzi, R. Modulation of the oxidative stress and inflammatory response by PPAR-gamma agonists in the hippocampus of rats exposed to cerebral ischemia/reperfusion. *Eur. J. Pharmacol.* **2006**, *530*, 70–80. [CrossRef] [PubMed]
19. Barron, M.; Gartlon, J.; Dawson, L.A.; Atkinson, P.J.; Pardon, M.C. A state of delirium: Deciphering the effect of inflammation on tau pathology in Alzheimer's disease. *Exp. Gerontol.* **2017**, *94*, 103–107. [CrossRef] [PubMed]
20. Wu, Z.; Nakanishi, H. Connection between periodontitis and Alzheimer's disease: Possible roles of microglia and leptomeningeal cells. *J. Pharmacol. Sci.* **2014**, *126*, 8–13. [CrossRef] [PubMed]
21. Clodfelder-Miller, B.J.; Zmijewska, A.A.; Johnson, G.V.; Jope, R.S. Tau is hyperphosphorylated at multiple sites in mouse brain in vivo after streptozotocin-induced insulin deficiency. *Diabetes* **2006**, *55*, 3320–3325. [CrossRef] [PubMed]
22. Aimone, J.B.; Li, Y.; Lee, S.W.; Clemenson, G.D.; Deng, W.; Gage, F.H. Regulation and function of adult neurogenesis: From genes to cognition. *Physiol. Rev.* **2014**, *94*, 991–1026. [CrossRef] [PubMed]

23. Guo, J.; Yu, C.; Li, H.; Liu, F.; Feng, R.; Wang, H.; Meng, Y.; Li, Z.; Ju, G.; Wang, J. Impaired neural stem/progenitor cell proliferation in streptozotocin-induced and spontaneous diabetic mice. *Neurosci. Res.* **2010**, *68*, 329–336. [CrossRef] [PubMed]
24. Maher, P.; Dargusch, R.; Ehren, J.L.; Okada, S.; Sharma, K.; Schubert, D. Fisetin lowers methylglyoxal dependent protein glycation and limits the complications of diabetes. *PLoS ONE* **2011**, *6*, e21226. [CrossRef] [PubMed]
25. Qi, Z.; Xu, Y.; Liang, Z.; Li, S.; Wang, J.; Wei, Y.; Dong, B. Naringin ameliorates cognitive deficits via oxidative stress, proinflammatory factors and the PPARγ signaling pathway in a type 2 diabetic rat model. *Mol. Med. Rep.* **2015**, *12*, 7093–7101. [CrossRef] [PubMed]
26. Takahashi, N.; Senda, M.; Lin, S.; Goto, T.; Yano, M.; Sasaki, T.; Murakami, S.; Kawada, T. Auraptene regulates gene expression involved in lipid metabolism through PPARα activation in diabetic obese mice. *Mol. Nutr. Food Res.* **2011**, *55*, 1791–1797. [CrossRef] [PubMed]
27. Infante-Garcia, C.; Jose Ramos-Rodriguez, J.; Marin-Zambrana, Y.; Teresa Fernandez-Ponce, M.; Casas, L.; Mantell, C.; Garcia-Alloza, M. Mango leaf extract improves central pathology and cognitive impairment in a type 2 diabetes mouse model. *Brain Pathol.* **2017**, *27*, 499–507. [CrossRef] [PubMed]
28. Zheng, Y.; Yang, Y.; Dong, B.; Zheng, H.; Lin, X.; Du, Y.; Li, X.; Zhao, L.; Gao, H. Metabonomic profiles delineate potential role of glutamate-glutamine cycle in db/db mice with diabetes-associated cognitive decline. *Mol. Brain* **2016**, *9*, 40. [CrossRef] [PubMed]
29. Webster, K.M.; Sun, M.; Crack, P.; O'Brien, T.J.; Shultz, S.R.; Semple, B.D. Inflammation in epileptogenesis after traumatic brain injury. *J. Neuroinflamm.* **2017**, *14*, 10. [CrossRef] [PubMed]
30. Okuyama, S.; Shinoka, W.; Nakamura, K.; Kotani, M.; Sawamoto, A.; Sugawara, K.; Sudo, M.; Nakajima, M.; Furukawa, Y. Suppressive effects of the peel of *Citrus kawachiensis* (*Kawachi Bankan*) on astroglial activation, tau phosphorylation, and inhibition of neurogenesis in the hippocampus of type 2 diabetic db/db mice. *Biosci. Biotechnol. Biochem.* **2018**, *82*, 1216–1224. [CrossRef] [PubMed]
31. Kuroyanagi, K.; Kang, M.S.; Goto, T.; Hirai, S.; Ohyama, K.; Kusudo, T.; Yu, R.; Yano, M.; Sasaki, T.; Takahashi, N.; et al. Citrus auraptene acts as an agonist for PPARs and enhances adiponectin production and MCP-1 reduction in 3T3-L1 adipocytes. *Biochem. Biophys. Res. Commun.* **2008**, *366*, 219–225. [CrossRef] [PubMed]
32. Medeiros, R.; Baglietto-Vargas, D.; LaFerla, F.M. The role of tau in Alzheimer's disease and related disorders. *CNS Neurosci. Ther.* **2011**, *17*, 514–524. [CrossRef] [PubMed]
33. Kim, B.; Backus, C.; Oh, S.; Hayes, J.M.; Feldman, E.L. Increased tau phosphorylation and cleavage in mouse models of type 1 and type 2 diabetes. *Endocrinology* **2009**, *150*, 5294–5301. [CrossRef] [PubMed]
34. Ballatore, C.; Lee, V.M.; Trojanowski, J.Q. Tau-mediated neurodegeneration in Alzheimer's disease and related disorders. *Nat. Rev. Neurosci.* **2007**, *8*, 663–672. [CrossRef] [PubMed]
35. Winocur, G.; Wojtowicz, J.M.; Sekeres, M.; Snyder, J.S.; Wang, S. Inhibition of neurogenesis interferes with hippocampus-dependent memory function. *Hippocampus* **2006**, *16*, 296–304. [CrossRef] [PubMed]
36. Shors, T.J.; Miesegaes, G.; Beylin, A.; Zhao, M.; Rydel, T.; Gould, E. Neurogenesis in the adult is involved in the formation of trace memories. *Nature* **2001**, *410*, 372–376. [CrossRef] [PubMed]
37. Yi, S.S.; Hwang, I.K.; Choi, J.W.; Won, M.H.; Seong, J.K.; Yoon, Y.S. Effects of hypothyroidism on cell proliferation and neuroblasts in the hippocampal dentate gyrus in a rat model of type 2 diabetes. *Anat. Cell Biol.* **2010**, *43*, 185–193. [CrossRef] [PubMed]
38. Hamilton, A.; Patterson, S.; Porter, D.; Gault, V.A.; Holscher, C. Novel GLP-1 mimetics developed to treat type 2 diabetes promote progenitor cell proliferation in the brain. *J. Neurosci. Res.* **2011**, *89*, 481–489. [CrossRef] [PubMed]

13

Fruit and Vegetable By-Products to Fortify Spreadable Cheese

Annalisa Lucera, Cristina Costa, Valeria Marinelli, Maria Antonietta Saccotelli, Matteo Alessandro Del Nobile * and Amalia Conte

Department of Agricultural Sciences, Food and Environment, University of Foggia, Via Napoli, 25–71121 Foggia, Italy; annalisa.lucera@unifg.it (A.L.); cristina.costa@unifg.it (C.C.); valeria.marinelli@unifg.it (V.M.); mariantoniettasaccotelli@gmail.com (M.A.S.); amalia.conte@unifg.it (A.C.)
* Correspondence: matteo.delnobile@unifg.it

Abstract: In this work, spreadable cheese was enriched with flours from by-products (red and white grape pomace, tomato peel, broccoli, corn bran, and artichokes) as sources of fibres and antioxidant compounds. The physicochemical and the sensory properties of all the cheese samples were analysed. Results revealed that total phenolic content, flavonoids, and antioxidant activity of samples containing grape pomace significantly increased, followed by broccoli, artichoke, corn bran, and tomato peel by-products, compared to the control cheese. Specifically, cheeses containing white and red grape pomace recorded high phenolic content (2.74 $\pm$ 0.04 and 2.34 $\pm$ 0.15 mg GAEs/g dw, respectively) compared to the control (0.66 mg GAEs/g dw).

Keywords: by-products; bioactive compounds; spreadable cheese; functional food; waste reduction

1. Introduction

Nowadays, about one-third of fruit and vegetables in the form of peels, pips, and skins can be discarded during preparation and processing, thus producing significant wastes that represent one of the major problems of the food industry. Fruit and vegetable by-products can also be promising sources of functional compounds, being rich in carotenoids, dietary fibres, polyphenols, tocopherols, vitamins, and other substances [1]. For this reason, several works deal with the use of vegetable by-products to enhance the nutritional value or the technological properties of food. For example, mango peel powders were used to enhance the antioxidant properties of macaroni [2]. Sudha et al. [3] reported that the incorporation of apple pomace into wheat flour as a fibre source improved the rheological characteristics of cake. Grape marc extract was used in substitution of water to produce spaghetti, obtaining a food characterized by high content of phenolic compounds, flavonoids, and consequently high antioxidant activity [4]. Boubaker et al. [5] used artichoke stem powder as a source of dietary fibre and polyphenols to partially substitute wheat flour during bread making. Moreover, broccoli by-products were added in gluten-free mini sponge cakes to increase the polyphenolic and glucosinolates content [6].

In the dairy industry, there has been an increasing demand for healthy cheese, even though there are still very few studies available dealing with the use of fruit and vegetable by-products to fortify dairy products. Some valid examples about the use of wine grape pomace as antioxidant dietary fibre to enhance the nutritional value of yogurt and ice cream are reported [7,8]. Bertolino et al. [9] also demonstrated that the addition of hazelnut skins improved functional properties of yogurt. Marchiani et al. [10] assessed the physicochemical and nutritional quality of grape pomace powder to fortify semi-hard cheese. Abd Elhamid [11] proposed the incorporation of wheat bran in Kariesh cheese.

In this context, by-products from broccoli, artichoke, tomato peel, red and white grape pomace, and corn bran are taken into account, being interesting sources of healthy compounds (anthocyanins, catechins, flavonols, fibres, and phenolic acids) for spreadable cheese fortification [1]. This cheese is a soft, mild cheese, with slightly acidic tasting and diacetyl flavour. It is usually manufactured by the coagulation of milk mixed with cream by acidification with starter culture. It is used as spread on bagels, as salad dressing, and as ingredient for dessert. Generally, it is not a significant source of polyphenols and dietary fibres.

The objective of the present study was to evaluate the influence of the supplementation of different by-products (i.e., broccoli, artichoke, tomato peel, red and white grape pomaces by-products, and corn bran) on physicochemical and sensory quality of spreadable cheese. Cheese moisture content, pH, total phenolic compounds, total flavonoids, antioxidant activity, and sensory characterization were carried out for each cheese sample.

2. Materials and Methods

2.1. *Raw Materials*

White and red grape pomace (made up of skins, seeds, and stalks), tomato peels, broccoli stems and leaves, and artichoke external leaves were provided by Foggia, a local company (Southern Italy). The samples were dried at 30–35 °C in a dryer (SG600, Namad, Rome, Italy) for 48 h. The dried vegetables were reduced to fine powder by a hammer mill (16/BV-Beccaria s.r.l., Cuneo, Italy) and then stored at 4 °C until further utilization. The commercial corn bran was purchased from Limagrain Cereales Ingredients (Ennezat, France).

2.2. *Chemicals*

Folin-Ciocalteu reagent, gallic acid monohydrate, methanol, hydrochloric acid, ABTS (2,2-azino-bis(3-ethylbenzothiazoline-6-sulfonic acid) diammonium salt), potassium persulfate ($K_2S_2O_8$), Trolox (6-hydroxy-2,5,7,8-tetramethylchroman-2-carboxylic acid) aluminium chloride ($AlCl_3$), sodium nitrite ($NaNO_2$), sodium hydroxide solution (NaOH), quercetin, sodium acetate trihydrate ($CH_3COONa{\cdot}3H_2O$), glacial acetic acid (CH_3COOH), 2,4,6-Tripyridyl-s-Triazine (TPTZ), ferric chloride ($FeCl_3$), and ferrous sulphate heptahydrate ($FeSO_4{\cdot}7H_2O$) were supplied from Sigma-Aldrich (Milan, Italy). Anhydrous sodium carbonate (Na_2CO_3) was supplied from Carlo Erba (Milan, Italy). For the preparation of the phosphate buffered saline (PBS), the following salts were used: sodium phosphate dibasic heptahydrate ($HNa_2O_4P{\cdot}7H_2O$) and sodium phosphate monobasic monohydrate ($H_2NaO_4P{\cdot}H_2O$). These were purchased from Sigma-Aldrich (Milan, Italy). All reagents were of analytical grade.

2.3. *Cheese Manufacture*

Spreadable cheese was made from pasteurised skimmed cow milk (0.1% fat) (Granarolo spa, branch office of Gioia del Colle, Italy). First, the starter composed by mesophilic aromatic culture (CHN-22 CHR Hansen) was added at 27 °C and incubated until complete acid coagulation (pH = 4.5–4.6). The formed curd was than mixed and placed into baskets lined with a cotton cloth and left to drain overnight under refrigerated conditions (4 ± 1 °C). The resulting cheese was mixed with salt (0.2% *w*/*w*) and fructo-oligosaccharide (FOS) (3% *w*/*w*) (Orafti beneo P95). After, the spreadable cheese was divided into portions of 100 g and the different by-products flours, such as broccoli (Br), artichoke (Art), tomato peel (TP), red (RGP) and white (WGP) grape pomaces, and corn bran (CB), were added at a concentration of 5% (*w*/*w*). The control cheese (CNT) without any substance was also prepared. For clarity, the cheeses supplemented with by-products are labelled as following: Br-SC (spreadable cheese enriched with broccoli), Art-SC (artichoke), TP-SC (tomato peel), RGP-SC and WGP-SC (red and white grape marc flour, respectively), and CB-SC (corn bran). All cheeses were subjected to physicochemical evaluation and sensory characterization right after their production.

2.4. Extraction and Determination of Total Phenolic Compounds and Total Flavonoids

The extraction of phenolic compounds from each flour and cheese sample was performed as described by Rashidinejad et al. [12] with slight modifications. Briefly, 1 g of sample was mixed with 50 mL of acidified methanol (95% MeOH containing 1% HCl) and extracted for 30 min at 50 °C in a water bath (Grant OLS200, Cambridge, UK) at 200 rpm. The mixture was cooled and filtered by cheese cloth; the residues were washed with 2 mL of the same solvent. The obtained extracts were immediately analysed. Extraction was carried out in triplicate for each sample.

Total phenolic compounds were determined in triplicate by UV-vis spectrophotometry according to the Folin-Ciocalteu method [13]. The total phenolic content was expressed as mg of gallic acid equivalents (GAEs) per g of dry weight (dw).

Total flavonoids content both in vegetable flours and in fortified cheeses was determined by the aluminium chloride colorimetric method, according to Huang et al. [14] with modifications. Each extract (0.5 mL), prepared as previously described, was mixed with 2 mL of distilled water and 150 μL of a 5% sodium nitrite ($NaNO_2$) solution. After 6 min, 150 μL of a 10% aluminium chloride ($AlCl_3$) solution was added and the mixture was left to rest for 6 min. Finally, 1 mL of 1 M sodium hydroxide was added and total volume was made up to 5 mL with distilled water. Then, the solutions were mixed and for each sample the absorbance was read in triplicate against blank at 415 nm. The calibration curve was prepared using quercetin as standard in the range 6.25–500 mg/L (R^2 = 0.9985) and total amount of flavonoids was expressed in mg of quercetin equivalents (QEs) per g of dry weight (dw).

2.5. Antioxidant Activity

The antioxidant activity in vegetable by-products flours and cheeses was assessed using two methods: ABTS (2,2-azino-bis (3-ethylbenzothiazoline-6-sulfonic acid diammonium salt) and FRAP (ferric reducing antioxidant power) assays. The first test is based on the ability of antioxidants to interact with the radical cation $ABTS^{\bullet+}$ (2,2-azinobis-(3-ethylbenzothiazoline-6-sulfonic acid) inhibiting its absorption at 734 nm. The antioxidant activity was determinate according to Marinelli et al. [4] and was expressed as mg Trolox equivalents per g of dry weight. All analyses were carried out in triplicate.

The FRAP assay was carried out according to the procedure described by Benzie et al. [15] with slight modifications. The FRAP reagent was prepared by mixing 100 mL of 300 mM acetate buffer at pH = 3.6 (consisting of 3.1 g of sodium acetate trihydrate and 16 mL of acetic acid glacial per litre of buffer solution), 10 mL of 10 mM TPTZ solution (0.031 g TPTZ in 10 mL of 40 mM HCl dissolved at 50 °C) and 10 mL of 20 mM $FeCl_3$ aqueous solution. The FRAP solution was prepared on the day of analysis and held at 37 °C. An amount of 3 mL of FRAP reagent was added to 200 μL of each properly diluted extract. The mixture was left to react for 30 min at 37 °C and then the absorbance was read at 593 nm. The calibration curve was obtained using as standard $FeSO_4{\cdot}7H_2O$ at concentrations from 0.0125 mM to 0.6 mM (R^2 = 0.9981). The antioxidant activity was expressed as μmols of ferrous equivalent Fe (II) per gram of dried sample. All tests were carried out in triplicate.

2.6. Moisture Content and pH

Moisture content was determined using a thermal balance (Sartorius, Göttingen, Germany). Five grams of homogenised sample was distributed uniformly on an aluminium pan and placed in the thermal balance set at 130 °C. For each cheese sample two replicates were measured.

The pH of the processed spreadable cheese was measured, after direct insertion of an electrode into the sample, using a previously calibrated digital pH meter (Hanna Instruments, Milan, Italy). Each measure was made twice on two different samples.

2.7. Sensory Characterization

The sensory characteristics of all spreadable cheese samples were evaluated by a panel of seven experienced judges (four females and three males aged between 25 years and 45 years) who were members of the Laboratory of Food Packaging. The panellists had at least several years of experience in sensory evaluation prior to this study; however, they were retrained for this study in a session of 2 h to be experienced in the products and terminology. Appropriate descriptive terms for sensory evaluation were decided during the retraining sessions. The evaluated attributes comprised six terms for flavour and aroma (overall intensity, sweetness, salty, acid, bitter, and astringent), two terms describing aftertaste (intensity and persistence), and six attributes encompassing texture and mouth feel (spreadability, fibrous, adhesiveness, solubility, graininess, juiciness). Each sensory attribute was described as reported in the publication of Niro et al. [16]. Cheese samples were rated for their spreadability on a cracker. The intensity of each attribute was evaluated on the scale from 0 to 7 (0 = not detected; 7 = very detected) [16]. The spreadable cheeses were prepared on the day of the analysis and stored at room temperature until 1 h before the evaluation.

2.8. Statistical Analysis

The results were compared by a one-way analysis of variance (ANOVA). A Duncan's multiple range test, with the option of homogeneous groups ($p < 0.05$), was carried out to determine significant differences between cheese samples. The scores from the descriptive sensory analysis were used to construct a principal component analysis (PCA). STATISTICA 7.1 for Windows (StatSoft, Inc, Tulsa, OK, USA) was used for all analyses.

3. Results and Discussion

3.1. Chemical Quality

Chemical characterization of flours from by-products and of fortified spreadable cheese, in terms of total phenolic content, flavonoids, and antioxidant activity measured by ABTS and FRAP (μmol $FeSO_4 \cdot 7H_2O$/g dw) assays, is shown respectively in Tables 1 and 2.

Table 1. Total phenolic content (TPC), total flavonoids content (TFC), and antioxidant activity measured by ABTS (2,2-azino-bis(3-ethylbenzothiazoline-6-sulfonic acid) diammonium salt) and FRAP (ferric reducing antioxidant power) assays of different by-products.

	TPC (mg GAEs/g dw)	TFC (mg QEs/g dw)	ABTS (mg TEs/g dw)	FRAP (μMol $FeSO_4 \cdot 7H_2O$/g dw)
Broccoli by-products	14.59 ± 0.14 [b]	5.55 ± 0.16 [c]	23.70 ± 1.29 [d]	212.40 ± 12.60 [b]
Corn Bran	5.01 ± 0.08 [a]	3.71 ± 0.02 [b]	7.73 ± 0.30 [b]	64.50 ± 2.68 [a]
Artichokes by-products	21.15 ± 0.24 [c]	9.83 ± 0.14 [e]	16.76 ± 0.16 [c]	267.20 ± 2.29 [b]
Tomato peel	4.90 ± 0.48 [a]	2.21 ± 0.02 [a]	4.21 ± 0.27 [a]	23.30 ± 0.63 [a]
Red grape pomace	107.40 ± 2.08 [e]	12.99 ± 0.39 [f]	127.36 ± 2.89 [f]	1886.00 ± 156.70 [d]
White grape pomace	90.51 ± 0.36 [d]	8.84 ± 0.10 [d]	110.13 ± 2.90 [e]	1619.00 ± 85.30 [c]

[a–f]: Data in columns with different superscripts are significantly different ($p < 0.05$). Results are expressed as means ± Standard Deviation for $n = 3$.

As can be seen in Table 1, the red grape pomace powder was the by-product with the highest amount of total phenols (107.4 ± 2.08 mg GAEs/g dw), flavonoids (12.9 ± 0.39 mg QEs/g dw), and antioxidant activity (127.36 ± 2.89 mg TEs/g dw and 1886 ± 156.7 μmol $FeSO_4 \cdot 7H_2O$/g dw for ABTS and FRAP, respectively) among the by-products investigated in this work, followed by the white grape pomace.

As it can be inferred from data listed in Table 2, the addition of by-products to cheese significantly increased the total phenolic content and the flavonoids, compared to the control sample, except in cheese enriched with tomato peel, probably due to the scarce source of bioactive compounds. Specifically, cheese containing white and red grape pomace recorded high phenolic content (2.74 ± 0.04 and 2.34 ± 0.15 mg GAEs/g dw, respectively) followed by broccoli (1.78 ± 0.02 mg GAEs/g dw), artichoke (1.20 ± 0.22 mg GAEs/g dw), and corn bran (0.90 ± 0.04 mg GAEs/g dw). Some unexpected results were observed, because the TPC of WGP-SC was slightly higher than that of RGP-SC. This experimental finding could be ascribed to more than one reason, for example, their stability or more simply to the method used for total phenols determination (i.e., the Folin-Ciocalteu method). As a fact, this method is not selective and therefore it can detect other reducing compounds reacting with the Folin-Ciocalteu reagent [10,12]. On the contrary, Gonzàlez-Centeno et al. [17], who studied the phenolic composition and the antioxidant activity of by-products of 10 different cultivars of *Vitis vinifera*, both white and red, observed that there was no significant difference among varieties.

Table 2. Total phenolic content (TPC), total flavonoids content (TFC), and antioxidant activity measured by ABTS and FRAP assays of spreadable cheese enriched with 5% by-products.

	TPC (mg GAEs/g dw)	TFC (mg QEs/g dw)	ABTS (mg TEs/g dw)	FRAP (μMol $FeSO_4 \cdot 7H_2O$/g dw)
CNT	0.66 ± 0.06 [a]	0.47 ± 0.00 [a]	0.96 ± 0.08 [a]	1.52 ± 0.05 [a]
Br-SC	1.78 ± 0.02 [d]	0.79 ± 0.07 [c]	2.09 ± 0.06 [d]	6.65 ± 0.20 [d]
CB-SC	0.90 ± 0.04 [b]	0.49 ± 0.03 [a]	1.71 ± 0.09 [c]	4.53 ± 0.47 [c]
Art-SC	1.20 ± 0.22 [c]	0.06 ± 0.03 [b]	1.71 ± 0.20 [c]	4.74 ± 0.13 [c]
TP-SC	0.72 ± 0.02 [a]	0.47 ± 0.00 [a]	1.51 ± 0.07 [b]	2.58 ± 0.12 [b]
RGP-SC	2.34 ± 0.15 [e]	0.86 ± 0.08 [d]	3.95 ± 0.19 [e]	26.17 ± 0.72 [e]
WGP-SC	2.74 ± 0.04 [f]	0.89 ± 0.03 [d]	4.00 ± 0.06 [e]	26.45 ± 0.25 [e]

CNT: control spreadable cheese; Br-SC: broccoli spreadable cheese; CB-SC: corn bran spreadable cheese; Art-SC: artichoke spreadable cheese; TP-SC: tomato peel spreadable cheese; RGP-SC: red grape pomace spreadable cheese; WGP-SC: white grape pomace spreadable cheese. [a–f]: Data in columns with different superscripts are significantly different ($p < 0.05$). Results are expressed as means ± Standard Deviation for $n = 3$.

From the antioxidant activity point of view, cheese fortification involved a significant increase in all the cases. The same result has been confirmed by both the ABTS and the FRAP assay. According to Alonso et al. [18], there is a positive correlation between the antioxidant activity and the total polyphenolic content of samples. In this work, best results were obtained for cheese enriched with red and white grape pomace. Other authors tried to enrich dairy products, in particular yogurt, with bioactive compounds from red grape pomace [7,10]. Tseng et Zhao [7] used wine grape pomace as a source of dietary fibre and polyphenols in yogurt and salad dressing for enhancing nutritional value and improving storability of the products. They noted a higher amount of dietary fibre and polyphenol contents and a slower lipid oxidation of samples during refrigeration storage.

Marchiani et al. [10] fortified yogurt with grape skin powder and observed a significantly higher total phenolic content and antioxidant activity than the control. Rashidinejad et al. [19] incorporated green tea extract into full-fat cheese to investigate the effect of green tea catechins on antioxidant properties and also noticed a significant increase of TPC and antioxidant activity at all concentrations.

3.2. Moisture Content and pH

Figure 1a reports the pH values of each cheese added with vegetable by-products and of the control cheese right after production. As can be observed, the pH value was 4.53 for the CNT cheese and it did not change significantly after the addition of corn bran and tomato peel by-product. Contrary, for samples with red and white grape pomace powders added, a decrease of pH from 4.53 to 4.34 and 4.42, respectively, was observed. Similar results were obtained by Tseng et al. [7], who detected a decrease of pH in yogurt immediately after the addition of wine grape pomace. For the Br-SC and Art-SC, a slight pH increase was found.

Concerning the percentage of moisture, it was observed that all tested spreadable cheese with vegetable by-products presented a moisture reduction compared to the control (Figure 1b). Probably, the addition of the by-product flours increased the total solids content in the formulation and consequently the moisture percentage decreased. In the literature, several examples confirmed a decrease of moisture content in cheese with different flours added. In particular, Safaa [20] observed that the total solid content in yogurt and soft cheese increased by increasing chia flour addition and contextually the moisture content decreased compared to control. Also, Arunkumar et al. [21] observed that the incorporation of 5%, 10%, and 15% soy flour significantly decreased the moisture of filled spreads by about 61.4%, 59.5%, and 57.7%, respectively. This redaction may be due to the relevant increase in total solid content of spreads by flour incorporation. According to El-Aziz et al. [22], the addition of food by-products increased the total solid content in cheese formulation, thus leading to a moisture decrease.

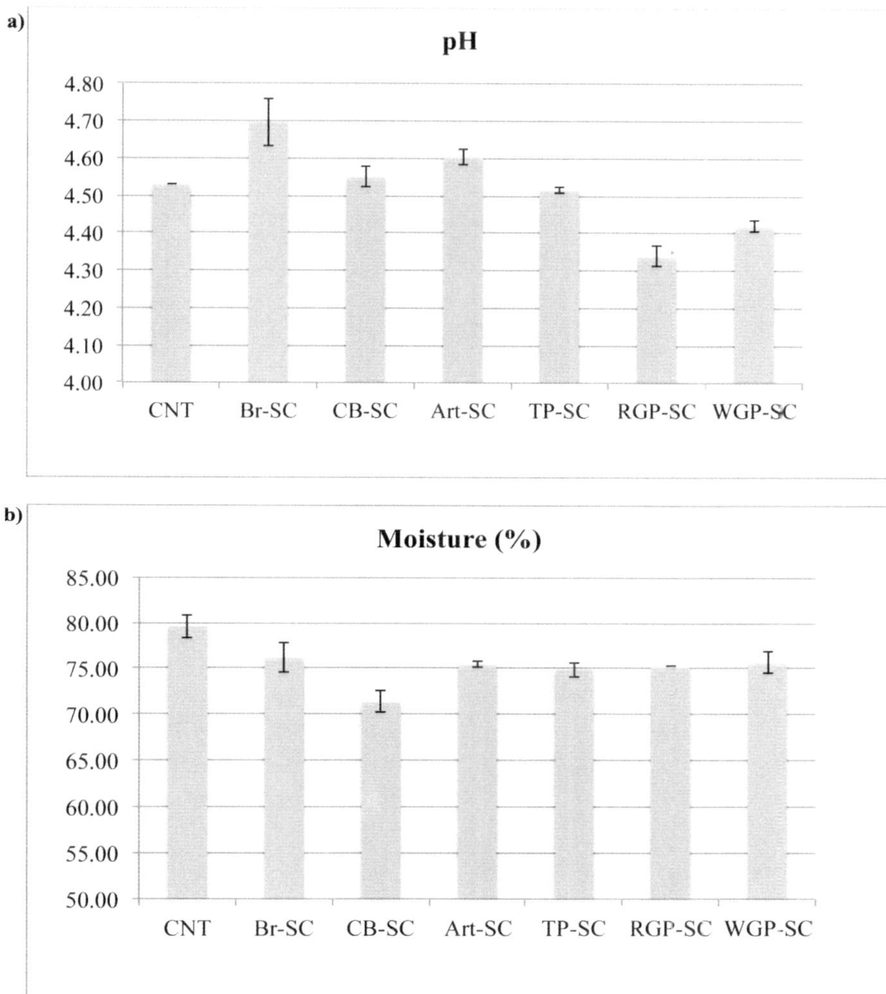

Figure 1. pH (**a**) and moisture content (**b**) of spreadable cheese enriched with different by-products.

3.3. Sensory Quality

Ratings for flavour and textural attributes of spreadable cheeses are presented in Tables 3 and 4, respectively.

Table 3. Ratings for flavour attributes of seven spreadable cheeses investigated.

	Flavour Attributes (0–7)							
Samples	Overall Intensity	Sweetness	Salty	Acid	Bitter	Astringent	Aftertaste Intensity	Aftertaste Persistence
CNT	6.0 ± 0.3 [b]	1.2 ± 0.4 [a]	1.0 ± 0.0 [a,b]	4.6 ± 0.4 [b]	n.d.	n.d.	6.0 ± 0.0 [b]	6.0 ± 0.0 [c]
Br-SC	7.0 ± 0.0 [c]	n.d.	1.4 ± 0.4 [b]	5.1 ± 0.2 [b]	n.d.	1.2 ± 0.4 [a]	7.0 ± 0.2 [c]	6.7 ± 0.4 [d]
CB-SC	5.6 ± 0.3 [a]	2.0 ± 0.0 [b]	0.7 ± 0.3 [a]	4.0 ± 0.2 [a]	n.d.	2.0 ± 0.0 [b]	5.6 ± 0.3 [b]	5.4 ± 0.2 [b]

Table 3. *Cont.*

Samples	Flavour Attributes (0–7)							
	Overall Intensity	Sweetness	Salty	Acid	Bitter	Astringent	Aftertaste Intensity	Aftertaste Persistence
Art-SC	6.9 ± 0.2^{c}	n.d.	1.6 ± 0.4^{b}	4.9 ± 0.4^{b}	6.0 ± 0.0	0.8 ± 0.4^{a}	6.6 ± 0.4^{c}	6.2 ± 0.3^{c}
TP-SC	5.5 ± 0.3^{a}	n.d.	0.5 ± 0.5^{a}	6.0 ± 0.0^{c}	n.d.	0.9 ± 0.4^{a}	5.0 ± 0.3^{a}	4.1 ± 0.2^{a}
RGP-SC	7.0 ± 0.0^{c}	n.d.	n.d.	7.0 ± 0.0^{d}	n.d.	3.0 ± 0.0^{c}	7.0 ± 0.0^{d}	7.0 ± 0.0^{d}
WGP-SC	6.9 ± 0.2^{c}	n.d.	n.d.	6.9 ± 0.2^{d}	n.d.	3.0 ± 0.3^{c}	7.0 ± 0.2^{d}	6.2 ± 0.3^{c}

$^{a–d}$: Data in each column with different superscripts are significantly different ($p < 0.05$). Results are expressed as means ± Standard Deviation. n.d.: not detected; CNT: control spreadable cheese; Br-SC: broccoli spreadable cheese; CB-SC: corn bran spreadable cheese; Art-SC: artichoke spreadable cheese; TP-SC: tomato peel spreadable cheese; RGP-SC: red grape pomace spreadable cheese; WGP-SC: white grape pomace spreadable cheese.

Table 4. Rating for textural attributes of spreadable cheeses investigated.

Samples	Textural Attributes (0–7)					
	Spreadability	Fibrous	Adhesiveness	Graininess	Solubility	Juiciness
CNT	7.0 ± 0.0^{d}	n.d.	4.0 ± 0.0^{a}	n.d.	6.0 ± 0.3^{d}	6.0 ± 0.0^{c}
Br-SC	4.5 ± 0.4^{a}	6.0 ± 0.0^{b}	5.5 ± 0.3^{d}	5.1 ± 0.2^{b}	3.0 ± 0.3^{a}	3.9 ± 0.2^{a}
CB-SC	6.3 ± 0.2^{c}	4.5 ± 0.4^{a}	4.5 ± 0.4^{b}	3.9 ± 0.2^{a}	5.0 ± 0.3^{c}	4.5 ± 0.4^{b}
Art-SC	5.5 ± 0.3^{b}	6.3 ± 0.2^{c}	5.5 ± 0.0^{d}	5.5 ± 0.0^{c}	3.9 ± 0.2^{b}	4.0 ± 0.0^{a}
TP-SC	6.0 ± 0.0^{c}	6.5 ± 0.0^{c}	5.1 ± 0.2^{c}	5.1 ± 0.2^{b}	4.0 ± 0.0^{b}	4.0 ± 0.3^{a}
RGP-SC	5.3 ± 0.2^{b}	7.0 ± 0.2^{d}	5.0 ± 0.0^{c}	6.0 ± 0.0^{d}	4.5 ± 0.4^{c}	4.0 ± 0.3^{a}
WGP-SC	5.1 ± 0.2^{b}	7.0 ± 0.0^{d}	5.1 ± 0.2^{c}	6.0 ± 0.3^{d}	4.6 ± 0.4^{c}	4.0 ± 0.3^{a}

$^{a–d}$: Data in each column with different superscripts are significantly different ($p < 0.05$). Results are expressed as means ± Standard Deviation. n.d.: not detected; CNT: control spreadable cheese; Br-SC: broccoli spreadable cheese; CB-SC: corn bran spreadable cheese; Art-SC: artichoke spreadable cheese; TP-SC: tomato peel spreadable cheese; RGP-SC: red grape pomace spreadable cheese; WGP-SC: white grape pomace spreadable cheese.

The intensity scores for different flavours ranged among the investigated cheeses from 4 to 7 for overall intensity, acid, aftertaste intensity, and aftertaste persistence, whereas less variation (from 0 to 2) was observed for sweetness and salty. An acid taste was detected in all spreadable cheese samples, caused by the increase in acidity and by the pH decrease during the coagulation process. However, for the cheese added with red and white grape pomace powders, the acid value was higher, as confirmed by their final pH value (see Figure 1a). A pH reduction for yogurt with wine grape pomace powders added was also confirmed by Tseng and Zhao [7]. Contrary, sweetness parameter was detected only for CNT and CB-SC samples; no bitter taste was detected, except for the cheese containing the artichoke flour. This is not surprising, as it is well known that artichoke is popular for its pleasant bitter taste, which is mostly attributed to the cynarin found in the green parts of the plant [23]. Moreover, a greater astringent sensation was perceived for RGP-SC and WGP-SC samples, probably due to the presence of polyphenol substances, such as tannins, that are generally found in grape skins [24]. Regarding the textural attributes (Table 4), the CNT showed high spreadability value (score 7), while the Br-SC sample was the least spreadable among the investigated samples (score 4.5); the Art-SC, RGP-SC, and WGP-SC cheeses showed similar scores (between 5.0 and 5.5). They were found to be less spreadable with respect to the TP-SC and CB-SC samples that exhibited values of 6.0 and 6.35, respectively. The spreadability reduction may be associated to the change in moisture content and to the increase in total solid content of cheese by flour incorporation [8,10]. Fibrous, adhesiveness, and graininess attributes were also influenced by the vegetable flours; in fact, except for the CNT and the CB-SC cheese, their values ranged from 5 to 7 for all the samples. The less soluble samples like Br-SC, Art-SC, and the two grape pomace powder cheeses investigated were also the least juicy (scores from 3 to 4.5). In the literature, several examples of the effects of the water binding capacity of by-products on texture parameters and tactile sensation when incorporated into different foods (i.e., bakery, dairy, and meat products) have been reported [11,25–27].

To study the variability of the sensory attributes of cheese, the principal component analysis was carried out (Figure 2).

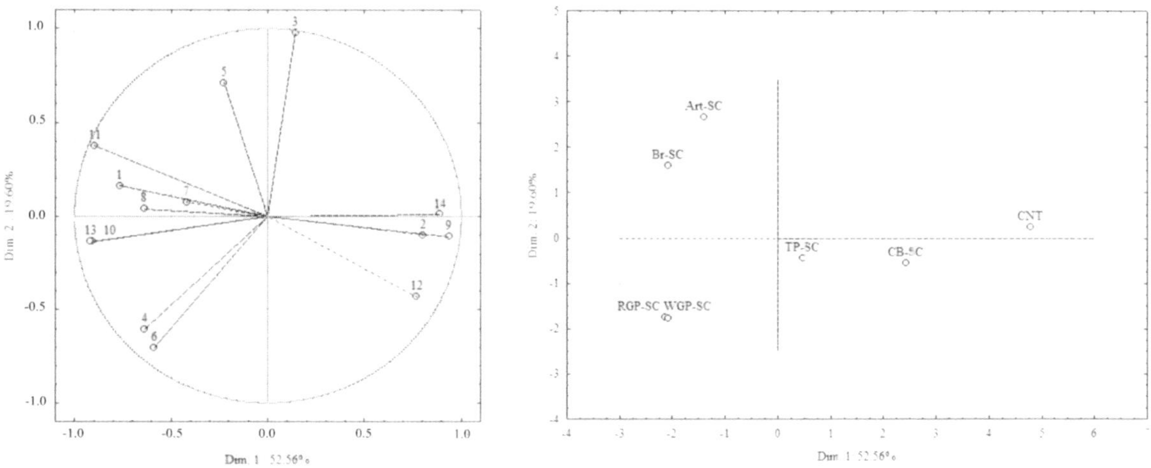

Figure 2. Principal components analysis of the sensory attributes of cheese (sample plot: **right**, variable plot: **left**). CNT: control spreadable cheese; CB-SC: corn bran spreadable cheese; Br-SC: broccoli spreadable cheese; WGP-SC: white grape pomace spreadable cheese; RGP-SC: red grape pomace spreadable cheese; Art-SC: artichoke spreadable cheese; TP-SC: tomato peel spreadable cheese. Attributes 1 (Overall intensity), 2 (Sweetness), 3 (Salty), 4 (Acid), 5 (Bitter), 6 (Astringent), 7 (Aftertaste Intensity), 8 (Aftertaste Persistence), 9 (Spreadability), 10 (Fibrous), 11 (Adhesiveness), 12 (Solubility), 13 (Graininess), 14 (Juiciness).

The first dimension (Dim 1) and the second dimension (Dim 2) explained 52.56% and 19.60% of the total variability, respectively. Salty, juiciness, sweetness, spreadability, and solubility are on the right side of the plot, while all the other sensory attributes are on the left side. The first axis explains 52.56% of the total variance and separates the seven cheeses into two groups. CNT, CB-SC, and TP-SC were different from the other four cheeses on the basis of the salty, juiciness, sweetness, solubility, and spreadability sensory attributes. The other cheeses were mostly described with attributes like bitter, aftertaste, adhesiveness, overall intensity, graininess, fibrous, acid, and astringent. Within this group of four cheeses, the second axis, which explains 19.60% of the total variance, distinguished RGP-SC and WGP-SC from the other cheeses. The acid and astringent attributes on the negative part of the second axis can explain the separation of those cheeses from the other ones.

4. Conclusions

In this work, the influence of by-products addition on physicochemical and sensory properties of spreadable cheese was investigated. The results highlighted that the best results from a nutritional point of view were obtained for the cheese samples with red and white wine grape pomace added, followed by broccoli, artichoke, and corn bran. Generally, the addition of vegetable flour to cheese significantly increased the total phenolic content and flavonoids compared to the control sample. However, technological options could be optimized with red and white wine grape pomace added to spreadable cheese in order to increase antioxidant compounds without compromising the sensory properties.

Author Contributions: Annalisa Lucera, Cristina Costa, Amalia Conte, and Matteo Alessandro Del Nobile designed the study and elaborated data; Annalisa Lucera, Cristina Costa, Valeria Marinelli, and Maria Antonietta Saccotelli conducted the experiments; Annalisa Lucera, Cristina Costa, and Valeria Marinelli drafted the paper; Amalia Conte and Matteo Alessandro Del Nobile wrote the paper.

Conflicts of Interest: Any conflict of interest needs to be declared.

References

1. Schieber, A.; Stintzing, F.C.; Carle, R. By-products of plant food processing as a source of functional compounds—Recent developments. *Trends Food Sci. Technol.* **2001**, *12*, 401–413. [CrossRef]
2. Ajila, C.M.; Aalami, M.; Leelavathi, K.; Prasada Rao, U.J.S. Mango peel powder: A potential source of antioxidant and dietary fiber in macaroni preparations. *Innov. Food Sci. Emerg. Technol.* **2010**, *11*, 219–224. [CrossRef]
3. Sudha, M.L.; Baskaran, V.; Leelavathi, K. Apple pomace as a source of dietary fiber and polyphenols and its effect on the rheological characteristics and cake making. *Food Chem.* **2007**, *104*, 686–692. [CrossRef]
4. Marinelli, V.; Padalino, L.; Nardiello, D.; Del Nobile, M.A.; Conte, A. New Approach to Enrich Pasta with Polyphenols from Grape Marc. *J. Chem.* **2015**. [CrossRef]
5. Boubaker, M.; Omri, A.E.L.; Blecker, C.; Bouzouita, N. Fibre concentrate from artichoke (*Cynara scolymus* L.) stem by-products: Characterization and application as a bakery product ingredient. *Food Sci. Technol. Int.* **2016**, *22*, 759–768. [CrossRef] [PubMed]
6. Drabinska, N.; Ciska, E.; Szmatowicz, B.; Krupa-Kozak, U. Broccoli by-products improve the nutraceutical potential of gluten-free mini sponge cakes. *Food Chem.* **2017**. [CrossRef]
7. Tseng, A.; Zhao, Y. Wine grape pomace as antioxidant dietary fibre for enhancing nutritional value and improving storability of yogurt and salad dressing. *Food Chem.* **2013**, *138*, 356–365. [CrossRef] [PubMed]
8. Hwang, J.-Y.; Shyu, Y.-S.; Hsu, C.-K. Grape wine lees improves the rheological and adds antioxidant properties to ice cream. *LWT* **2009**, *42*, 312–318. [CrossRef]
9. Bertolino, M.; Belviso, S.; Dal Bello, B.; Ghirardello, D.; Giordano, M.; Rolle, L.; Gerbi, V.; Zeppa, G. Influence of the addition of different hazelnut skins on the physicochemical, antioxidant, polyphenol and sensory properties of yogurt. *LWT* **2015**, *63*, 1145–1154. [CrossRef]
10. Marchiani, R.; Bertolino, M.; Ghirardello, D.; McSweeney, P.L.H.; Zeppa, G. Physicochemical and nutritional qualities of grape pomace powder-fortified semi-hard cheeses. *J. Food Sci. Technol.* **2015**. [CrossRef] [PubMed]
11. Abd Elhamid, A.M. Physicochemical, rheological and sensory properties of Egyptian Kariesh cheese containing wheat bran. *Int. J. Dairy Technol.* **2016**. [CrossRef]
12. Rashidinejad, A.; Birch, E.J.; Sun-Waterhouse, D.; Everett, D.W. Effects of catechin on the phenolic content and antioxidant properties of low-fat cheese. *Int. J. Food Sci. Technol.* **2013**, *48*, 2448–2455. [CrossRef]
13. Spinelli, S.; Conte, A.; Lecce, L.; Incoronato, A.L.; Del Nobile, M.A. Microencapsulated propolis to enhance the antioxidant properties of fresh fish burgers. *J. Food Process Eng.* **2015**, *38*, 527–535. [CrossRef]
14. Huang, Y.-S.; Ho, S.-C. Polymethoxy flavones are responsible for the anti-inflammatory activity of citrus fruit peel. *Food Chem.* **2010**, *119*, 868–873. [CrossRef]
15. Benzie, I.F.F.; Strain, J.J. The Ferric Reducing Ability of Plasma (FRAP) as a Measure of "Antioxidant Power": The FRAP Assay. *Anal. Biochem.* **1996**, *239*, 70–76. [CrossRef] [PubMed]
16. Niro, S.; Fratianni, A.; Tremonte, P.; Sorrentino, E.; Tipaldi, L.; Panfili, G.; Coppola, R. Innovative Caciocavallo cheeses made from a mixture of cow milk with ewe or goat milk. *J. Dairy Sci.* **2014**, *97*, 1296–1304. [CrossRef] [PubMed]
17. Gonzàlez-Centeno, M.R.; Jourdes, M.; Femenia, A.; Simal, S.; Rosselló, C.; Teissedre, P.-L. Proanthocyanidin Composition and Antioxidant Potential of the Stem Winemaking By-products from 10 Different Grape Varieties (*Vitis vinifera* L.). *J. Agric. Food Chem.* **2012**, *60*, 11850–11858. [CrossRef] [PubMed]
18. Alonso, A.M.; Guillèn, D.A.; Barroso, C.G.; Puertas, B.; Garcìa, A. Determination of antioxidant activity of wine by products and its correlation with polyphenolic content. *J. Agric. Food Chem.* **2002**, *50*, 5832–5836. [CrossRef] [PubMed]
19. Rashidinejad, A.; Birch, E.J.; Everett, D.W. A novel functional full-fat hard cheese containing liposomal nanoencapsulated green tea catechins: Manufacture and recovery following simulated digestion. *Food Funct.* **2016**, *7*, 3283–3294. [CrossRef] [PubMed]
20. Safaa, M.A.F. Evaluation of Yogurt and Soft Cheese Fortified with Chia Seeds. *World J. Dairy Food Sci.* **2017**, *12*, 1–12.
21. Arunkumar, H. Effect of soy flour and soy oil on the composition and sensory characteristics of paneer spread. *J. Res. Agric. Anim. Sci.* **2014**, *6*, 1–5.
22. El-Aziz, M.A.; Mohamed, S.H.S.; Seleet, F.T. Production and Evaluation of Soft Cheese Fortified with Ginger Extract as a Functional Dairy Food. *Pol. J. Food Nutr. Sci.* **2012**, *62*, 77–83. [CrossRef]

23. Nasser, A.M.A.G. Phytochemical Study of *Cynara scolymus* L. (Artichoke) (Asteraceae) Cultivated in Iraq, Detection and Identification of Phenolic Acid Compounds Cynarin and Chlorogenic Acid. *Iraqi J. Pharm Sci.* **2012**, *21*, 6–13.
24. Ky, I.; Crozier, A.; Cros, G.; Teissedre, P.-L. Polyphenols composition of wine and grape sub-products and potential effects on chronic diseases. *Nutr. Aging* **2014**, *2*, 165–177.
25. Savadkoohi, S.; Hoogenkamp, H.; Shamsi, K.; Farahnaky, A. Colour, sensory and textural attributes of beef frankfurter, beef ham and meat-free sausage containing tomato pomace. *Meat Sci.* **2014**, *97*, 410–418. [CrossRef] [PubMed]
26. Özvural, E.B.; Vural, H. Grape seed flour is a viable ingredient to improve the nutritional profile and reduce lipid oxidation of frankfurters. *Meat Sci.* **2011**, *88*, 179–183. [CrossRef] [PubMed]
27. O'Shea, N.; Arendt, E.; Gallagher, E. Dietary fibre and phytochemical characteristics of fruit and vegetable by-products and their recent applications as novel ingredients in food products. *Innov. Food Sci. Emerg. Technol.* **2012**, *16*, 1–10. [CrossRef]

14

Reactive Oxygen Species and Mitochondrial Dynamics: The Yin and Yang of Mitochondrial Dysfunction and Cancer Progression

Jan Ježek, Katrina F. Cooper * and Randy Strich

Department of Molecular Biology, Rowan University Graduate School of Biomedical Sciences, Stratford, NJ 08084, USA; jezekj6@rowan.edu (J.J.); strichra@rowan.edu (R.S.)

* Correspondence: cooperka@rowan.edu

Abstract: Mitochondria are organelles with a highly dynamic ultrastructure maintained by a delicate equilibrium between its fission and fusion rates. Understanding the factors influencing this balance is important as perturbations to mitochondrial dynamics can result in pathological states. As a terminal site of nutrient oxidation for the cell, mitochondrial powerhouses harness energy in the form of ATP in a process driven by the electron transport chain. Contemporaneously, electrons translocated within the electron transport chain undergo spontaneous side reactions with oxygen, giving rise to superoxide and a variety of other downstream reactive oxygen species (ROS). Mitochondrially-derived ROS can mediate redox signaling or, in excess, cause cell injury and even cell death. Recent evidence suggests that mitochondrial ultrastructure is tightly coupled to ROS generation depending on the physiological status of the cell. Yet, the mechanism by which changes in mitochondrial shape modulate mitochondrial function and redox homeostasis is less clear. Aberrant mitochondrial morphology may lead to enhanced ROS formation, which, in turn, may deteriorate mitochondrial health and further exacerbate oxidative stress in a self-perpetuating vicious cycle. Here, we review the latest findings on the intricate relationship between mitochondrial dynamics and ROS production, focusing mainly on its role in malignant disease.

Keywords: mitochondrial dynamics; mitochondrial ultrastructure; redox signaling; oxidative stress; reactive oxygen species; superoxide; cancer

---

1. Introduction

1.1. From Bean to Interconnected Web

In textbooks, mitochondria are classically depicted as round, bean-like organelles [1]. The oval shape of mitochondria observed by electron microscopy is consistent with the endosymbiotic theory that mitochondria evolved from a bacterial ancestor [2–4]. However, in living cells, mitochondria typically display dynamic networks of interconnected tubules with many branching points (Movie S1). The fluctuating nature of mitochondrial ultrastructure affords these organelles flexibility in regulating the bioenergetic flux of key molecular elements such as ATP, lipids, proteins, mitochondrial DNA (mtDNA), metabolites, cofactors, and ions throughout the entire mitochondrial network [5,6]. Small guanosine 5′-triphosphatase (GTPase) proteins like Miro help provide a high degree of homeostatic heterogeneity within the mitochondrial matrix by trafficking mitochondria along cytoskeletal filaments within [7,8] or between cells [9], thereby exposing mitochondria to distinct biochemical milieus [10]. Although mitochondrial motility was predominantly studied in neurons where mitochondria serve a specialized function [11], recent literature has revealed molecular players of the neuronal mitochondrial transport machinery that may be deregulated in cancers [12]. In this scenario, these molecular motors hijack mitochondria and transfer them into cancer cell peripheries as a localized energy supply for increased mobility and metastasis of the tumor. Accordingly, mitochondrial fragmentation is believed to facilitate repositioning of mitochondria in cancer cells [13].

1.2. The Fission/Fusion Machinery

The overall steady-state morphological appearance of the mitochondrial reticulum is governed by the opposing activities of large GTPases directing either fission or fusion. Fusion of the outer and inner mitochondrial membrane (OMM and IMM) is mediated by mitofusins Mfn1 [14] or Mfn2 [15] and optic atrophy 1 (Opa1) [16,17], respectively. Profusion activity has also been reported for mitochondrial phospholipase D (PLD) [18] and mitofilin [19], which is part of the newly-discovered mitochondrial contact site and cristae organizing system (MICOS) [20,21]. In response to oxidative stress [22–24] or during cell division [25], the recruitment and activation of the mitochondrial fission GTPase, dynamin-related protein 1 (Drp1), shifts the balance toward the fragmented phenotype [26–28]. Oligomerization of Drp1 into a spiral-shaped filament around a mitochondrial tubule precedes the simultaneous constriction of both OMM and IMM, which occurs in a GTP-dependent manner [29]. Mitochondrial fission factor (Mff), mitochondrial fission 1 (Fis1), or mitochondrial dynamic proteins 49 and 51 (MiD49 and MiD51) are receptor-adapters that actively facilitate Drp1 interaction with the OMM during mitochondrial division [30–32]. Drp1 is post-translationally regulated via phosphorylation, ubiquitination, SUMOylation, and *S*-nitrosylation. For example, phosphorylation at Ser616 by the protein kinase C isoform δ (PKCδ) is activating, whereas phosphorylation at Ser637 by protein kinase A (PKA) inhibits Drp1 function [33]. Moreover, activity of the classic GTPase dynamin 2 (Dyn2) is required for final mitochondrial scission, indicating that this process is complex, requiring multiple steps and contributing factors [34].

1.3. Linking Mitochondrial Dynamics to Cell Death Pathways

Fragmentation of the mitochondrial network is linked with several physiological indicators of mitochondrial dysfunction, including loss of mitochondrial membrane potential ($\Delta\Psi_m$), decreased respiration and oxidative phosphorylation (OXPHOS), metabolic shift towards glycolysis, and increased mitochondrial ROS formation [33]. Glucose or fatty acid catabolism may also give rise to fragmented mitochondria, albeit with hyperpolarized $\Delta\Psi_m$ and augmented OXPHOS [35]. Collapse of the reticular form of mitochondria into fragments represents a key intermediate accompanying the activation of either salvaging or pro-death pathways depending on the stimulus. Resultant fragments of dysfunctional mitochondria can be selectively targeted for mitophagy to promote cell survival [36] or, in severe oxidative stress, trigger the intrinsic pathway of apoptosis (Figure 1) [37]. A common denominator for apoptotic and mitophagic stress response is the involvement of mitochondrial fission, perhaps triggered by mitochondrial ROS [38,39].

Intrinsic, or mitochondrial, apoptosis is characterized by increased association of the pro-apoptotic protein Bcl-2-associated X (Bax) with the OMM [40]. Bax, and its close homolog Bcl-2 homologous antagonist/killer (Bak), which constitutively resides in OMM, oligomerize to induce mitochondrial outer membrane permeabilization (MOMP). MOMP is accompanied by the release of pro-apoptotic factors, including cytochrome C, apoptosis-inducing factor (AIF), second mitochondria-derived activator of caspase/direct inhibitor of apoptosis-binding protein with low pI (Smac/DIABLO), Omi/high temperature requirement protein A2 (Omi/HtrA2), and other second-messengers that initiate either caspase-dependent or caspase-independent cell death [41,42]. Although regulation of MOMP by mitochondrial dynamics is still elusive, considerable progress has been made towards visualizing Bax-mediated OMM pore formation in cells by means of super-resolution microscopy [43–45]. Consistent with a positive role for fission in programmed cell death (PCD), promoting fusion or inhibiting fragmentation prevents or delays the onset of apoptosis [46] or mitophagy [47]. Given that evading apoptosis is a hallmark of cancer, correct control of mitochondrial dynamics is critical for slowing or inhibiting tumor progression [22,36,48–50]. In addition, failure of these mitochondrial quality control check-points can contribute to the development of degenerative pathologies such as type 2 diabetes [51–53], heart and brain ischemia-reperfusion (I/R) injury [54], cardiovascular disorders [55–59], and neuropathies [59–61] such as Parkinson's [62] and Alzheimer's disease [63]. Mitochondrial dysregulation is also thought to contribute to physiological processes associated with aging [64,65]. Are fragmented mitochondria a cause or consequence of ROS overproduction? Is it the severity of mitochondrial dysfunction that discriminates between redox signaling and oxidative stress? Can oxidative stress be regulated by mitochondrial morphology? Are there different mitochondrial fission phenotypes? Can we therapeutically treat mitochondrial dynamics? This review focuses on the interplay between mitochondrial dynamics and ROS homeostasis relevant to the etiology of malignant neoplastic diseases.

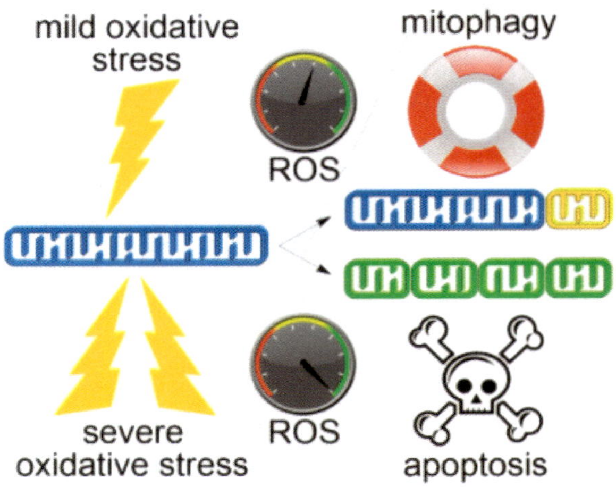

Figure 1. Changing cell fates depending on oxidative damage extent and mitochondrial dynamics. Under mild oxidative stress conditions (top), clearance of defective mitochondrion (yellow) by mitophagy reduces ROS levels and enhances cell survival. Acute oxidative stress (bottom) promotes extensive mitochondrial fission and dysfunction that ultimately leads to elevated ROS, loss of mitochondrial integrity (green) and apoptotic cell death.

2. Modulation of Mitochondrial Dynamics by Reactive Oxygen Species

2.1. Mitochondria Are a Prime Source of ROS

A primary function of mitochondria is to generate proton-motive force, required for ATP synthesis during OXPHOS to support cellular processes. As such, mitochondria constitute a major metabolic hub, or a "molecular furnace", in which catabolic pathways intersect to oxidize nutrients. Along the electron transport chain (ETC), up to 2% of electrons leak before reaching Complex IV, incompletely reacting with oxygen in a one-electron reduction to produce superoxide (anion radical) instead of a water molecule [66]. Mitochondria are the major producer of superoxide and other downstream ROS in the cell [67], the main source of mitochondrially-derived superoxide being Complex I and III [68]. Additionally, mitochondrial superoxide is generated by electron-transferring flavoprotein-ubiquinone oxidoreductase during fatty acid oxidation, glycerol-3-phosphate dehydrogenase, and other IMM-associated oxidoreductases [69]. Superoxide is membrane-impermeant and is readily dismutated to non-radical, membrane-diffusible, H_2O_2 by superoxide dismutase (SOD) or non-enzymatic mechanisms [70,71]. As a membrane-diffusible species, mitochondrially-generated H_2O_2 has been implicated in cell-wide redox signal transduction [72–77]. H_2O_2 can be further reduced by divalent metal ions or superoxide in the Fenton [78] or Haber-Weiss reactions [79], respectively, to produce the hydroxyl radical ($^{\bullet}OH$). This highly toxic molecule promiscuously reacts with a broad range of metabolites, thus inducing oxidative damage [80]. Depending on the physiological context, NADPH oxidases (NOX) and dual oxidases (DUOX) can further contribute to cellular superoxide formation [81].

2.2. Mitochondrial ROS and Cancer, a Double-Edged Sword

ROS are well known activators of apoptosis [82,83]. Due to oncogenic mutations, increased metabolic activity, or decreased mitochondrial function, many cancer types are intrinsically associated with elevated ROS generation [84–86] and mitochondrial fragmentation [33,87]. In addition to being a mutagenic motor that can drive a cell out of senescence, conventional anti-cancer strategies utilize pro-oxidant drugs to push the ROS levels beyond a death-inducing threshold specifically in cancer but not normal cells [88–91]. A typical example is cisplatin, which stimulates both nuclear DNA and mtDNA damage with concomitant mitochondrial fission [22] and increased mitochondrial ROS generation [92]. As proof of concept, antioxidants interfere with the therapeutic mechanism of cisplatin [93]. In addition to chemical pro-oxidants, singlet oxygen ($^1O_2$) itself is a ROS molecule that has gained particular attention in the treatment of shallow tumors such as skin melanoma by photodynamic therapy (PDT). In PDT, $^1O_2$ and free radicals are generated by irradiation of a pre-administered photosensitizing drug to induce apoptotic or necrotic cell death in cancer cells [94,95].

Dwelling in close proximity to the epicenter of oxidative metabolism, mtDNA is considered particularly vulnerable to free radicals and oxidative damage. The free radical theory of ageing is defined by the positive correlation between accumulated ROS and mtDNA mutations [96]. Considering that the mitochondrial genome encodes subunits of four out of five ETC Complexes (Complex I and III–V), mutations in mtDNA predispose ageing cells to mitochondrial dysfunction in a self-perpetuating vicious cycle [97]. Intramitochondrial mixing by coordinated mitochondrial fission and fusion cycles could represent an important complementary mechanism to preserve mtDNA integrity against oxidative injury [98]. Taken together, observations that ageing is associated with the fragmented mitochondrial phenotype and mtDNA damage would seem to suggest mitochondrial dynamics and ROS formation are mutually intertwined physiological processes that contribute to a slow decay of mitochondrial function during ageing.

2.3. Antioxidant Defense Systems

In order to cope with elevated ROS production, cells utilize a host of intricate antioxidant-defense mechanisms. The most abundant intracellular antioxidant, glutathione (GSH), participates in H_2O_2 detoxification through thiol-disulfide interchange catalyzed by glutathione peroxidase (GPX), yielding oxidized glutathione (GSSG) [99,100]. Glutathione reductase, in turn, plays a key role in maintaining the reduced form of glutathione [101]. In addition to its direct antioxidant capacity, GSSG contributes to antioxidant defense by inducing mitochondrial hyper-fusion in an Mfn1- and Mfn2-dependent manner [102]. Other H_2O_2 scavengers include catalase, which is mainly located in the peroxisomes where it converts H_2O_2 to water and oxygen [103], and the peroxiredoxin (PRX) system [104], relying upon the thioredoxin (TRX) and thioredoxin reductase catalytic cycle [105,106]. Stable peroxiredoxin 3 depletion in transformed mesothelioma cells leads to a hyper-fused mitochondrial phenotype, which is rescued by overexpression of mitochondrially-targeted or cytosolic catalase [107]. Additionally, antioxidant action is inherent in the activity of the uncoupling protein (UCP) family [108,109] and DJ-1 [110]. Ectopic overexpression of SET, an inhibitor of protein phosphatase 2A, in human embryonic kidney cancer cells increases UCP2 and UCP3 levels in parallel with Drp1- and Fis1-dependent mitochondrial fragmentation and diminished autophagic flux [111]. In the mouse model of I/R injury, DJ-1 elicits cardioprotection by preventing excessive mitochondrial fission [112]. Although antioxidant systems are recognized therapeutic targets, they are prone to transcriptional activation by oncogenes and thereby enhance tumorigenesis and chemoresistance [113,114].

3. Signaling Pathways Controlling Mitochondrial Dynamics

ROS-generating stimuli that induce mitochondrial network fragmentation can be divided into either external insults such as during treatment with pro-oxidants or chemotherapeutic agents, PDT, ionizing radiation, immune response, or viral infection that incur cell injury, or be part of physiological redox signaling, for example during hypoxia. In general, stress response signaling pathways convey both external and internal cues between a redox-sensitive receptor and the downstream effectors of the mitochondrial fission machinery (Figure 2). How these signals regulate mitochondrial fission and converge upon the apoptotic stress response is still rather enigmatic and therefore an area of active research. This section will review the current trends and paradigms of ROS-mediated signaling that form a link between redox-sensing elements and mitochondrial dynamics and their role in cancer invasiveness, tumor progression, and metastasis.

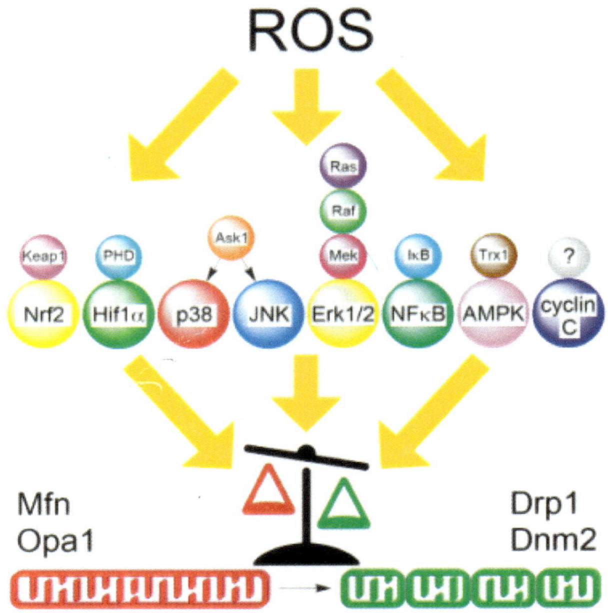

Figure 2. Simplified relationship between ROS-induced redox signaling and mitochondrial dynamics. ROS stimuli are recognized by redox sensors (top), which transduce the signal to their respective effector kinases (center). Phosphorylation by these kinases can either inhibit mitochondrial fusion (red) or stimulate fission (green) proteins that results in the shift of the overall balance from elongated to fragmented morphology (bottom). As indicated, Ras/ERK MAPK signaling involves multiple kinases. Redox sensor for mammalian cyclin C pathway has not yet been determined.

3.1. Nrf2/Keap1 Signaling

The master regulator of cellular stress response is the transcription factor nuclear factor (erythroid-derived 2)-like 2 (Nrf2), which reacts to exogenous stimuli by translocating from the cytosol to nucleus and initiating the expression of a broad range of antioxidant-defense and cytoprotective genes [115,116]. Since Nrf2 is upregulated in numerous tumors, it has been viewed as a promising target for cancer chemoprevention and therapy [117]. Kelch-like ECH-associated protein 1 (Keap1) is an E3 ubiquitin ligase and a redox-sensor for Nrf2 signaling that in the absence of oxidative stress targets Nrf2 for ubiquitin-mediated destruction [118]. Nrf2 is stabilized in the cytosol upon oxidative or electrophilic stress. Although Nrf2 was demonstrated to influence mitochondrial bioenergetics [119], the underlying mechanism is poorly understood. For example, mutant Huntingtin interferes with Nrf2 signaling, which resulted in increased fragmentation of mitochondrial network in response to low-level H_2O_2 treatment and increased susceptibility to oxidative stress in striatal cells [120]. Furthermore, Nrf2 mediates the redox-dependent effect of sulforaphane, an isothiocyanate found in cruciferous vegetables, on increased mitochondrial fragmentation, Bax induction, and the ensuing apoptosis in prostate cancer cells [121]. This response was specific to tumor cells as sulforaphane behaved as an antioxidant and promoted mitochondrial fusion and nephroprotection in parallel experiments using a non-transformed kidney cell line. Altogether, these studies imply that activation of the Nrf2 antioxidant response can be a prospective therapeutic strategy in both neurodegenerative and malignant diseases.

3.2. *HIF1α-Mediated Response to Hypoxia*

The classic example of redox sensing in cancer is the stabilization of the transcription factor hypoxia-inducible factor 1α (HIF1α) that allows solid tumors to adapt to low-oxygen stress by promoting aerobic glycolysis (Warburg's effect), angiogenesis, and tumor invasion [122,123]. Under normoxia, hydroxylation of HIF1α by the prolyl hydroxylase domain (PHD) family of dioxygenases results in its binding to the von Hippel-Lindau protein followed by ubiquitin-dependent destruction [124]. HIF1α is stabilized in the cytosol under hypoxia due to the limited availability of oxygen for the PHD-mediated hydroxylation step. Stabilized HIF1α binds to the oxygen-insensitive subunit HIF1β and the heterodimer subsequently translocates to the nucleus to initiate the transcription of a myriad of hypoxia-response genes to promote metabolic reprogramming stimulating aerobic glycolysis while suppressing OXPHOS activity [125]. HIF1α induction stimulates expression of several glycolytic genes including phosphofructokinase, pyruvate kinase, and lactate dehydrogenase. Paradoxically, hypoxic exposure is accompanied by an initial oxidative burst of superoxide generated by mitochondria [126,127] or NOX enzymes [128]. The hypoxia-induced superoxide burst can originate from Complex I [129] or the outer Complex III ubiqinone-binding site [130]. Chandel hypothesized that the Complex III-derived superoxide signal, which is released into the mitochondrial intermembrane space, is necessary for PHD inactivation and consequent stabilization of HIF1α at the onset of hypoxia. This model implicates mitochondria as active oxygen sensors [131].

There is a distinct association between oxygen deprivation and mitochondrial fragmentation in malignant cells. Hypoxia-induced Drp1 overexpression and mitochondrial fission have been linked to increased migration and metastatic activity in breast cancer MDA-MB-231 [132] and U251 glioblastoma cell lines [133]. Importantly, HIF1α stabilization is required for hypoxia-induced mitochondrial fission [134]. Bioenergetic profiling identified an ovarian cell line (OVCA420) that exhibited fragmented mitochondria due to increased Drp1 expression [135]. These cells also displayed reduced respiration and increased glycolysis. In addition, OVCA420 cells failed to stabilize HIF1α in a 1% oxygen environment reducing cellular fitness to hypoxic conditions. These findings are consistent with the model that mitochondrial dynamics not only play an important role in cellular energetics, but may also serve as a sensor for the hypoxic response. Taken together, these studies suggest that HIF1α can act as a fundamental driver of both mitochondrial fission and cancer progression.

3.3. *ASK1/p38 MAPK Pathway*

The p38 mitogen-activated protein kinase (MAPK) is stimulated by the apoptosis signal-regulating kinase 1 (ASK1) protein kinase to transduce redox signals as well as other types of stress, to stimulate stress response programs, growth or differentiation depending on the signal [136,137]. Cytosolic thioredoxin 1 (Trx1) and mitochondrial thioredoxin 2 (Trx2) act as redox sensors for ASK1-mediated apoptosis signaling [138]. In their reduced form, TRXs sequester ASK1 from inducing stress- and cytokine-regulated apoptosis. This inhibition is relieved upon a pro-oxidant stimulus, which is sensed by intramolecular disulfide bond formation between Cys32 and Cys35 in TRX and this leads to the dissociation of the free kinase [139]. One role for the p38 MAPK signaling is in the adaptation of mitochondrial morphology to hypoxia. In response to hypoxia, p38 MAPK induces mitochondrial fragmentation by upregulating Siah2, which mediates derepression of Drp1 by the mitochondrial scaffolding protein AKAP121 [140]. Siah2 is an E3 ubiquitin ligase that targets AKAP121 for proteasomal degradation. In addition to p38 MAPK [141], Siah2 is upregulated by hypoxia-induced Akt signaling most likely through indirect mechanisms [142]. PKCδ-activated p38 MAPK was demonstrated to directly phosphorylate Drp1 to induce its mitochondrial translocation and subsequent mitochondrial fission in response to succinate challenge [143]. This change in mitochondrial network ultrastructure was required for promoting human mesenchymal stem cell (hMSC) motility via upregulation and redistribution of F-actin. Moreover, pharmacological inhibition of p38 MAPK prevented mitochondrial fragmentation and the onset of mitophagy in a rat brain I/R (stroke) model [144]. In addition to p38 MAPK, c-Jun N-terminal kinase (JNK) can also be activated by ASK1 in response to oxidative stress [145]. JNK has mitochondrial substrates including those important for apoptosis [146] but a role in stress-induced fission/fusion has yet to be elucidated. These data indicate that p38-driven mitochondrial fission may represent an important cytological cue to promote tumorigenesis and metastasis.

3.4. Ras/ERK1/2 MAPK Pathway

The small GTPase Ras, is a well-known effector of the redox-mediated stress response [147] as well as a potent driver of malignant transformation when constitutively activated by mutation [148]. Collectively with three isoforms (Kras, Nras, and Hras), Ras is one of the most frequently mutated oncogenes occurring in approximately 25% of human tumors. When tethered to the plasma membrane through farnesyl and palmitoyl lipid moieties, Ras functions as a molecular switch oscillating between an active (GTP-bound) and inactive (GDP-bound) state. The GTP and GDP status of Ras is directed by the activity of guanine nucleotide exchange factors and GTPase-activating proteins, respectively [149,150]. Normally, Ras transduces external cues such as growth factor and cytokine stimulation to downstream MAPK cascade effectors composed of rapidly accelerated fibrosarcoma (Raf) (MAP3K), MAPK/extracellular signal-regulated kinase (MAPK/ERK) kinase 1 and 2 (MEK1/2) (MAP2K), and ERK1/2 (MAPK), to promote cell proliferation, differentiation, and motility [151]. In addition, Ras directly mediates redox signaling or initiates the oxidative stress response that can trigger apoptotic cell death [152]. Mechanistically, Ras senses ROS and RNS changes through its redox-sensitive cysteine found within a conserved consensus signature sequence NKXD, where X indicates redox-sensitive cysteine (not conserved). The reaction mechanism is thought to involve either one- or two-electron cysteine oxidation, the former being considered more common and proceeding through a thiyl radical intermediate $RS^{\bullet}$, where R denotes an alkyl group. $RS^{\bullet}$ promotes oxidation of the bound guanine nucleotide resulting in its release and rapid turnover.

Numerous reports implicate Ras in modulating mitochondrial ultrastructure [153]. For example, Kashatus and Nascimento et al. reported that ERK2-mediated activating phosphorylation of Drp1 at Ser616 was required for mitochondrial fragmentation and tumor cell proliferation [154]. Similar effects of oncogenic Ras activation on the dynamics of mitochondria and tumor progression have been observed in cells and human melanoma cell lines [155]. In this setting, ERK1/2-dependent Drp1 activation promotes mitochondrial fission, $\Delta\Psi_m$ loss, and mitochondrial ROS generation during Ras^{G12V}-driven tumor transformation. This phosphorylation mark is also used by cyclin B-Cdk1 to simulate fission at mitosis to allow the efficient partitioning of mitochondria in daughter cells [156]. Overexpression of constitutively-active $Hras^{G12V}$ mutant or MAPK activation was associated with increased mitochondrial fission and tumor growth in both in vitro human pancreatic cancer and mouse xenograft models. This fission may be stimulating cell division by generating enough ROS to serve as both a growth catalysis and mitochondrial segregation. Drp1 depletion by shRNA-mediated knockdown or expression of phosphorylation-defective mutant prevented mitochondrial fission and Ras-induced growth. Similarly, pharmacological inhibition of the MAPK pathway led to Drp1 downregulation, increased mitochondrial fusion, and metabolic activity. These findings suggest that mitochondrial dynamics could be a viable therapeutic strategy for Ras-driven neoplasia.

3.5. The Canonical NF-κB Pathway

The redox-sensitive transcription factor nuclear factor κB (NF-κB) plays a major role in inflammation but is also commonly overexpressed and aberrantly activated in a variety of cancers. NF-κB activation is associated with evasion of apoptosis and tumor inflammatory or immune responses [157,158]. NF-κB is a common name for a dimeric complex formed by the members of the Rel family including p50, p52, RelA (p65), RelB and c-Rel [159]. NF-κB normally resides in the cytosol where it forms inhibitory complexes with members of the IκB protein family (IκBα, IκBβ, IκBγ, IκBε, IκBζ, p100, p105, and Bcl-3) [160,161]. Upon activation by pro-inflammatory or redox stimuli, the IκB kinase (IKK) complex composed of IKKα, IKKβ, and NF-κB essential modulator (NEMO) targets IκB proteins for ubiquitin/proteasome-mediated degradation. This frees NF-κB allowing nuclear translocation and the execution of inflammatory programs [162,163]. IKKα- and IKKαβ-deficient mouse embryonic fibroblast (MEF) cells, but not those lacking IKKβ, exhibit a fragmented mitochondrial network that positively correlate with reduced OPA1 expression [161]. In addition, both effects could be rescued by ectopic overexpression of IKKα. Curiously, PGC-1α-dependent mitochondrial biogenesis and ROS production, as well as improved mitochondrial function and antioxidant capacity, were noted in peripheral blood mononuclear cells obtained from professional football players who underwent an eight week period of active training, all of which was attributed to NF-κB activation [164].

Importantly, ROS-dependent NF-κB activation was observed in parallel with increased mitochondrial Ca^{2+} levels and mitochondrial fission in immortalized mouse kidney epithelial cells and mouse splenocytes lacking the mitochondrial tumor suppressor Fus1 [165]. Accordingly, Fus1-deficient splenocytes exerted increased $\Delta\Psi_m$ and mitochondrial ROS production. Furthermore, NF-κB and Nrf2 were implicated in cigarette smoke-induced mitochondrial fragmentation, dysfunction, and ROS generation in human airway smooth muscle (ASM) cells [166]. This was accompanied by increased Drp1 and decreased Mfn2 expression at both protein and mRNA level. In summary, these results highlight the central role of NF-κB in regulating mitochondrial structure dynamics.

3.6. AMPK Redox Sensing

As an energy-sensing enzyme, AMP-activated protein kinase (AMPK) is the central gatekeeper of redox and bioenergetic homeostasis [167–169]. Upon nutrient deprivation, AMPK induces the activation of catabolic (glycolysis, amino acid and fatty acid oxidation) and inhibition of anabolic pathways (gluconeogenesis, fatty acid biosynthesis) to restore depleted ATP levels [170]. AMPK can be allosterically activated by an increased AMP:ATP ratio or directly by low glucose levels [171]. Structurally, AMPK is a heterotrimeric protein composed of catalytic α subunit as well as regulatory β and γ subunits, each of which has distinct isoforms (two isoforms exist for subunit α and β, three for γ) [172]. AMPK is frequently downregulated during tumorigenesis, which contributes to the Warburg phenotype, tumor adaptation, and cancer progression [173]. This is consistent with a tumor suppressor function for AMPK. However, AMPK activation has been observed in a subset of tumors, which may represent a survival mechanism for poorly vascularized tumors [174,175]. Apart from being a core energy-sensor, AMPK is also implicated in redox sensing. Indeed, the presence of H_2O_2 [176], superoxide [177], or reactive nitrogen species (RNS), such as NO [178], can stimulate AMPK. AMPK activity is induced by Trx1-dependent reduction of cysteine residues serving as a redox regulator [179]. An alternative hypothesis claims that oxidative stress stimulates AMPK activity indirectly by elevating the AMP:ATP ratio [180]. These mechanisms are not mutually exclusive and both may contribute to AMPK regulation depending on the context.

Mitochondrial ROS levels are kept in check by peroxisome proliferator-activated receptor-gamma coactivator-1α (PGC-1α)-dependent induction of antioxidant defense mechanisms [181]. AMPK stimulates PGC-1α-dependent mitochondrial biogenesis [182], which may be important as fusion prevents mitochondrial dysfunction and ROS formation [183]. Conversely, AMPK mediates energy deprivation-induced mitochondrial fission following Complex I (rotenone) and III (antimycin A) inhibition by directly phosphorylating Mff [184]. This fragmented mitochondrial phenotype was observed following mitochondrial stress and is believed to predispose cells to mitophagy [185–187]. A recent study revealed a role for AMPK downstream of Drp1-mediated mitochondrial fission. Drp1 activity was augmented in brain tumor initiating (BTI) cells due to enhanced activating phosphorylation status leading to fragmented mitochondrial network morphology and increased cell survival [188]. Pharmacological inhibition or genetic knockdown of Drp1 was sufficient to induce apoptosis, which was reversed in Drp1 and AMPK double-knockdown cells, implying a modulatory role of Drp1 on AMPK function. In another report, AMPK was stimulated by the concerted activity of the oncogene Myc and an OMM phospholipase PLD6 resulting in net mitochondrial fusion [189]. The indirect, myc-driven activation of AMPK led to the repression of the transcriptional regulators Yap and Taz, whose functions are associated with tumor resistance and metastasis, resulting in poor therapeutic outcome and patient survival [190,191]. Collectively, these investigations identify AMPK as another key player in integrating oncogenic transformation events to mitochondrial morphology changes during tumorigenesis. Moreover, manipulating mitochondrial dynamics can influence basic cancer metabolism, providing a new avenue to attack this disease.

3.7. Cyclin C Connects Oxidative Stress-Induced Fission to Apoptosis

Cyclin C is a highly conserved and ubiquitously expressed transcription factor that serves as a stress signaling effector that functions in the nucleus and at the mitochondria. Together with cyclin-dependent kinase 8 (Cdk8), cyclin C normally resides in the nucleus as part of the Mediator complex to regulate Cdk8 and polymerase II-dependent transcription. In the nucleus, cyclin C-Cdk8 function as co-activators with p53 to induce a subset of stress response genes [192]. Independent of transcription, cyclin C re-localizes to the mitochondria where it stimulates mitochondrial fission in response to oxidative stress in both mammalian [22] and yeast [23,24] models. In the cytoplasm, cyclin C directly activates Drp1 at OMM to facilitate mitochondrial fission. Intriguingly, oxidative stress-induced mitochondrial fragmentation did not require the Ser616 activating phosphorylation. This finding indicates that the cell recognizes stress-activated fission differently than that occurring during mitotic cell division. Furthermore, cyclin C is required for mitochondrial-dependent intrinsic, but not extrinsic, apoptosis [22]. This role for cyclin C at the mitochondria does not require Cdk8, suggesting that transcriptional regulation is not involved. In yeast cells, deletion of the mediator component *MED13* released cyclin C into the cytoplasm [193], revealing that cyclin C was necessary and sufficient to induce complete mitochondrial fragmentation. In stressed yeast cells, cyclin C release is facilitated by Med13 destruction mediated by the Skp, Cullin, F-box-containing complex (SCF) ubiquitin ligase and activating phosphorylation by the Slt2/Mpk1 MAPK [194]. Heterozygous deletion of cyclin C gene (*CCNC*) has been linked to the progression of acute lymphoblastic leukemia [195], osteosarcoma [196], and thyroid [197] cancer, suggesting that cyclin C is a bona fide tumor suppressor. Nevertheless, due to its utility, the cyclin C-mitochondrial axis is emerging as a prospective therapeutic target for both cancer and neurodegenerative diseases.

3.8. Other Redox Sensing Systems

Other redox signaling proteins including p53 [198], forkhead box O (FOXO) [199,200], Notch [201], PTEN [202], apurinic/apyrimidinic endonuclease 1/redox factor 1 (APE1/Ref-1) [203], ataxia-telangiectasia mutated (ATM) [204], activator protein 1 (AP-1), cAMP response element binding protein (CREB), heat shock factor 1 (HSF1), and specificity protein 1 (SP1) [205,206] have also been tangentially associated with control of mitochondrial shape and structure. How mitochondrial dynamics control by these factors is coupled to their redox sensing function remains to be clarified.

4. Modulation of Reactive Oxygen Species by Mitochondrial Dynamics

An increasing body of evidence suggests a reciprocal link between mitochondrial morphology and ROS formation [207]. According to this hypothesis, mitochondrial shape and structure are intimately linked to the control of redox homeostasis by modulating ROS as a downstream signal (Figure 3). We will summarize recent observations of how mitochondrial fission and fusion influence mitochondrial ROS generation and how mitochondrial dynamics could be exploited as a potential therapeutic target for medical interventions.

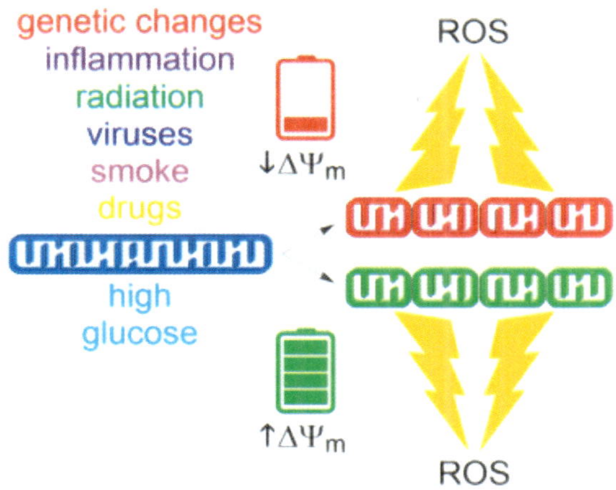

Figure 3. Drivers of fission-induced mitochondrial ROS production. Mitochondrial network fragmentation can occur at both extremes of $\Delta\Psi_m$. Whereas low $\Delta\Psi_m$ values result from insults causing mitochondrial dysfunction (top), high $\Delta\Psi_m$ values can be achieved by metabolic stimulation such as with high glucose (bottom). Both stimuli result in fragmented organelles and subsequent generation of superoxide by ETC.

4.1. Mitochondrial-Derived ROS and Fission, the Vicious Cycle

Increased mitochondrial fragmentation corresponded to an unfavorable prognosis for hepatocellular carcinoma (HCC) patients presumably due to concurrent Drp1 upregulation and downregulation of Mfn1 [208]. The fragmented mitochondrial phenotype observed after Drp1 overexpression or Mfn1 knockdown in several HCC cell lines was associated with ROS overproduction, Akt (also known as protein kinase B) activation, evasion of apoptosis, and induction of general autophagy pathway [208]. Conversely, Drp1 knockdown or Mfn1 overexpression attenuated ROS generation. Mechanistically, mitochondrial fission-induced redox activation of Akt promoted Mdm2-dependent ubiquitin-proteasomal degradation of p53 and IKK-dependent NF-κB activation [208]. Promisingly, mdivi-1, an allosteric and reversible Drp1 inhibitor, induced apoptosis and suppressed the growth of xenograft HCC tumors in immunodeficient mouse model [208]. Overexpression of Mff in human immortalized fibroblasts was reported to induce extensive mitochondrial fragmentation and concomitant mitochondrial dysfunction characterized by $\Delta\Psi_m$ loss, inefficient OXPHOS, and subsequent ATP depletion, giving rise to increased oxidative stress along with concomitant activation of mitophagy and NF-κB-dependent autophagy [209]. Consequently, Mff-overexpressing fibroblasts exhibited metabolic reprogramming towards aerobic glycolysis and excessive lactate secretion, which supported the growth of breast cancer cells in a paracrine-like manner when co-injected into nude mice. Mitochondrial dynamics in cancer-associated stromal cells could therefore be an important driver of early tumorigenesis in neighboring cancer cells as well as an eventual therapeutic target. Recent work has shed more light on the role of NF-κB-inducing kinase (NIK), a principal component of the non-canonical NF-κB pathway, in controlling mitochondrial network dynamics and subcellular localization of mitochondria in relation to tumor malignancy and invasiveness [210]. Using loss- and gain-of-function approaches, Jung and Ravi et al. have shown that NIK relies on Drp1 to mediate mitochondrial fission. This was observed in MEF cells, several cancer cell lines, as well as patient glioblastoma tissue samples. NIK recruits Drp1 to OMM, facilitates its phosphorylation-dependent activation, and consequent mitochondrial fragmentation independently of IKKα, IKKβ, and NF-κB. Consistently, intracellular ROS levels were decreased in both NIK- or Drp1-deficient glioma BT25 cells. Apart from regulating mitochondrial shape, these authors also revealed the ability of NIK to promote mitochondrial migration and motility towards cell periphery and this coincided with increased tumor invasiveness.

Dynamic changes in mitochondrial network morphology were recognized to participate in the reprogramming of somatic cells into induced pluripotent stem cells (iPSCs) [211]. Mfn1- or

Mfn2-deficient MEF cells transduced with the pluripotency factor cocktail containing Oct4, Sox2, Klf4, and c-Myc (OSKM) displayed fragmented mitochondria and increased ROS formation [212]. Such redox stimulus induced HIF1α stabilization even in the absence of hypoxia. In addition, Mfn1 or Mfn2 depletion in OSKM-treated MEF cells downregulated p53 and p21 and activated Ras and Raf. Altogether, this contributed to a genetic switch causing metabolic reprogramming from OXPHOS to glycolysis, which was identified in MEF-derived iPSCs. Analogically, mitochondrial dynamics has been implicated in the regulation of neural stem cell (NSC) maintenance and self-renewal [213]. Depletion of both Mfn1 and Mfn2 or Opa1 increased mitochondrial fragmentation and superoxide production without causing oxidative damage, consistent with the signaling role of mitochondrial fission-induced ROS. When assessed by a neurosphere formation assay, Opa1-deficient NSCs displayed compromised self-renewal capacity, which was reversed by antioxidant treatments. Conversely, Drp1-deficient NSCs showed opposite effects. In addition, employing rotenone or genetic deletion of AIF to specifically induce Complex I-mediated superoxide generation phenocopied the effect of Opa1 loss on neurosphere formation. Further supporting the role of mitochondrial dynamics in determining the fate of NSCs, mitochondrial morphology-regulated redox signaling was necessary for the execution of Nrf2-dependent developmental program responsible for the differentiation of NSCs into neurons.

4.2. Metabolic Stimulation

The outcome that metabolic changes have on mitochondrial function and dynamic responses can be different than those observed following genetic mutation. For example, in a cardiovascular injury model, hyperglycemic conditions trigger Drp1-mediated mitochondrial fragmentation and concomitant ROS formation that resulted in mitochondrial permeability transition (MPT)-dependent apoptosis [214]. This was observed in both rat heart myoblast H9c2 cell line and primary neonatal cardiomyocytes. In H9c2 cells, mitochondrial fission induced by high glucose levels (20 mM) stems from elevated mitochondrial metabolism and therefore cannot be associated with defective mitochondrial function [215]. In analogy, succinate induced Drp1-dependent mitochondrial fission in hMSC that stimulated ROS generation at high $\Delta\Psi_m$ and OXPHOS activity [143]. These results indicate that sufficient ROS can be generated by accelerated metabolism to push the cell past the cell death threshold. An interesting study found that in a model of diabetic nephropathy (DN), exposure of kidney glomerular mesangial cells to high glucose levels leads to mitochondrial translocation of Drp1, and subsequent mitochondrial fragmentation, increased ROS production, lipid peroxidation, p38 MAPK activation, and collagen IV synthesis [216]. Mdivi-1 abolished these effects including the translocation of Drp1 to mitochondria. Moreover, treatment with the antioxidant *N*-acetyl-L-cysteine (NAC) attenuated p38 MAPK phosphorylation, suggesting that Drp1-induced ROS activate p38 MAPK in a feed-forward regulatory loop. Inquiries into the spatial behavior of mitochondria during metabolic overload and/or reprogramming deserve further scientific attention not only in cancer but also in other metabolic disorders such as type 2 diabetes.

4.3. Inflammatory Stimulation

Exposure of mouse embryonic endothelial (MEE) or COS-7 cells to transforming growth factor beta (TGFβ) led to increased mitochondrial fragmentation, which positively correlated with mitochondrial superoxide overproduction [217]. Treatment with the TGFβ receptor I (TβRI) kinase inhibitor SB431542 reversed both effects in control MEE cells but not upon knockdown of the TβRI kinase substrate Smad2. Indeed, the authors went on to show that Smad2 promotes mitochondrial fusion by directly interacting with Mfn2 and recruiting the Rab and Ras interactor 1 (RIN1) as the guanine nucleotide exchange factor for Mfn2. Furthermore, an elegant study investigated the molecular underpinnings of osteogenic dysfunction during TNFα-induced inflammation [218]. TNFα treatment led to increased mitochondrial ROS formation and Drp1 expression followed by excessive mitochondrial fragmentation. Strikingly, both symptoms of mitochondrial dysfunction were inhibited by NAC or mdivi-1 treatment, thus further supporting the notion that superoxide generation and Drp1-mediated fission are intimately interlinked phenomena. Furthermore, T cell activation by cluster of differentiation 3 (CD3) antibodies has been reported to induce mitochondrial fission and ROS production in a Drp1-dependent manner [219]. The activation of Drp1 proceeded through T cell receptor (TCR)-dependent NO signaling and resulted in production of interleukin 2 (IL-2) and the CD95 via ROS-activated NF-κB. Increased levels of IL-2 and CD95 led to simultaneously augmented rates of proliferation and extrinsic apoptosis in CD3-activated T cells.

Lipopolysaccharide (LPS), a surface glycolipid of Gram-negative bacteria and an inflammatory endotoxin, has been found to stimulate mitochondrial fission, mitochondria- and NOX-derived superoxide production in immortalized microglial cell line [220]. As a regulated event, the observed ROS formation occurred downstream of the change in mitochondrial morphology since the effects were abolished by treatment with the antioxidant oleuropein, a secoiridoid glycoside abundant in olive leaf, which inhibited Drp1 Ser637 dephosphorylation as well as LPS-induced inflammation. To summarize, mitochondrial dynamics is an essential component for the inflammatory response that directs proliferation or cell death depending on the immune signal.

4.4. Anticancer Drugs

In addition to endogenous metabolites and compounds, several chemotherapeutic agents are proposed to generate ROS through altered mitochondrial morphology. Inhibitor of the hedgehog signaling pathway, cyclopamine tartrate, elicited antiproliferative and pro-apoptotic behavior in non-small-cell lung cancer cell lines by inducing mitochondrial fission accompanied by decreased respiration, increased $\Delta\Psi_m$, and ROS formation [221]. Cambogin, a naturally-occurring polycyclic polyprenylated acylphloroglucinol, displayed cytostatic and apoptosis-inducing effects in breast cancer cell lines. Increased mitochondrial superoxide as well as cytosolic NADPH oxidase 1 (Nox1)-mediated ROS generation paralleled elevated mitochondrial fission and diminished $\Delta\Psi_m$ following cambogin treatment [222]. The mechanism of action of cambogin may involve the release of ASK1 from inhibition by Trx1. Activated ASK1 is then free to stimulate apoptosis via JNK signaling. Nox1 inhibition or siRNA-mediated knockdown restored normal mitochondrial morphology and ROS production to basal values. The authors concluded that mitochondrial ROS may converge upon mitochondrial dynamics downstream of Nox1 activation. This interpretation is again consistent with the feed-forward regulatory mechanism of mitochondrial ROS-induced ROS generation during structural remodeling of mitochondria. Moreover, silica nanoparticles were reported to induce mitochondrial fragmentation in human umbilical vein endothelial cells, which was caused by dysregulation of the fission machinery proteins, $\Delta\Psi_m$ loss, and accompanied by increased mitochondrial ROS formation and decreased mtDNA copy number [223]. These studies underscore the fact that mitochondrial ultrastructure changes can be inherently part of the mechanism of action of ROS-generating chemotherapeutics.

4.5. Ionizing Radiation

Ionizing radiation composed of α particles (${}^{4}_{2}He^{2+}$) has been documented to upregulate Drp1 expression, induce mitochondrial fission, and cause damage to Complex II and IV in immortalized human small airway epithelial (SAE) cells [224]. Elevated levels of mitochondrial superoxide were one of the characteristics associated with α particle radiation-induced mitochondrial dysfunction. Whereas mdivi-1 pretreatment preserved the integrity of mitochondrial network after exposure of SAE cells to α radiation, it did not immediately rescue mitochondrial function implying that α particles cause direct damage to ETC components.

4.6. Viral Infection

Simultaneously increased ROS and mitochondrial fragmentation due to perturbed mitochondrial function were observed during the infection of astrocytoma U-87MG (glioma) cells by the vaccine strain of Venezuelan equine encephalitis virus (VEEV) [225]. Mdivi-1 treatment prevented VEEV-induced mitochondrial fission and doxorubicin-induced apoptosis in U-87MG cells. Although the exact mechanism of VEEV infection is unknown, these data confirm that viruses are capable of impacting on the fission/fusion machinery to predispose infected cells towards cell death.

4.7. Cigarette Smoke

Cigarette smoke can be regarded as oxidative insult [226]. Cigarette smoke-induced mitochondrial ROS production that was observed in ASM cells [166] was prevented by Drp1 siRNA-mediated knockdown. Conversely, Mfn2 knockdown elevated mitochondrial ROS levels in the presence or absence of cigarette smoke. These results further support the role of mitochondrial dynamics in modulating mitochondria-generated ROS.

5. Conclusions

Mitochondrial network dynamics has important consequences for physiological homeostasis as well as in disease states. A vital determinant of mitochondrial structure is the mitochondrial membrane potential. Within physiological values of $\Delta\Psi_m$, mitochondria are interconnected and elongated. However, at both low (mitochondrial dysfunction) and high (metabolic saturation) extremes of $\Delta\Psi_m$, mitochondria display a fragmented phenotype accompanied by increased ROS generation. Given that mitochondrial fission represents an early step in apoptosis, mitochondrial ROS play a fundamental role at the intersection between these two processes. Although visually similar in appearance, two types of fragmented state should be distinguished—reversible and irreversible. Whether fragmentation of mitochondrial network commits cells to cell death is likely to be indicated by the presence of the latter phenotype. Structurally, this may be the terminal state of ROS-induced ROS vicious cycle that may involve escalating mitochondrial fission as a core component of this mechanism (Figure 4) [227]. Hence, manipulating mitochondrial morphology towards fission by pro-oxidants or towards fusion by antioxidants or mdivi-1 seems to be a viable therapeutic strategy in combating cancer and degenerative diseases, respectively [228].

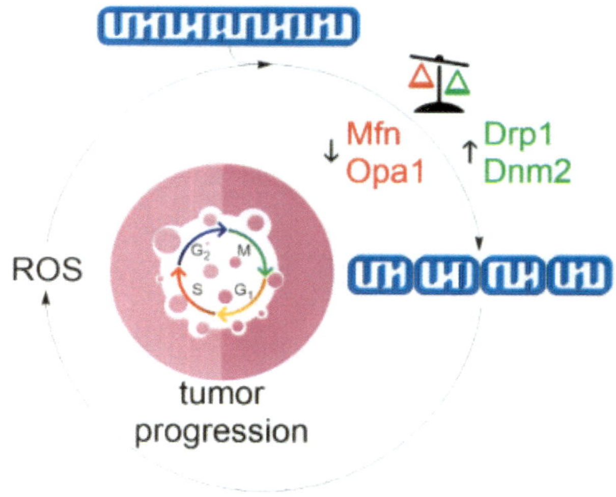

Figure 4. The vicious cycle of mitochondrial fragmentation and ROS production. Fission of the mitochondrial network, such as during oxidative stress (Figure 2), induces mitochondrial ROS generation (Figure 3) initiating a self-perpetuating cycle promoting mitochondrial dysfunction, cell cycle progression and genetic mutation that stimulates neoplastic growth and tumor initiation.

Acknowledgments: The authors acknowledge Zachary A. C. Kiss for help with the manuscript. This work was supported by NIH grant GM R15-113196 and GM RO1-113052 awarded to Katrina F. Cooper and Randy Strich, respectively.

Author Contributions: Jan Ježek wrote the manuscript and drew the figures. Randy Strich and Katrina F. Cooper edited the manuscript.

Conflicts of Interest: The authors declare no conflict of interest.

References

1. Nicholls, D.G.; Ferguson, S.J. *Bioenergetics*, 4th ed.; Academic Press, Elsevier: Amsterdam, The Netherlands, 2013; 419p.
2. Rongvaux, A. Innate immunity and tolerance toward mitochondria. *Mitochondrion* **2017**. [CrossRef] [PubMed]
3. Munoz-Gomez, S.A.; Wideman, J.G.; Roger, A.J.; Slamovits, C.H. The origin of mitochondrial cristae from alphaproteobacteria. *Mol. Biol. Evol.* **2017**, *34*, 943–956. [CrossRef] [PubMed]
4. Zorov, D.B.; Plotnikov, E.Y.; Silachev, D.N.; Zorova, L.D.; Pevzner, I.B.; Zorov, S.D.; Babenko, V.A.; Jankauskas, S.S.; Popkov, V.A.; Savina, P.S. Microbiota and mitobiota. Putting an equal sign between mitochondria and bacteria. *Biochemistry* **2014**, *79*, 1017–1031. [CrossRef] [PubMed]
5. Willems, P.H.; Rossignol, R.; Dieteren, C.E.; Murphy, M.P.; Koopman, W.J. Redox homeostasis and mitochondrial dynamics. *Cell Metab.* **2015**, *22*, 207–218. [CrossRef] [PubMed]
6. Mishra, P.; Chan, D.C. Metabolic regulation of mitochondrial dynamics. *J. Cell Biol.* **2016**, *212*, 379–387. [CrossRef] [PubMed]
7. Melkov, A.; Abdu, U. Regulation of long-distance transport of mitochondria along microtubules. *Cell. Mol. Life Sci.* **2017**. [CrossRef] [PubMed]
8. Wu, M.; Kalyanasundaram, A.; Zhu, J. Structural and biomechanical basis of mitochondrial movement in eukaryotic cells. *Int. J. Nanomed.* **2013**, *8*, 4033–4042. [CrossRef]
9. Berridge, M.V.; Neuzil, J. The mobility of mitochondria: Intercellular trafficking in health and disease. *Clin. Exp. Pharmacol. Physiol.* **2017**. [CrossRef] [PubMed]
10. Tang, B.L. MIRO GTPases in mitochondrial transport, homeostasis and pathology. *Cells* **2016**, *5*, 1. [CrossRef] [PubMed]
11. Harbauer, A.B. Mitochondrial health maintenance in axons. *Biochem. Soc. Trans.* **2017**, *45*, 1045–1052. [CrossRef] [PubMed]
12. Altieri, D.C. Mitochondria on the move: Emerging paradigms of organelle trafficking in tumour plasticity and metastasis. *Br. J. Cancer* **2017**, *117*, 301–305. [CrossRef] [PubMed]
13. Pendin, D.; Filadi, R.; Pizzo, P. The concerted action of mitochondrial dynamics and positioning: New characters in cancer onset and progression. *Front. Oncol.* **2017**, *7*, 102. [CrossRef] [PubMed]
14. Cao, Y.L.; Meng, S.; Chen, Y.; Feng, J.X.; Gu, D.D.; Yu, B.; Li, Y.J.; Yang, J.Y.; Liao, S.; Chan, D.C.; et al. Mfn1 structures reveal nucleotide-triggered dimerization critical for mitochondrial fusion. *Nature* **2017**, *542*, 372–376. [CrossRef] [PubMed]
15. Schrepfer, E.; Scorrano, L. Mitofusins, from mitochondria to metabolism. *Mol. Cell.* **2016**, *61*, 683–694. [CrossRef] [PubMed]
16. Pagliuso, A.; Cossart, P.; Stavru, F. The ever-growing complexity of the mitochondrial fission machinery. *Cell. Mol. Life Sci.* **2017**. [CrossRef] [PubMed]
17. MacVicar, T.; Langer, T. Opa1 processing in cell death and disease—The long and short of it. *J. Cell Sci.* **2016**, *129*, 2297–2306. [CrossRef] [PubMed]
18. Adachi, Y.; Itoh, K.; Yamada, T.; Cerveny, K.L.; Suzuki, T.L.; Macdonald, P.; Frohman, M.A.; Ramachandran, R.; Iijima, M.; Sesaki, H. Coincident phosphatidic acid interaction restrains Drp1 in mitochondrial division. *Mol. Cell* **2016**, *63*, 1034–1043. [CrossRef] [PubMed]
19. Van Laar, V.S.; Berman, S.B.; Hastings, T.G. Mic60/mitofilin overexpression alters mitochondrial dynamics and attenuates vulnerability of dopaminergic cells to dopamine and rotenone. *Neurobiol. Dis.* **2016**, *91*, 247–261. [CrossRef] [PubMed]

20. Schorr, S.; van der Laan, M. Integrative functions of the mitochondrial contact site and cristae organizing system. *Semin. Cell Dev. Biol.* **2017**. [CrossRef] [PubMed]
21. Wollweber, F.; von der Malsburg, K.; van der Laan, M. Mitochondrial contact site and cristae organizing system: A central player in membrane shaping and crosstalk. *Biochim. Biophys. Acta* **2017**, *1864*, 1481–1489. [CrossRef] [PubMed]
22. Wang, K.; Yan, R.; Cooper, K.F.; Strich, R. Cyclin C mediates stress-induced mitochondrial fission and apoptosis. *Mol. Biol. Cell* **2015**, *26*, 1030–1043. [CrossRef] [PubMed]
23. Strich, R.; Cooper, K.F. The dual role of cyclin C connects stress regulated gene expression to mitochondrial dynamics. *Microb. Cell* **2014**, *1*, 318–324. [CrossRef] [PubMed]
24. Cooper, K.F.; Khakhina, S.; Kim, S.K.; Strich, R. Stress-induced nuclear-to-cytoplasmic translocation of cyclin C promotes mitochondrial fission in yeast. *Dev. Cell* **2014**, *28*, 161–173. [CrossRef] [PubMed]
25. Horbay, R.; Bilyy, R. Mitochondrial dynamics during cell cycling. *Apoptosis* **2016**, *21*, 1327–1335. [CrossRef] [PubMed]
26. Ramachandran, R. Mitochondrial dynamics: The dynamin superfamily and execution by collusion. *Semin. Cell Dev. Biol.* **2017**. [CrossRef] [PubMed]
27. Hu, C.; Huang, Y.; Li, L. Drp1-dependent mitochondrial fission plays critical roles in physiological and pathological progresses in mammals. *Int. J. Mol. Sci.* **2017**, *18*, 144. [CrossRef] [PubMed]
28. Antonny, B.; Burd, C.; De Camilli, P.; Chen, E.; Daumke, O.; Faelber, K.; Ford, M.; Frolov, V.A.; Frost, A.; Hinshaw, J.E.; et al. Membrane fission by dynamin: What we know and what we need to know. *EMBO J.* **2016**, *35*, 2270–2284. [CrossRef] [PubMed]
29. Kraus, F.; Ryan, M.T. The constriction and scission machineries involved in mitochondrial fission. *J. Cell Sci.* **2017**, *130*, 2953–2960. [CrossRef] [PubMed]
30. Atkins, K.; Dasgupta, A.; Chen, K.H.; Mewburn, J.; Archer, S.L. The role of Drp1 adaptor proteins MiD49 and MiD51 in mitochondrial fission: Implications for human disease. *Clin. Sci.* **2016**, *130*, 1861–1874. [CrossRef] [PubMed]
31. Osellame, L.D.; Singh, A.P.; Stroud, D.A.; Palmer, C.S.; Stojanovski, D.; Ramachandran, R.; Ryan, M.T. Cooperative and independent roles of the Drp1 adaptors Mff, MiD49 and MiD51 in mitochondrial fission. *J. Cell Sci.* **2016**, *129*, 2170–2181. [CrossRef] [PubMed]
32. Liu, R.; Chan, D.C. The mitochondrial fission receptor Mff selectively recruits oligomerized Drp1. *Mol. Biol. Cell* **2015**, *26*, 4466–4477. [CrossRef] [PubMed]
33. Nagdas, S.; Kashatus, D.F. The interplay between oncogenic signaling networks and mitochondrial dynamics. *Antioxidants* **2017**, *6*, 33. [CrossRef]
34. Lee, J.E.; Westrate, L.M.; Wu, H.; Page, C.; Voeltz, G.K. Multiple dynamin family members collaborate to drive mitochondrial division. *Nature* **2016**, *540*, 139–143. [CrossRef] [PubMed]
35. Liesa, M.; Shirihai, O.S. Mitochondrial dynamics in the regulation of nutrient utilization and energy expenditure. *Cell Metab.* **2013**, *17*, 491–506. [CrossRef] [PubMed]
36. Bordi, M.; Nazio, F.; Campello, S. The close interconnection between mitochondrial dynamics and mitophagy in cancer. *Front. Oncol.* **2017**, *7*, 81. [CrossRef] [PubMed]
37. Martinez-Carreres, L.; Nasrallah, A.; Fajas, L. Cancer: Linking powerhouses to suicidal bags. *Front. Oncol.* **2017**, *7*, 204. [CrossRef] [PubMed]
38. Ciccarese, F.; Ciminale, V. Escaping death: Mitochondrial redox homeostasis in cancer cells. *Front. Oncol.* **2017**, *7*, 117. [CrossRef] [PubMed]
39. Wang, Y.; Nartiss, Y.; Steipe, B.; McQuibban, G.A.; Kim, P.K. ROS-induced mitochondrial depolarization initiates park2/parkin-dependent mitochondrial degradation by autophagy. *Autophagy* **2012**, *8*, 1462–1476. [CrossRef] [PubMed]
40. Pena-Blanco, A.; Garcia-Saez, A.J. Bax, Bak and beyond-mitochondrial performance in apoptosis. *FEBS J.* **2017**. [CrossRef] [PubMed]
41. Kim, H.J.; Maiti, P.; Barrientos, A. Mitochondrial ribosomes in cancer. *Semin. Cancer Biol.* **2017**, *47*, 67–81. [CrossRef] [PubMed]
42. Rathore, R.; McCallum, J.E.; Varghese, E.; Florea, A.M.; Busselberg, D. Overcoming chemotherapy drug resistance by targeting inhibitors of apoptosis proteins (IAPS). *Apoptosis* **2017**, *22*, 898–919. [CrossRef] [PubMed]

43. Sahl, S.J.; Hell, S.W.; Jakobs, S. Fluorescence nanoscopy in cell biology. *Nat. Rev. Mol. Cell Biol.* **2017**, *18*, 685–701. [CrossRef] [PubMed]
44. Grosse, L.; Wurm, C.A.; Bruser, C.; Neumann, D.; Jans, D.C.; Jakobs, S. Bax assembles into large ring-like structures remodeling the mitochondrial outer membrane in apoptosis. *EMBO J.* **2016**, *35*, 402–413. [CrossRef] [PubMed]
45. Salvador-Gallego, R.; Mund, M.; Cosentino, K.; Schneider, J.; Unsay, J.; Schraermeyer, U.; Engelhardt, J.; Ries, J.; Garcia-Saez, A.J. Bax assembly into rings and arcs in apoptotic mitochondria is linked to membrane pores. *EMBO J.* **2016**, *35*, 389–401. [CrossRef] [PubMed]
46. Kalkavan, H.; Green, D.R. Momp, cell suicide as a BCL-2 family business. *Cell Death Differ.* **2018**, *25*, 46–55. [CrossRef] [PubMed]
47. Suarez-Rivero, J.M.; Villanueva-Paz, M.; de la Cruz-Ojeda, P.; de la Mata, M.; Cotan, D.; Oropesa-Avila, M.; de Lavera, I.; Alvarez-Cordoba, M.; Luzon-Hidalgo, R.; Sanchez-Alcazar, J.A. Mitochondrial dynamics in mitochondrial diseases. *Diseases* **2016**, *5*, 1. [CrossRef] [PubMed]
48. Simula, L.; Nazio, F.; Campello, S. The mitochondrial dynamics in cancer and immune-surveillance. *Semin. Cancer Biol.* **2017**, *47*, 29–42. [CrossRef] [PubMed]
49. Srinivasan, S.; Guha, M.; Kashina, A.; Avadhani, N.G. Mitochondrial dysfunction and mitochondrial dynamics-the cancer connection. *Biochim. Biophys. Acta* **2017**, *1858*, 602–614. [CrossRef] [PubMed]
50. Trotta, A.P.; Chipuk, J.E. Mitochondrial dynamics as regulators of cancer biology. *Cell. Mol. Life Sci.* **2017**, *74*, 1999–2017. [CrossRef] [PubMed]
51. Gonzalez-Franquesa, A.; Patti, M.E. Insulin resistance and mitochondrial dysfunction. *Adv. Exp. Med. Biol.* **2017**, *982*, 465–520. [CrossRef] [PubMed]
52. Rovira-Llopis, S.; Banuls, C.; Diaz-Morales, N.; Hernandez-Mijares, A.; Rocha, M.; Victor, V.M. Mitochondrial dynamics in type 2 diabetes: Pathophysiological implications. *Redox Biol.* **2017**, *11*, 637–645. [CrossRef] [PubMed]
53. Wada, J.; Nakatsuka, A. Mitochondrial dynamics and mitochondrial dysfunction in diabetes. *Acta Med. Okayama* **2016**, *70*, 151–158. [CrossRef] [PubMed]
54. Anzell, A.R.; Maizy, R.; Przyklenk, K.; Sanderson, T.H. Mitochondrial quality control and disease: Insights into ischemia-reperfusion injury. *Mol. Neurobiol.* **2017**. [CrossRef] [PubMed]
55. Nan, J.; Zhu, W.; Rahman, M.S.; Liu, M.; Li, D.; Su, S.; Zhang, N.; Hu, X.; Yu, H.; Gupta, M.P.; et al. Molecular regulation of mitochondrial dynamics in cardiac disease. *Biochim. Biophys. Acta* **2017**, *1864*, 1260–1273. [CrossRef] [PubMed]
56. Tong, M.; Sadoshima, J. Mitochondrial autophagy in cardiomyopathy. *Curr. Opin. Genet. Dev.* **2016**, *38*, 8–15. [CrossRef] [PubMed]
57. Marin-Garcia, J.; Akhmedov, A.T. Mitochondrial dynamics and cell death in heart failure. *Heart Fail. Rev.* **2016**, *21*, 123–136. [CrossRef] [PubMed]
58. Vasquez-Trincado, C.; Garcia-Carvajal, I.; Pennanen, C.; Parra, V.; Hill, J.A.; Rothermel, B.A.; Lavandero, S. Mitochondrial dynamics, mitophagy and cardiovascular disease. *J. Physiol.* **2016**, *594*, 509–525. [CrossRef] [PubMed]
59. Chiang, S.; Kalinowski, D.S.; Jansson, P.J.; Richardson, D.R.; Huang, M.L. Mitochondrial dysfunction in the neuro-degenerative and cardio-degenerative disease, friedreich's ataxia. *Neurochem. Int.* **2017**. [CrossRef] [PubMed]
60. Gao, J.; Wang, L.; Liu, J.; Xie, F.; Su, B.; Wang, X. Abnormalities of mitochondrial dynamics in neurodegenerative diseases. *Antioxidants* **2017**, *6*, 25. [CrossRef] [PubMed]
61. Wu, Q.; Luo, C.L.; Tao, L.Y. Dynamin-related protein 1 (Drp1) mediating mitophagy contributes to the pathophysiology of nervous system diseases and brain injury. *Histol. Histopathol.* **2017**, *32*, 551–559. [CrossRef] [PubMed]
62. Bose, A.; Beal, M.F. Mitochondrial dysfunction in parkinson's disease. *J. Neurochem.* **2016**, *139* (Suppl. S1), 216–231. [CrossRef] [PubMed]
63. Cai, Q.; Tammineni, P. Alterations in mitochondrial quality control in alzheimer's disease. *Front. Cell Neurosci.* **2016**, *10*, 24. [CrossRef] [PubMed]
64. Boengler, K.; Kosiol, M.; Mayr, M.; Schulz, R.; Rohrbach, S. Mitochondria and ageing: Role in heart, skeletal muscle and adipose tissue. *J. Cachexia Sarcopenia Muscle* **2017**, *8*, 349–369. [CrossRef] [PubMed]

65. Lopez-Lluch, G. Mitochondrial activity and dynamics changes regarding metabolism in ageing and obesity. *Mech. Ageing Dev.* **2017**, *162*, 108–121. [CrossRef] [PubMed]
66. Wang, W.; Gong, G.; Wang, X.; Wei-LaPierre, L.; Cheng, H.; Dirksen, R.; Sheu, S.S. Mitochondrial flash: Integrative reactive oxygen species and ph signals in cell and organelle biology. *Antioxid. Redox Signal.* **2016**, *25*, 534–549. [CrossRef] [PubMed]
67. Bae, Y.S.; Oh, H.; Rhee, S.G.; Yoo, Y.D. Regulation of reactive oxygen species generation in cell signaling. *Mol. Cells* **2011**, *32*, 491–509. [CrossRef] [PubMed]
68. Brand, M.D. Mitochondrial generation of superoxide and hydrogen peroxide as the source of mitochondrial redox signaling. *Free Radic. Biol. Med.* **2016**, *100*, 14–31. [CrossRef] [PubMed]
69. Wong, H.S.; Dighe, P.A.; Mezera, V.; Monternier, P.A.; Brand, M.D. Production of superoxide and hydrogen peroxide from specific mitochondrial sites under different bioenergetic conditions. *J. Biol. Chem.* **2017**, *292*, 16804–16809. [CrossRef] [PubMed]
70. Zou, X.; Ratti, B.A.; O'Brien, J.G.; Lautenschlager, S.O.; Gius, D.R.; Bonini, M.G.; Zhu, Y. Manganese superoxide dismutase (SOD2): Is there a center in the universe of mitochondrial redox signaling? *J. Bioenerg. Biomembr.* **2017**, *49*, 325–333. [CrossRef] [PubMed]
71. Mondola, P.; Damiano, S.; Sasso, A.; Santillo, M. The Cu, Zn superoxide dismutase: Not only a dismutase enzyme. *Front. Physiol.* **2016**, *7*, 594. [CrossRef] [PubMed]
72. Gao, X.; Schottker, B. Reduction-oxidation pathways involved in cancer development: A systematic review of literature reviews. *Oncotarget* **2017**, *8*, 51888–51906. [CrossRef] [PubMed]
73. Scialo, F.; Fernandez-Ayala, D.J.; Sanz, A. Role of mitochondrial reverse electron transport in ros signaling: Potential roles in health and disease. *Front. Physiol.* **2017**, *8*, 428. [CrossRef] [PubMed]
74. Kuksal, N.; Chalker, J.; Mailloux, R.J. Progress in understanding the molecular oxygen paradox-function of mitochondrial reactive oxygen species in cell signaling. *Biol. Chem.* **2017**, *398*, 1209–1227. [CrossRef] [PubMed]
75. Roy, J.; Galano, J.M.; Durand, T.; Le Guennec, J.Y.; Lee, J.C. Physiological role of reactive oxygen species as promoters of natural defenses. *FASEB J.* **2017**, *31*, 3729–3745. [CrossRef] [PubMed]
76. Sies, H.; Berndt, C.; Jones, D.P. Oxidative stress. *Annu. Rev. Biochem.* **2017**, *86*, 715–748. [CrossRef] [PubMed]
77. Sies, H. Hydrogen peroxide as a central redox signaling molecule in physiological oxidative stress: Oxidative eustress. *Redox Biol.* **2017**, *11*, 613–619. [CrossRef] [PubMed]
78. Mahaseth, T.; Kuzminov, A. Potentiation of hydrogen peroxide toxicity: From catalase inhibition to stable DNA-iron complexes. *Mutat. Res.* **2017**, *773*, 274–281. [CrossRef] [PubMed]
79. Leitao, E.F.V.; Ventura, E.; de Souza, M.A.F.; Riveros, J.M.; do Monte, S.A. Spin-forbidden branching in the mechanism of the intrinsic haber-weiss reaction. *ChemistryOpen* **2017**, *6*, 360–363. [CrossRef] [PubMed]
80. Gammella, E.; Recalcati, S.; Cairo, G. Dual role of ROS as signal and stress agents: Iron tips the balance in favor of toxic effects. *Oxid. Med. Cell. Longev.* **2016**, *2016*, 8629024. [CrossRef] [PubMed]
81. Little, A.C.; Sulovari, A.; Danyal, K.; Heppner, D.E.; Seward, D.J.; Van der Vliet, A. Paradoxical roles of dual oxidases in cancer biology. *Free Radic. Biol. Med.* **2017**, *110*, 117–132. [CrossRef] [PubMed]
82. Zou, Z.; Chang, H.; Li, H.; Wang, S. Induction of reactive oxygen species: An emerging approach for cancer therapy. *Apoptosis* **2017**, *22*, 1321–1335. [CrossRef] [PubMed]
83. Vakifahmetoglu-Norberg, H.; Ouchida, A.T.; Norberg, E. The role of mitochondria in metabolism and cell death. *Biochem. Biophys. Res. Commun.* **2017**, *482*, 426–431. [CrossRef] [PubMed]
84. Rodic, S.; Vincent, M.D. Reactive oxygen species (ROS) are a key determinant of cancer's metabolic phenotype. *Int. J. Cancer* **2018**, *142*, 440–448. [CrossRef] [PubMed]
85. Idelchik, M.; Begley, U.; Begley, T.J.; Melendez, J.A. Mitochondrial ROS control of cancer. *Semin. Cancer Biol.* **2017**, *47*, 57–66. [CrossRef] [PubMed]
86. Liu, J.; Wang, Z. Increased oxidative stress as a selective anticancer therapy. *Oxid. Med. Cell. Longev.* **2015**, *2015*, 294303. [CrossRef] [PubMed]
87. Chen, H.; Chan, D.C. Mitochondrial dynamics in regulating the unique phenotypes of cancer and stem cells. *Cell Metab.* **2017**, *26*, 39–48. [CrossRef] [PubMed]
88. Raza, M.H.; Siraj, S.; Arshad, A.; Waheed, U.; Aldakheel, F.; Alduraywish, S.; Arshad, M. ROS-modulated therapeutic approaches in cancer treatment. *J. Cancer Res. Clin. Oncol.* **2017**. [CrossRef] [PubMed]
89. Galadari, S.; Rahman, A.; Pallichankandy, S.; Thayyullathil, F. Reactive oxygen species and cancer paradox: To promote or to suppress? *Free Radic. Biol. Med.* **2017**, *104*, 144–164. [CrossRef] [PubMed]

90. Milkovic, L.; Siems, W.; Siems, R.; Zarkovic, N. Oxidative stress and antioxidants in carcinogenesis and integrative therapy of cancer. *Curr. Pharm. Des.* **2014**, *20*, 6529–6542. [CrossRef] [PubMed]
91. Cabello, C.M.; Bair, W.B., 3rd; Wondrak, G.T. Experimental therapeutics: Targeting the redox achilles heel of cancer. *Curr. Opin. Investig. Drugs* **2007**, *8*, 1022–1037. [PubMed]
92. Marullo, R.; Werner, E.; Degtyareva, N.; Moore, B.; Altavilla, G.; Ramalingam, S.S.; Doetsch, P.W. Cisplatin induces a mitochondrial-ROS response that contributes to cytotoxicity depending on mitochondrial redox status and bioenergetic functions. *PLoS ONE* **2013**, *8*, e81162. [CrossRef] [PubMed]
93. Mut-Salud, N.; Alvarez, P.J.; Garrido, J.M.; Carrasco, E.; Aranega, A.; Rodriguez-Serrano, F. Antioxidant intake and antitumor therapy: Toward nutritional recommendations for optimal results. *Oxid. Med. Cell. Longev.* **2016**, *2016*, 6719534. [CrossRef] [PubMed]
94. Abo-Neima, S.E. Treatment of cancer by low intensity laser radiation therapy. *Prog Biophys. Mol. Biol.* **2017**. [CrossRef] [PubMed]
95. Deng, K.; Li, C.; Huang, S.; Xing, B.; Jin, D.; Zeng, Q.; Hou, Z.; Lin, J. Recent progress in near infrared light triggered photodynamic therapy. *Small* **2017**, *13*. [CrossRef] [PubMed]
96. Luo, H.; Chiang, H.H.; Louw, M.; Susanto, A.; Chen, D. Nutrient sensing and the oxidative stress response. *Trends Endocrinol. Metab.* **2017**, *28*, 449–460. [CrossRef] [PubMed]
97. Wang, C.H.; Wu, S.B.; Wu, Y.T.; Wei, Y.H. Oxidative stress response elicited by mitochondrial dysfunction: Implication in the pathophysiology of aging. *Exp. Biol. Med.* **2013**, *238*, 450–460. [CrossRef] [PubMed]
98. Yang, L.; Long, Q.; Liu, J.; Tang, H.; Li, Y.; Bao, F.; Qin, D.; Pei, D.; Liu, X. Mitochondrial fusion provides an 'initial metabolic complementation' controlled by mtdna. *Cell. Mol. Life Sci.* **2015**, *72*, 2585–2598. [CrossRef] [PubMed]
99. Enns, G.M.; Cowan, T.M. Glutathione as a redox biomarker in mitochondrial disease-implications for therapy. *J. Clin. Med.* **2017**, *6*, 50. [CrossRef]
100. Jiao, Y.; Wang, Y.; Guo, S.; Wang, G. Glutathione peroxidases as oncotargets. *Oncotarget* **2017**, *8*, 80093–80102. [CrossRef] [PubMed]
101. Couto, N.; Wood, J.; Barber, J. The role of glutathione reductase and related enzymes on cellular redox homoeostasis network. *Free Radic. Biol. Med.* **2016**, *95*, 27–42. [CrossRef] [PubMed]
102. Shutt, T.; Geoffrion, M.; Milne, R.; McBride, H.M. The intracellular redox state is a core determinant of mitochondrial fusion. *EMBO Rep.* **2012**, *13*, 909–915. [CrossRef] [PubMed]
103. Glorieux, C.; Calderon, P.B. Catalase, a remarkable enzyme: Targeting the oldest antioxidant enzyme to find a new cancer treatment approach. *Biol. Chem.* **2017**, *398*, 1095–1108. [CrossRef] [PubMed]
104. Rhee, S.G.; Kil, I.S. Multiple functions and regulation of mammalian peroxiredoxins. *Annu. Rev. Biochem.* **2017**, *86*, 749–775. [CrossRef] [PubMed]
105. Zhang, J.; Li, X.; Han, X.; Liu, R.; Fang, J. Targeting the thioredoxin system for cancer therapy. *Trends Pharmacol. Sci.* **2017**, *38*, 794–808. [CrossRef] [PubMed]
106. Monteiro, H.P.; Ogata, F.T.; Stern, A. Thioredoxin promotes survival signaling events under nitrosative/oxidative stress associated with cancer development. *Biomed. J.* **2017**, *40*, 189–199. [CrossRef] [PubMed]
107. Cunniff, B.; Wozniak, A.N.; Sweeney, P.; DeCosta, K.; Heintz, N.H. Peroxiredoxin 3 levels regulate a mitochondrial redox setpoint in malignant mesothelioma cells. *Redox Biol.* **2014**, *3*, 79–87. [CrossRef] [PubMed]
108. Baffy, G. Mitochondrial uncoupling in cancer cells: Liabilities and opportunities. *Biochim. Biophys. Acta* **2017**, *1858*, 655–664. [CrossRef] [PubMed]
109. Jezek, J.; Dlaskova, A.; Zelenka, J.; Jaburek, M.; Jezek, P. H_2O_2-activated mitochondrial phospholipase iPLA(2)gamma prevents lipotoxic oxidative stress in synergy with UCP2, amplifies signaling via G-protein-coupled receptor GPR40, and regulates insulin secretion in pancreatic beta-cells. *Antioxid. Redox Signal.* **2015**, *23*, 958–972. [CrossRef] [PubMed]
110. Oh, S.E.; Mouradian, M.M. Cytoprotective mechanisms of DJ-1 against oxidative stress through modulating ERK1/2 and ASK1 signal transduction. *Redox Biol.* **2018**, *14*, 211–217. [CrossRef] [PubMed]
111. Almeida, L.O.; Goto, R.N.; Neto, M.P.; Sousa, L.O.; Curti, C.; Leopoldino, A.M. Set overexpression in HEK293 cells regulates mitochondrial uncoupling proteins levels within a mitochondrial fission/reduced autophagic flux scenario. *Biochem. Biophys. Res. Commun.* **2015**, *458*, 300–306. [CrossRef] [PubMed]

112. Shimizu, Y.; Lambert, J.P.; Nicholson, C.K.; Kim, J.J.; Wolfson, D.W.; Cho, H.C.; Husain, A.; Naqvi, N.; Chin, L.S.; Li, L.; et al. Dj-1 protects the heart against ischemia-reperfusion injury by regulating mitochondrial fission. *J. Mol. Cell. Cardiol.* **2016**, *97*, 56–66. [CrossRef] [PubMed]
113. Benfeitas, R.; Uhlen, M.; Nielsen, J.; Mardinoglu, A. New challenges to study heterogeneity in cancer redox metabolism. *Front. Cell Dev. Biol.* **2017**, *5*, 65. [CrossRef] [PubMed]
114. Moloney, J.N.; Cotter, T.G. ROS signalling in the biology of cancer. *Semin. Cell Dev. Biol.* **2017**. [CrossRef] [PubMed]
115. Basak, P.; Sadhukhan, P.; Sarkar, P.; Sil, P.C. Perspectives of the NRF-2 signaling pathway in cancer progression and therapy. *Toxicol. Rep.* **2017**, *4*, 306–318. [CrossRef] [PubMed]
116. Holmstrom, K.M.; Kostov, R.V.; Dinkova-Kostova, A.T. The multifaceted role of Nrf2 in mitochondrial function. *Curr. Opin. Toxicol.* **2016**, *1*, 80–91. [CrossRef] [PubMed]
117. Krajka-Kuzniak, V.; Paluszczak, J.; Baer-Dubowska, W. The NRF2-are signaling pathway: An update on its regulation and possible role in cancer prevention and treatment. *Pharmacol. Rep.* **2017**, *69*, 393–402. [CrossRef] [PubMed]
118. Holmstrom, K.M.; Baird, L.; Zhang, Y.; Hargreaves, I.; Chalasani, A.; Land, J.M.; Stanyer, L.; Yamamoto, M.; Dinkova-Kostova, A.T.; Abramov, A.Y. Nrf2 impacts cellular bioenergetics by controlling substrate availability for mitochondrial respiration. *Biol. Open* **2013**, *2*, 761–770. [CrossRef] [PubMed]
119. Suzuki, T.; Yamamoto, M. Stress-sensing mechanisms and the physiological roles of the keap1-Nrf2 system during cellular stress. *J. Biol. Chem.* **2017**, *292*, 16817–16824. [CrossRef] [PubMed]
120. Jin, Y.N.; Yu, Y.V.; Gundemir, S.; Jo, C.; Cui, M.; Tieu, K.; Johnson, G.V. Impaired mitochondrial dynamics and Nrf2 signaling contribute to compromised responses to oxidative stress in striatal cells expressing full-length mutant huntingtin. *PLoS ONE* **2013**, *8*, e57932. [CrossRef] [PubMed]
121. Negrette-Guzman, M.; Huerta-Yepez, S.; Vega, M.I.; Leon-Contreras, J.C.; Hernandez-Pando, R.; Medina-Campos, O.N.; Rodriguez, E.; Tapia, E.; Pedraza-Chaverri, J. Sulforaphane induces differential modulation of mitochondrial biogenesis and dynamics in normal cells and tumor cells. *Food Chem. Toxicol.* **2017**, *100*, 90–102. [CrossRef] [PubMed]
122. Schito, L.; Semenza, G.L. Hypoxia-inducible factors: Master regulators of cancer progression. *Trends Cancer* **2016**, *2*, 758–770. [CrossRef] [PubMed]
123. Masoud, G.N.; Li, W. Hif-1alpha pathway: Role, regulation and intervention for cancer therapy. *Acta Pharm. Sin. B* **2015**, *5*, 378–389. [CrossRef] [PubMed]
124. Nguyen, T.L.; Duran, R.V. Prolyl hydroxylase domain enzymes and their role in cell signaling and cancer metabolism. *Int. J. Biochem. Cell Biol.* **2016**, *80*, 71–80. [CrossRef] [PubMed]
125. Ivan, M.; Kaelin, W.G., Jr. The EGLN-HIF O2-sensing system: Multiple inputs and feedbacks. *Mol. Cell* **2017**, *66*, 772–779. [CrossRef] [PubMed]
126. Plecita-Hlavata, L.; Jezek, J.; Jezek, P. Aglycemia keeps mitochondrial oxidative phosphorylation under hypoxic conditions in HepG2 cells. *J. Bioenerg. Biomembr.* **2015**, *47*, 467–476. [CrossRef] [PubMed]
127. Hernansanz-Agustin, P.; Izquierdo-Alvarez, A.; Sanchez-Gomez, F.J.; Ramos, E.; Villa-Pina, T.; Lamas, S.; Bogdanova, A.; Martinez-Ruiz, A. Acute hypoxia produces a superoxide burst in cells. *Free Radic. Biol. Med.* **2014**, *71*, 146–156. [CrossRef] [PubMed]
128. Smith, K.A.; Waypa, G.B.; Schumacker, P.T. Redox signaling during hypoxia in mammalian cells. *Redox Biol.* **2017**, *13*, 228–234. [CrossRef] [PubMed]
129. Fernandez-Aguera, M.C.; Gao, L.; Gonzalez-Rodriguez, P.; Pintado, C.O.; Arias-Mayenco, I.; Garcia-Flores, P.; Garcia-Perganeda, A.; Pascual, A.; Ortega-Saenz, P.; Lopez-Barneo, J. Oxygen sensing by arterial chemoreceptors depends on mitochondrial complex I signaling. *Cell Metab.* **2015**, *22*, 825–837. [CrossRef] [PubMed]
130. Guzy, R.D.; Schumacker, P.T. Oxygen sensing by mitochondria at complex III: The paradox of increased reactive oxygen species during hypoxia. *Exp. Physiol.* **2006**, *91*, 807–819. [CrossRef] [PubMed]
131. Chandel, N.S. Mitochondrial regulation of oxygen sensing. *Adv. Exp. Med. Biol.* **2010**, *661*, 339–354. [CrossRef] [PubMed]
132. Han, X.J.; Yang, Z.J.; Jiang, L.P.; Wei, Y.F.; Liao, M.F.; Qian, Y.; Li, Y.; Huang, X.; Wang, J.B.; Xin, H.B.; et al. Mitochondrial dynamics regulates hypoxia-induced migration and antineoplastic activity of cisplatin in breast cancer cells. *Int. J. Oncol.* **2015**, *46*, 691–700. [CrossRef] [PubMed]

133. Wan, Y.Y.; Zhang, J.F.; Yang, Z.J.; Jiang, L.P.; Wei, Y.F.; Lai, Q.N.; Wang, J.B.; Xin, H.B.; Han, X.J. Involvement of Drp1 in hypoxia-induced migration of human glioblastoma u251 cells. *Oncol. Rep.* **2014**, *32*, 619–626. [CrossRef] [PubMed]
134. Salminen, A.; Kaarniranta, K.; Kauppinen, A. AMPK and HIF signaling pathways regulate both longevity and cancer growth: The good news and the bad news about survival mechanisms. *Biogerontology* **2016**, *17*, 655–680. [CrossRef] [PubMed]
135. Dier, U.; Shin, D.H.; Hemachandra, L.P.; Uusitalo, L.M.; Hempel, N. Bioenergetic analysis of ovarian cancer cell lines: Profiling of histological subtypes and identification of a mitochondria-defective cell line. *PLoS ONE* **2014**, *9*, e98479. [CrossRef] [PubMed]
136. Ryuno, H.; Naguro, I.; Kamiyama, M. ASK family and cancer. *Adv. Biol. Regul.* **2017**, *66*, 72–84. [CrossRef] [PubMed]
137. Latimer, H.R.; Veal, E.A. Peroxiredoxins in regulation of MAPK signalling pathways; sensors and barriers to signal transduction. *Mol. Cells* **2016**, *39*, 40–45. [CrossRef] [PubMed]
138. Lu, J.; Holmgren, A. Thioredoxin system in cell death progression. *Antioxid. Redox Signal.* **2012**, *17*, 1738–1747. [CrossRef] [PubMed]
139. Matsuzawa, A. Thioredoxin and redox signaling: Roles of the thioredoxin system in control of cell fate. *Arch Biochem. Biophys.* **2017**, *617*, 101–105. [CrossRef] [PubMed]
140. Kim, H.; Scimia, M.C.; Wilkinson, D.; Trelles, R.D.; Wood, M.R.; Bowtell, D.; Dillin, A.; Mercola, M.; Ronai, Z.A. Fine-tuning of Drp1/Fis1 availability by akap121/siah2 regulates mitochondrial adaptation to hypoxia. *Mol. Cell* **2011**, *44*, 532–544. [CrossRef] [PubMed]
141. Tormos, A.M.; Talens-Visconti, R.; Nebreda, A.R.; Sastre, J. P38 MAPK: A dual role in hepatocyte proliferation through reactive oxygen species. *Free Radic. Res.* **2013**, *47*, 905–916. [CrossRef] [PubMed]
142. Nakayama, K.; Qi, J.; Ronai, Z. The ubiquitin ligase siah2 and the hypoxia response. *Mol. Cancer Res.* **2009**, *7*, 443–451. [CrossRef] [PubMed]
143. Ko, S.H.; Choi, G.E.; Oh, J.Y.; Lee, H.J.; Kim, J.S.; Chae, C.W.; Choi, D.; Han, H.J. Succinate promotes stem cell migration through the gpr91-dependent regulation of Drp1-mediated mitochondrial fission. *Sci. Rep.* **2017**, *7*, 12582. [CrossRef] [PubMed]
144. Zhang, X.M.; Zhang, L.; Wang, G.; Niu, W.; He, Z.; Ding, L.; Jia, J. Suppression of mitochondrial fission in experimental cerebral ischemia: The potential neuroprotective target of p38 MAPK inhibition. *Neurochem. Int.* **2015**, *90*, 1–8. [CrossRef] [PubMed]
145. Obsil, T.; Obsilova, V. Structural aspects of protein kinase ASK1 regulation. *Adv. Biol. Regul.* **2017**, *66*, 31–36. [CrossRef] [PubMed]
146. Dhanasekaran, D.N.; Reddy, E.P. JNK signaling in apoptosis. *Oncogene* **2008**, *27*, 6245–6251. [CrossRef] [PubMed]
147. Ferro, E.; Goitre, L.; Baldini, E.; Retta, S.F.; Trabalzini, L. Ras gtpases are both regulators and effectors of redox agents. *Methods Mol. Biol.* **2014**, *1120*, 55–74. [CrossRef] [PubMed]
148. Papke, B.; Der, C.J. Drugging Ras: Know the enemy. *Science* **2017**, *355*, 1158–1163. [CrossRef] [PubMed]
149. Simanshu, D.K.; Nissley, D.V.; McCormick, F. Ras proteins and their regulators in human disease. *Cell* **2017**, *170*, 17–33. [CrossRef] [PubMed]
150. Schopel, M.; Potheraveedu, V.N.; Al-Harthy, T.; Abdel-Jalil, R.; Heumann, R.; Stoll, R. The small gtpases ras and rheb studied by multidimensional nmr spectroscopy: Structure and function. *Biol. Chem.* **2017**, *398*, 577–588. [CrossRef] [PubMed]
151. Tanimura, S.; Takeda, K. ERK signalling as a regulator of cell motility. *J. Biochem* **2017**, *162*, 145–154. [CrossRef] [PubMed]
152. Mitchell, L.; Hobbs, G.A.; Aghajanian, A.; Campbell, S.L. Redox regulation of Ras and Rho GTPases: Mechanism and function. *Antioxid. Redox Signal.* **2013**, *18*, 250–258. [CrossRef] [PubMed]
153. Cook, S.J.; Stuart, K.; Gilley, R.; Sale, M.J. Control of cell death and mitochondrial fission by ERK1/2 map kinase signalling. *FEBS J.* **2017**, *284*, 4177–4195. [CrossRef] [PubMed]
154. Kashatus, J.A.; Nascimento, A.; Myers, L.J.; Sher, A.; Byrne, F.L.; Hoehn, K.L.; Counter, C.M.; Kashatus, D.F. ERK2 phosphorylation of Drp1 promotes mitochondrial fission and MAPK-driven tumor growth. *Mol. Cell* **2015**, *57*, 537–551. [CrossRef] [PubMed]

155. Serasinghe, M.N.; Wieder, S.Y.; Renault, T.T.; Elkholi, R.; Asciolla, J.J.; Yao, J.L.; Jabado, O.; Hoehn, K.; Kageyama, Y.; Sesaki, H.; et al. Mitochondrial division is requisite to ras-induced transformation and targeted by oncogenic MAPK pathway inhibitors. *Mol. Cell* **2015**, *57*, 521–536. [CrossRef] [PubMed]
156. Taguchi, N.; Ishihara, N.; Jofuku, A.; Oka, T.; Mihara, K. Mitotic phosphorylation of dynamin-related GTPase Drp1 participates in mitochondrial fission. *J. Biol. Chem.* **2007**, *282*, 11521–11529. [CrossRef] [PubMed]
157. Colomer, C.; Marruecos, L.; Vert, A.; Bigas, A.; Espinosa, L. Nf-kappab members left home: Nf-kappab-independent roles in cancer. *Biomedicines* **2017**, *5*, 26. [CrossRef] [PubMed]
158. Darvishi, B.; Farahmand, L.; Eslami, S.Z.; Majidzadeh, A.K. Nf-kappab as the main node of resistance to receptor tyrosine kinase inhibitors in triple-negative breast cancer. *Tumour Biol.* **2017**, *39*. [CrossRef] [PubMed]
159. Begalli, F.; Bennett, J.; Capece, D.; Verzella, D.; D'Andrea, D.; Tornatore, L.; Franzoso, G. Unlocking the nf-kappab conundrum: Embracing complexity to achieve specificity. *Biomedicines* **2017**, *5*, 50. [CrossRef]
160. Capece, D.; Verzella, D.; Tessitore, A.; Alesse, E.; Capalbo, C.; Zazzeroni, F. Cancer secretome and inflammation: The bright and the dark sides of NF-κB. *Semin. Cell. Dev. Biol.* **2017**. [CrossRef] [PubMed]
161. Laforge, M.; Rodrigues, V.; Silvestre, R.; Gautier, C.; Weil, R.; Corti, O.; Estaquier, J. Nf-kappab pathway controls mitochondrial dynamics. *Cell Death Differ.* **2016**, *23*, 89–98. [CrossRef] [PubMed]
162. Mitchell, S.; Vargas, J.; Hoffmann, A. Signaling via the NF-κB system. *Wiley Interdiscip. Rev. Syst. Biol. Med.* **2016**, *8*, 227–241. [CrossRef] [PubMed]
163. Buelna-Chontal, M.; Zazueta, C. Redox activation of Nrf2 & NF-κB: A double end sword? *Cell Signal.* **2013**, *25*, 2548–2557. [CrossRef] [PubMed]
164. Busquets-Cortes, C.; Capo, X.; Martorell, M.; Tur, J.A.; Sureda, A.; Pons, A. Training and acute exercise modulates mitochondrial dynamics in football players' blood mononuclear cells. *Eur. J. Appl. Physiol.* **2017**, *117*, 1977–1987. [CrossRef] [PubMed]
165. Uzhachenko, R.; Ivanov, S.V.; Yarbrough, W.G.; Shanker, A.; Medzhitov, R.; Ivanova, A.V. Fus1/Tusc2 is a novel regulator of mitochondrial calcium handling, Ca^{2+}-coupled mitochondrial processes, and Ca^{2+}-dependent NFAT and NF-κB pathways in $CD4^{+}$ T cells. *Antioxid. Redox Signal.* **2014**, *20*, 1533–1547. [CrossRef] [PubMed]
166. Aravamudan, B.; Kiel, A.; Freeman, M.; Delmotte, P.; Thompson, M.; Vassallo, R.; Sieck, G.C.; Pabelick, C.M.; Prakash, Y.S. Cigarette smoke-induced mitochondrial fragmentation and dysfunction in human airway smooth muscle. *Am. J. Physiol. Lung Cell. Mol. Physiol.* **2014**, *306*, L840–L854. [CrossRef] [PubMed]
167. Cordero, M.D. *AMP-Activated Protein Kinase*; Springer: Berlin/Heidelberg, Germany; New York, NY, USA, 2016.
168. Herzig, S.; Shaw, R.J. AMPK: Guardian of metabolism and mitochondrial homeostasis. *Nat. Rev. Mol. Cell Biol.* **2017**. [CrossRef] [PubMed]
169. Carling, D. AMPK signalling in health and disease. *Curr. Opin. Cell Biol.* **2017**, *45*, 31–37. [CrossRef] [PubMed]
170. Garcia, D.; Shaw, R.J. AMPK: Mechanisms of cellular energy sensing and restoration of metabolic balance. *Mol. Cell* **2017**, *66*, 789–800. [CrossRef] [PubMed]
171. Hardie, D.G.; Lin, S.C. AMP-activated protein kinase—Not just an energy sensor. *F1000Research* **2017**, *6*, 1724. [CrossRef] [PubMed]
172. Ross, F.A.; MacKintosh, C.; Hardie, D.G. AMP-activated protein kinase: A cellular energy sensor that comes in 12 flavours. *FEBS J.* **2016**, *283*, 2987–3001. [CrossRef] [PubMed]
173. He, X.; Li, C.; Ke, R.; Luo, L.; Huang, D. Down-regulation of adenosine monophosphate-activated protein kinase activity: A driver of cancer. *Tumour Biol.* **2017**, *39*. [CrossRef] [PubMed]
174. Jeon, S.M.; Hay, N. The double-edged sword of AMPK signaling in cancer and its therapeutic implications. *Arch. Pharm. Res.* **2015**, *38*, 346–357. [CrossRef] [PubMed]
175. Faubert, B.; Vincent, E.E.; Poffenberger, M.C.; Jones, R.G. The amp-activated protein kinase (AMPK) and cancer: Many faces of a metabolic regulator. *Cancer Lett.* **2015**, *356*, 165–170. [CrossRef] [PubMed]
176. Zmijewski, J.W.; Banerjee, S.; Bae, H.; Friggeri, A.; Lazarowski, E.R.; Abraham, E. Exposure to hydrogen peroxide induces oxidation and activation of amp-activated protein kinase. *J. Biol. Chem.* **2010**, *285*, 33154–33164. [CrossRef] [PubMed]

177. Rabinovitch, R.C.; Samborska, B.; Faubert, B.; Ma, E.H.; Gravel, S.P.; Andrzejewski, S.; Raissi, T.C.; Pause, A.; St-Pierre, J.; Jones, R.G. AMPK maintains cellular metabolic homeostasis through regulation of mitochondrial reactive oxygen species. *Cell Rep.* **2017**, *21*, 1–9. [CrossRef] [PubMed]
178. Han, Y.; Wang, Q.; Song, P.; Zhu, Y.; Zou, M.H. Redox regulation of the amp-activated protein kinase. *PLoS ONE* **2010**, *5*, e15420. [CrossRef] [PubMed]
179. Shao, D.; Oka, S.; Liu, T.; Zhai, P.; Ago, T.; Sciarretta, S.; Li, H.; Sadoshima, J. A redox-dependent mechanism for regulation of AMPK activation by thioredoxin1 during energy starvation. *Cell Metab.* **2014**, *19*, 232–245. [CrossRef] [PubMed]
180. Auciello, F.R.; Ross, F.A.; Ikematsu, N.; Hardie, D.G. Oxidative stress activates AMPK in cultured cells primarily by increasing cellular amp and/or adp. *FEBS Lett.* **2014**, *588*, 3361–3366. [CrossRef] [PubMed]
181. Wu, S.B.; Wu, Y.T.; Wu, T.P.; Wei, Y.H. Role of ampk-mediated adaptive responses in human cells with mitochondrial dysfunction to oxidative stress. *Biochim. Biophys. Acta* **2014**, *1840*, 1331–1344. [CrossRef] [PubMed]
182. Cheng, J.; Zhang, T.; Ji, H.; Tao, K.; Guo, J.; Wei, W. Functional characterization of amp-activated protein kinase signaling in tumorigenesis. *Biochim. Biophys. Acta* **2016**, *1866*, 232–251. [CrossRef] [PubMed]
183. Kang, S.W.; Haydar, G.; Taniane, C.; Farrell, G.; Arias, I.M.; Lippincott-Schwartz, J.; Fu, D. AMPK activation prevents and reverses drug-induced mitochondrial and hepatocyte injury by promoting mitochondrial fusion and function. *PLoS ONE* **2016**, *11*, e0165638. [CrossRef] [PubMed]
184. Toyama, E.Q.; Herzig, S.; Courchet, J.; Lewis, T.L., Jr.; Loson, O.C.; Hellberg, K.; Young, N.P.; Chen, H.; Polleux, F.; Chan, D.C.; et al. Metabolism. AMP-activated protein kinase mediates mitochondrial fission in response to energy stress. *Science* **2016**, *351*, 275–281. [CrossRef] [PubMed]
185. Georgakopoulos, N.D.; Wells, G.; Campanella, M. The pharmacological regulation of cellular mitophagy. *Nat. Chem. Biol.* **2017**, *13*, 136–146. [CrossRef] [PubMed]
186. Senft, D.; Ronai, Z.A. Regulators of mitochondrial dynamics in cancer. *Curr. Opin. Cell Biol.* **2016**, *39*, 43–52. [CrossRef] [PubMed]
187. Escobar-Henriques, M.; Anton, F. Mechanistic perspective of mitochondrial fusion: Tubulation vs. Fragmentation. *Biochim. Biophys. Acta* **2013**, *1833*, 162–175. [CrossRef] [PubMed]
188. Xie, Q.; Wu, Q.; Horbinski, C.M.; Flavahan, W.A.; Yang, K.; Zhou, W.; Dombrowski, S.M.; Huang, Z.; Fang, X.; Shi, Y.; et al. Mitochondrial control by Drp1 in brain tumor initiating cells. *Nat. Neurosci.* **2015**, *18*, 501–510. [CrossRef] [PubMed]
189. Von Eyss, B.; Jaenicke, L.A.; Kortlever, R.M.; Royla, N.; Wiese, K.E.; Letschert, S.; McDuffus, L.A.; Sauer, M.; Rosenwald, A.; Evan, G.I.; et al. A MYC-driven change in mitochondrial dynamics limits YAP/TAZ function in mammary epithelial cells and breast cancer. *Cancer Cell* **2015**, *28*, 743–757. [CrossRef] [PubMed]
190. Panciera, T.; Azzolin, L.; Cordenonsi, M.; Piccolo, S. Mechanobiology of YAP and TAZ in physiology and disease. *Nat. Rev. Mol. Cell Biol.* **2017**, *18*, 758–770. [CrossRef] [PubMed]
191. Kim, M.H.; Kim, J. Role of YAP/TAZ transcriptional regulators in resistance to anti-cancer therapies. *Cell. Mol. Life Sci.* **2017**, *74*, 1457–1474. [CrossRef] [PubMed]
192. Donner, A.J.; Szostek, S.; Hoover, J.M.; Espinosa, J.M. CDK8 is a stimulus-specific positive coregulator of p53 target genes. *Mol. Cell* **2007**, *27*, 121–133. [CrossRef] [PubMed]
193. Khakhina, S.; Cooper, K.F.; Strich, R. Med13p prevents mitochondrial fission and programmed cell death in yeast through nuclear retention of cyclin C. *Mol. Biol. Cell* **2014**, *25*, 2807–2816. [CrossRef] [PubMed]
194. Stieg, D.C.; Willis, S.D.; Ganesan, V.; Ong, K.L.; Scurozo, J.; Song, M.; Grose, J.; Strich, R.; Cooper, K.F. A complex molecular switch directs stress-induced cyclin C nuclear release through SCF (Grr1) mediated degradation of Med13. *Mol. Biol. Cell* **2017**. [CrossRef] [PubMed]
195. Li, N.; Fassl, A.; Chick, J.; Inuzuka, H.; Li, X.; Mansour, M.R.; Liu, L.; Wang, H.; King, B.; Shaik, S.; et al. Cyclin C is a haploinsufficient tumour suppressor. *Nat. Cell Biol.* **2014**, *16*, 1080–1091. [CrossRef] [PubMed]
196. Ohata, N.; Ito, S.; Yoshida, A.; Kunisada, T.; Numoto, K.; Jitsumori, Y.; Kanzaki, H.; Ozaki, T.; Shimizu, K.; Ouchida, M. Highly frequent allelic loss of chromosome 6q16-23 in osteosarcoma: Involvement of cyclin C in osteosarcoma. *Int. J. Mol. Med.* **2006**, *18*, 1153–1158. [CrossRef] [PubMed]
197. Wreesmann, V.B.; Ghossein, R.A.; Patel, S.G.; Harris, C.P.; Schnaser, E.A.; Shaha, A.R.; Tuttle, R.M.; Shah, J.P.; Rao, P.H.; Singh, B. Genome-wide appraisal of thyroid cancer progression. *Am. J. Pathol.* **2002**, *161*, 1549–1556. [CrossRef]

198. Hafsi, H.; Hainaut, P. Redox control and interplay between p53 isoforms: Roles in the regulation of basal p53 levels, cell fate, and senescence. *Antioxid. Redox Signal.* **2011**, *15*, 1655–1667. [CrossRef] [PubMed]
199. Yao, S.; Fan, L.Y.; Lam, E.W. The FOXO3-FOXM1 axis: A key cancer drug target and a modulator of cancer drug resistance. *Semin. Cancer Biol.* **2017**. [CrossRef] [PubMed]
200. Klotz, L.O.; Sanchez-Ramos, C.; Prieto-Arroyo, I.; Urbanek, P.; Steinbrenner, H.; Monsalve, M. Redox regulation of foxo transcription factors. *Redox Biol.* **2015**, *6*, 51–72. [CrossRef] [PubMed]
201. Caliceti, C.; Nigro, P.; Rizzo, P.; Ferrari, R. ROS, Notch, and Wnt signaling pathways: Crosstalk between three major regulators of cardiovascular biology. *BioMed Res. Int.* **2014**, *2014*, 318714. [CrossRef] [PubMed]
202. Verrastro, I.; Tveen-Jensen, K.; Woscholski, R.; Spickett, C.M.; Pitt, A.R. Reversible oxidation of phosphatase and tensin homolog (PTEN) alters its interactions with signaling and regulatory proteins. *Free Radic. Biol. Med.* **2016**, *90*, 24–34. [CrossRef] [PubMed]
203. Laev, S.S.; Salakhutdinov, N.F.; Lavrik, O.I. Inhibitors of nuclease and redox activity of apurinic/apyrimidinic endonuclease 1/redox effector factor 1 (APE1/Ref-1). *Bioorg. Med. Chem.* **2017**, *25*, 2531–2544. [CrossRef] [PubMed]
204. Tang, S.; Hou, Y.; Zhang, H.; Tu, G.; Yang, L.; Sun, Y.; Lang, L.; Tang, X.; Du, Y.E.; Zhou, M.; et al. Oxidized ATM promotes abnormal proliferation of breast CAFs through maintaining intracellular redox homeostasis and activating the PI3K-AKT, MEK-ERK, and wnt-beta-catenin signaling pathways. *Cell Cycle* **2015**, *14*, 1908–1924. [CrossRef] [PubMed]
205. Espinosa-Diez, C.; Miguel, V.; Mennerich, D.; Kietzmann, T.; Sanchez-Perez, P.; Cadenas, S.; Lamas, S. Antioxidant responses and cellular adjustments to oxidative stress. *Redox Biol.* **2015**, *6*, 183–197. [CrossRef] [PubMed]
206. Marinho, H.S.; Real, C.; Cyrne, L.; Soares, H.; Antunes, F. Hydrogen peroxide sensing, signaling and regulation of transcription factors. *Redox Biol.* **2014**, *2*, 535–562. [CrossRef] [PubMed]
207. Kim, B.; Song, Y.S. Mitochondrial dynamics altered by oxidative stress in cancer. *Free Radic. Res.* **2016**, *50*, 1065–1070. [CrossRef] [PubMed]
208. Huang, Q.; Zhan, L.; Cao, H.; Li, J.; Lyu, Y.; Guo, X.; Zhang, J.; Ji, L.; Ren, T.; An, J.; et al. Increased mitochondrial fission promotes autophagy and hepatocellular carcinoma cell survival through the ROS-modulated coordinated regulation of the NFKB and TP53 pathways. *Autophagy* **2016**, *12*, 999–1014. [CrossRef] [PubMed]
209. Guido, C.; Whitaker-Menezes, D.; Lin, Z.; Pestell, R.G.; Howell, A.; Zimmers, T.A.; Casimiro, M.C.; Aquila, S.; Ando, S.; Martinez-Outschoorn, U.E.; et al. Mitochondrial fission induces glycolytic reprogramming in cancer-associated myofibroblasts, driving stromal lactate production, and early tumor growth. *Oncotarget* **2012**, *3*, 798–810. [CrossRef] [PubMed]
210. Jung, J.U.; Ravi, S.; Lee, D.W.; McFadden, K.; Kamradt, M.L.; Toussaint, L.G.; Sitcheran, R. NIK/MAP3k14 regulates mitochondrial dynamics and trafficking to promote cell invasion. *Curr. Biol.* **2016**, *26*, 3288–3302. [CrossRef] [PubMed]
211. Prieto, J.; Torres, J. Mitochondrial dynamics: In cell reprogramming as it is in cancer. *Stem Cells Int.* **2017**, *2017*, 8073721. [CrossRef] [PubMed]
212. Son, M.J.; Kwon, Y.; Son, M.Y.; Seol, B.; Choi, H.S.; Ryu, S.W.; Choi, C.; Cho, Y.S. Mitofusins deficiency elicits mitochondrial metabolic reprogramming to pluripotency. *Cell Death Differ.* **2015**, *22*, 1957–1969. [CrossRef] [PubMed]
213. Khacho, M.; Clark, A.; Svoboda, D.S.; Azzi, J.; MacLaurin, J.G.; Meghaizel, C.; Sesaki, H.; Lagace, D.C.; Germain, M.; Harper, M.E.; et al. Mitochondrial dynamics impacts stem cell identity and fate decisions by regulating a nuclear transcriptional program. *Cell Stem Cell* **2016**, *19*, 232–247. [CrossRef] [PubMed]
214. Yu, T.; Sheu, S.S.; Robotham, J.L.; Yoon, Y. Mitochondrial fission mediates high glucose-induced cell death through elevated production of reactive oxygen species. *Cardiovasc. Res.* **2008**, *79*, 341–351. [CrossRef] [PubMed]
215. Sedlic, F.; Muravyeva, M.Y.; Sepac, A.; Sedlic, M.; Williams, A.M.; Yang, M.; Bai, X.; Bosnjak, Z.J. Targeted modification of mitochondrial ros production converts high glucose-induced cytotoxicity to cytoprotection: Effects on anesthetic preconditioning. *J. Cell. Physiol.* **2017**, *232*, 216–224. [CrossRef] [PubMed]
216. Zhang, L.; Ji, L.; Tang, X.; Chen, X.; Li, Z.; Mi, X.; Yang, L. Inhibition to Drp1 translocation can mitigate p38 MAPK-signaling pathway activation in gmc induced by hyperglycemia. *Ren. Fail.* **2015**, *37*, 903–910. [CrossRef] [PubMed]

217. Kumar, S.; Pan, C.C.; Shah, N.; Wheeler, S.E.; Hoyt, K.R.; Hempel, N.; Mythreye, K.; Lee, N.Y. Activation of Mitofusin2 by Smad2-RIN1 complex during mitochondrial fusion. *Mol. Cell* **2016**, *62*, 520–531. [CrossRef] [PubMed]
218. Zhang, L.; Gan, X.; He, Y.; Zhu, Z.; Zhu, J.; Yu, H. Drp1-dependent mitochondrial fission mediates osteogenic dysfunction in inflammation through elevated production of reactive oxygen species. *PLoS ONE* **2017**, *12*, e0175262. [CrossRef] [PubMed]
219. Roth, D.; Krammer, P.H.; Gulow, K. Dynamin related protein 1-dependent mitochondrial fission regulates oxidative signalling in t cells. *FEBS Lett.* **2014**, *588*, 1749–1754. [CrossRef] [PubMed]
220. Park, J.; Min, J.S.; Chae, U.; Lee, J.Y.; Song, K.S.; Lee, H.S.; Lee, H.J.; Lee, S.R.; Lee, D.S. Anti-inflammatory effect of oleuropein on microglia through regulation of Drp1-dependent mitochondrial fission. *J. Neuroimmunol.* **2017**, *306*, 46–52. [CrossRef] [PubMed]
221. Alam, M.M.; Sohoni, S.; Kalainayakan, S.P.; Garrossian, M.; Zhang, L. Cyclopamine tartrate, an inhibitor of hedgehog signaling, strongly interferes with mitochondrial function and suppresses aerobic respiration in lung cancer cells. *BMC Cancer* **2016**, *16*, 150. [CrossRef] [PubMed]
222. Shen, K.; Lu, F.; Xie, J.; Wu, M.; Cai, B.; Liu, Y.; Zhang, H.; Tan, H.; Pan, Y.; Xu, H. Cambogin exerts anti-proliferative and pro-apoptotic effects on breast adenocarcinoma through the induction of nadph oxidase 1 and the alteration of mitochondrial morphology and dynamics. *Oncotarget* **2016**, *7*, 50596–50611. [CrossRef] [PubMed]
223. Guo, C.; Wang, J.; Jing, L.; Ma, R.; Liu, X.; Gao, L.; Cao, L.; Duan, J.; Zhou, X.; Li, Y.; et al. Mitochondrial dysfunction, perturbations of mitochondrial dynamics and biogenesis involved in endothelial injury induced by silica nanoparticles. *Environ. Pollut.* **2017**. [CrossRef] [PubMed]
224. Zhang, B.; Davidson, M.M.; Zhou, H.; Wang, C.; Walker, W.F.; Hei, T.K. Cytoplasmic irradiation results in mitochondrial dysfunction and Drp1-dependent mitochondrial fission. *Cancer Res.* **2013**, *73*, 6700–6710. [CrossRef] [PubMed]
225. Keck, F.; Brooks-Faulconer, T.; Lark, T.; Ravishankar, P.; Bailey, C.; Salvador-Morales, C.; Narayanan, A. Altered mitochondrial dynamics as a consequence of venezuelan equine encephalitis virus infection. *Virulence* **2017**, 1–18. [CrossRef] [PubMed]
226. Michaeloudes, C.; Bhavsar, P.K.; Mumby, S.; Chung, K.F.; Adcock, I.M. Dealing with stress: Defective metabolic adaptation in chronic obstructive pulmonary disease pathogenesis. *Ann. Am. Thorac. Soc.* **2017**, *14*, S374–S382. [CrossRef] [PubMed]
227. Galloway, C.A.; Yoon, Y. Perspectives on: SGP symposium on mitochondrial physiology and medicine: What comes first, misshape or dysfunction? The view from metabolic excess. *J. Gen. Physiol.* **2012**, *139*, 455–463. [CrossRef] [PubMed]
228. Rosdah, A.A.; Holien, J.H.; Delbridge, L.M.; Dusting, G.J.; Lim, S.Y. Mitochondrial fission—A drug target for cytoprotection or cytodestruction? *Pharmacol. Res. Perspect.* **2016**, *4*, e00235. [CrossRef] [PubMed]

Permissions

All chapters in this book were first published in ANTIOXIDANTS, by MDPI; hereby published with permission under the Creative Commons Attribution License or equivalent. Every chapter published in this book has been scrutinized by our experts. Their significance has been extensively debated. The topics covered herein carry significant findings which will fuel the growth of the discipline. They may even be implemented as practical applications or may be referred to as a beginning point for another development

The contributors of this book come from diverse backgrounds, making this book a truly international effort. This book will bring forth new frontiers with its revolutionizing research information and detailed analysis of the nascent developments around the world.

We would like to thank all the contributing authors for lending their expertise to make the book truly unique. They have played a crucial role in the development of this book. Without their invaluable contributions this book wouldn't have been possible. They have made vital efforts to compile up to date information on the varied aspects of this subject to make this book a valuable addition to the collection of many professionals and students.

This book was conceptualized with the vision of imparting up-to-date information and advanced data in this field. To ensure the same, a matchless editorial board was set up. Every individual on the board went through rigorous rounds of assessment to prove their worth. After which they invested a large part of their time researching and compiling the most relevant data for our readers.

The editorial board has been involved in producing this book since its inception. They have spent rigorous hours researching and exploring the diverse topics which have resulted in the successful publishing of this book. They have passed on their knowledge of decades through this book. To expedite this challenging task, the publisher supported the team at every step. A small team of assistant editors was also appointed to further simplify the editing procedure and attain best results for the readers.

Apart from the editorial board, the designing team has also invested a significant amount of their time in understanding the subject and creating the most relevant covers. They scrutinized every image to scout for the most suitable representation of the subject and create an appropriate cover for the book.

The publishing team has been an ardent support to the editorial, designing and production team. Their endless efforts to recruit the best for this project, has resulted in the accomplishment of this book. They are a veteran in the field of academics and their pool of knowledge is as vast as their experience in printing. Their expertise and guidance has proved useful at every step. Their uncompromising quality standards have made this book an exceptional effort. Their encouragement from time to time has been an inspiration for everyone.

The publisher and the editorial board hope that this book will prove to be a valuable piece of knowledge for researchers, students, practitioners and scholars across the globe.

List of Contributors

Gregory J. Fredericks, FuKun W. Hoffmann and Peter R. Hoffmann
Department of Cell and Molecular Biology, John A. Burns School of Medicine, University of Hawaii, 651 Ilalo Street, Honolulu, HI 96813, USA

Robert J. Hondal
Department of Biochemistry, University of Vermont, 89 Beaumont Ave, Given Building Room B413, Burlington, VT 05405, USA

Sharon Rozovsky
Department of Chemistry and Biochemistry, University of Delaware, 136 Brown Laboratory, Newark, DE 19716, USA

Johann Urschitz
Department of Anatomy, Biochemistry and Physiology, John A. Burns School of Medicine, University of Hawaii, 651 Ilalo Street, Honolulu, HI 96813, USA

Yan-Ting Shiu
Division of Nephrology and Hypertension, University of Utah, Salt Lake City, UT 84112, USA

Edgar A. Jaimes
Renal Service, Memorial Sloan Kettering Cancer Center, New York, NY 10065, USA
Renal Division, Weill Cornell Medical College, New York, NY 10065, USA

Athinoula L. Petrou, Theodoros Ntanos and Antonis Liapis
Laboratory of Inorganic Chemistry, Department of Chemistry, National and Kapodistrian University of Athens, Panepistimiopolis, 15771 Athens, Greece

Petros L. Petrou
Private practice in Cardiology, 6–8 Acheans Street, Nicosia 1101, Cyprus

Mirtha Navarro-Hoyos
Department of Chemistry, University of Costa Rica (UCR), Sede Rodrigo Facio,
San Pedro de Montes de Oca, San José 2060, Costa Rica

Diego Alvarado-Corella
Department of Biology, University of Costa Rica (UCR), Sede Rodrigo Facio, San Pedro de Montes de Oca, San Jose 2060, Costa Rica

Ileana Moreira-Gonzalez and Elizabeth Arnaez-Serrano
Department of Biology, Technological University of Costa Rica (TEC), Cartago 7050, Costa Rica

Maria Monagas-Juan
Institute of Food Science Research (CIAL), Spanish National Research Council (CSIC), C/Nicolás Cabrera 9, 28049 Madrid

Keneswary Ravichanthiran
Faculty of Food Science and Nutrition, Universiti Malaysia Sabah, Kota Kinabalu 2073, Sabah, Malaysia

Yifan Jin
Department of Public Health, Xi'an Jiaotong-Liverpool University, Suzhou 215123, China

Zheng Feei Ma
Department of Public Health, Xi'an Jiaotong-Liverpool University, Suzhou 215123, China
School of Medical Sciences, Universiti Sains Malaysia, Kota Bharu 15200, Kelantan, Malaysia

Hongxia Zhang
Department of Food Science, University of Otago, Dunedin 9016, New Zealand

Yang Cao
Department of Health Promotion, Pudong Maternal and Child Health Care Institution, Shanghai 201399, China

Chee Woon Wang
Department of Biochemistry, Faculty of Medicine, MAHSA University, Bandar Saujana Putra 42610, Jenjarom, Selangor, Malaysia

Shahzad Muhammad
Institute of Basic Medical Sciences, Khyber Medical University, Peshawar 25100, Pakistan

Elom K. Aglago
Joint Unit of Research in Nutrition and Food Science, Ibn Tofail University, Kenitra 14000, Morocco

Yihe Zhang
Division of Medicine, School of Life and Medical Sciences, University College London, London WC1E6BT, UK

Binyu Pan
Department of Clinical Nutrition, The First People's Hospital of Wujiang District, Suzhou 215200, China

Hamza El Hadi, Roberto Vettor and Marco Rossato
Internal Medicine 3, Department of Medicine—DIMED, University of Padova, Via Giustiniani 2, 35128 Padova, Italy

Roland Nemes
Faculty of Sports and Health Studies, Hosei University, Tokyo 194-0298, Japan

Erika Koltai
Research Institute of Sport Science, University of Physical Education, Alkotas u. 44, H-1123 Budapest, Hungary

Albert W. Taylor
Faculty of Health Sciences, The University of Western Ontario, London, ON N6G 1H1, Canada

Katsuhiko Suzuki
Faculty of Sport Sciences, Waseda University, Saitama 359-1192, Japan

Ferenc Gyori
Institute of Sport Science, University of Szeged, H-6726 Szeged, Hungary

Zsolt Radak
Research Institute of Sport Science, University of Physical Education, Alkotas u. 44, H-1123 Budapest, Hungary
Institute of Sport Science, University of Szeged, H-6726 Szeged, Hungary

Evangelos Zoidis
Department of Nutritional Physiology and Feeding, Faculty of Animal Science and Aquaculture, Agricultural University of Athens, 75 Iera Odos, 11855 Athens, Greece

Isidoros Seremelis, Nikolaos Kontopoulos and Georgios P. Danezis
Chemistry Laboratory, Department of Food Science and Human Nutrition, Agricultural University of Athens, 75 Iera Odos, 11855 Athens, Greece

Atul Dhall
Colleges of Nanoscale Science and Engineering, SUNY Polytechnic Institute, Albany, NY 12203, USA

William Self
Burnett School of Biomedical Sciences, College of Medicine, University of Central Florida, Orlando, FL 32816, USA

Rattanamanee Chomchan
Interdisciplinary Graduate School of Nutraceutical and Functional Food, Prince of Songkla University, Hat-Yai, Songkla 90112, Thailand

Panupong Puttarak
Department of Pharmaceutical Sciences, Prince of Songkla University, Hat-Yai, Songkla 90112, Thailand

Adelheid Brantner
Department of Pharmacognosy, Institute of Pharmaceutical Sciences, University of Graz, Graz 8010, Austria

Sunisa Siripongvutikorn
Department of Food Technology, Faculty of Agro-Industry, Prince of Songkla University, Hat-Yai, Songkla 90112, Thailand

Dina Cheaib
Faculty of Sciences, Beirut Arab University, Riad El Solh, Beirut 1107 2809, Lebanon

Nada El Darra and Iman El-Ghazzawi
Faculty of Health Sciences, Beirut Arab University, Tarik El Jedidah—Beirut, Riad El Solh, Beirut 1107 2809, Lebanon

Hiba N. Rajha, Richard G. Maroun and Nicolas Louka
Unité de Recherche Technologies et Valorisation Agro-alimentaire, Centre d'Analyses et de Recherche, Faculté des Sciences, Université Saint-Joseph de Beyrouth, B.P. 11-514 Riad El Solh, Beirut 1107 2050, Lebanon

Satoshi Okuyama, Tatsumi Nakashima, Kumi Nakamura, Wakana Shinoka, Maho Kotani, Atsushi Sawamoto, Mitsunari Nakajima and Yoshiko Furukawa
Department of Pharmaceutical Pharmacology, College of Pharmaceutical Sciences, Matsuyama University, 4-2 Bunkyo-cho, Matsuyama, Ehime 790-8578, Japan

Annalisa Lucera, Cristina Costa, Valeria Marinelli, Maria Antonietta Saccotelli, Matteo Alessandro Del Nobile and Amalia Conte
Department of Agricultural Sciences, Food and Environment, University of Foggia, Via Napoli, 25–71121 Foggia, Italy

Jan Ježek, Katrina F. Cooper and Randy Strich
Department of Molecular Biology, Rowan University Graduate School of Biomedical Sciences, Stratford, NJ 08084, USA

Index

S

T

U